NUTRITION AND METABOLISM: THEORY AND PRACTICES

Edited by
Rose Jean D. Capidlac

ArclerPress

Nutrition and Metabolism: Theory and Practices

Edited by Rose Jean D. Capidlac

Edition 2018

ArclerPress

Published by
Arcler Press LLC
708 3rd Avenue, 6th Floor
New York
NY 10017
United States of America
www.arclerpress.com

ISBN: 978-1-68094-580-5 (Hardback)

Printed in United States of America

Library of Congress Control Number: 2017933145

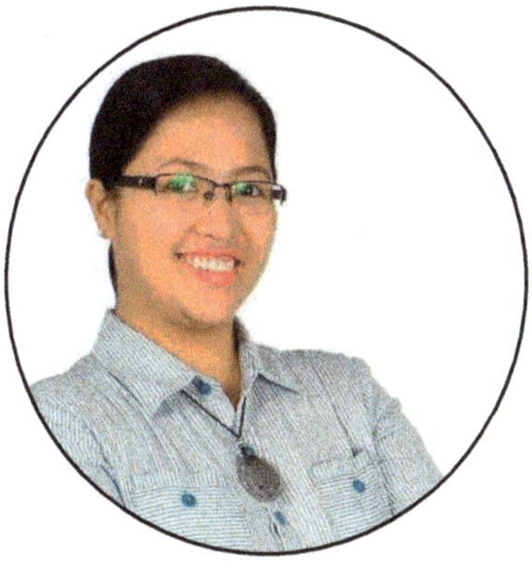

About the Editor

Rose Jean D. Capidlac

Rose Jean Capidlac obtained her bachelor's degree in nursing from Silliman University, Philippines, and ranked 7th in the national licensure examination. She is a copy editor and proofreader for four years now, with a focus on medical and scientific literature. She is also currently an online ESL teacher to Japanese businessmen and corporate employees.

Table of Contents

3 METABOLIC PATHWAYS

4 METABOLIC NETWORKS

5 CARBOHYDRATE METABOLISM

6 PROTEIN METABOLISM

7 LIPID METABOLISM

8 PURINE METABOLISM

List of Abbreviations

APRT	Adenine Phosphoribosyltransferase
ADP	Adenosine Diphosphate
ATP	Adenosine Triphosphate
ADI	Adequate Daily Intakes
ACEIs	Angiotensin Converting Enzyme Inhibitors
CMP	Cytidine Monophosphate
dCMP	Deoxycytidine Monophosphate
DM	Diabetes Mellitus
DMAPP	Dimethylallyl Pyrophosphate
EFSA	European Food Safety Authority
FVA	Flux Variability Analysis
FBA	Flux Balance Analysis
GPR	Gene-Protein-Reaction Expressions
GPP	Geranyl Pyrophosphate
GDM	Gestational Diabetes Mellitus
GDP	Guanosine Diphosphate
GTP	Guanosine Triphosphate
HGPRT	Hypoxanthine-Guanine Phosphoribosyltransferase
IPP	Intermediates Isopentenyl Pyrophosphate
IDF	International Diabetes Federation
IBS-D	Irritable Bowel Syndrome
KEGG	Kyoto Encyclopedia of Genes and Genomes
RDA	Recommended Dietary Allowance
UDCA	Ursodeoxycholic Acid

UMP	Uridine Monophosphate
WHO	World Health Organization

Preface

Metabolism is the chemical process your body uses to transform the food you eat into the fuel that keeps you alive. Nutrition (food) consists of proteins, carbohydrates, and fats. These substances are broken down by enzymes in your digestive system, and then carried to the cells where they can be used as fuel. Your body either uses these substances immediately, or stores them in the liver, body fat, and muscle tissues for later use. Metabolism is closely linked to nutrition and the availability of nutrients. Bioenergetics is a term which describes the biochemical or metabolic pathways by which the cell ultimately obtains energy. Energy formation is one of the vital components of metabolism. Nutrition is the key to metabolism. The pathways of metabolism rely upon nutrients that they breakdown in order to produce energy. This energy in turn is required by the body to synthesize new proteins, nucleic acids, etc. Nutrients in relation to metabolism encompass bodily requirement for various substances, individual functions in body, amount needed, level below which poor health results etc. Essential nutrients supply energy (calories) and supply the necessary chemicals which the body itself cannot synthesize. Food provides a variety of substances that are essential for the building, upkeep, and repair of body tissues, and for the efficient functioning of the body. The diet needs essential nutrients like carbon, hydrogen, oxygen, nitrogen, phosphorus, sulfur, and around 20 other inorganic elements. The major elements are supplied in carbohydrates, lipids, and protein. In addition, vitamins, minerals and water are necessary. Carbohydrates are the energy powerhouses in the body. They are pulled from the starches and sugars and cellulose we eat in our foods daily. Our metabolism will break down these nutrients and supply what we need for the day. People generally only consume around half of the daily need for these compounds. They are generally consumed from foods such as bread, cereal, rice, pasta, potatoes and wheat. Glucose is the main source of energy which is formed from metabolized starches and sugars combined. This takes place post-digestion. Proteins are what we need to build muscle and tissues. Proteins are an integral part of each cell in the human body. It is a life giving substance by which hemoglobin is formed. This is just as important as blood. Fat produces twice the energy than proteins or carbohydrates. Fat is essential in its healthy forms. It helps to produce cell structure, it protects the vital organs with a cushion, the fat soluble vitamins we take are absorbed through fats and fat will create storage for energy when we need it. Minerals are responsible for the regulation of bodily functions. The minerals found in food are not used for energy in a direct sense but they play an important role in metabolic processes.

Content Coverage

Chapters One and *Two* present figures about the nutrition and process of metabolism, respectively. It includes food intake, absorption, assimilation, biosynthesis, catabolism and excretion. The three main purposes of metabolism are the conversion of food/fuel to energy to run cellular processes, the conversion of food/fuel to building blocks for proteins, lipids, nucleic acids, and some carbohydrates, and the elimination of nitrogenous wastes.

Chapters Three and *Four* discuss the metabolic pathways and metabolic networks, respectively. A metabolic network is the complete set of metabolic and physical processes that determine the physiological and biochemical properties of a cell.

Chapter Five focuses on carbohydrate metabolism that signifies the various biochemical processes responsible for the formation, breakdown and interconversion of carbohydrates in living organisms.

Chapter Six emphasizes on protein metabolism that denotes the various biochemical processes responsible for the synthesis of proteins and amino acids, and the breakdown of proteins by catabolism.

Chapter Seven elucidates lipid metabolism; the process by which fatty acids are digested, broken down for energy, or stored in the human body for later energy use. These fatty acids are a component of triglycerides, which make up the bulk of the fat humans eat in foods like vegetable oils and animal products.

Chapter Eight is about purine metabolism which refers to the metabolic pathways to synthesize and break down purines that are present in many organisms.

CHAPTER 1

Core Concepts of Nutrition

Chapter Contents

- **Introduction**
- **History**
- **Nutrients**
- **Healthy Diets**
- **Environmental Nutrition**
- **Advice and Guidance**
- **Nutrition Literacy**
- **Malnutrition**

The essential nutrients for life include carbohydrates, proteins, and lipids (fats), as well as fiber, vitamins, minerals, and water—the solvent for all soluble ingredients in the blood and cells. The absorption of nutrients starts the moment we begin to digest our foods, as they are transported to assist all the metabolic processes in the human body.

Good nutrition means getting the right amount of nutrients from healthy foods in the right combinations. Having nutrition knowledge and making smart choices about the foods you eat can and will help you achieve optimum health over your lifetime, and be a key to avoiding obesity, illness, and many of today's most prevalent chronic diseases.

INTRODUCTION

Nutrition is the science that interprets the interaction of nutrients and other substances in food in relation to maintenance, growth, reproduction, health and disease of an organism. It includes food intake, absorption, assimilation, biosynthesis, catabolism and excretion.

The diet of an organism is what it eats, which is largely determined by the availability, the processing and palatability of foods. A healthy diet includes preparation of food and storage methods that preserve nutrients from oxidation, heat or leaching, and that reduce risk of foodborne illness.

Registered dietitian nutritionists (RDs or RDNs) are health professionals qualified to provide safe, evidence-based dietary advice which includes a review of what is eaten, a thorough review of nutritional health, and a personalized nutritional treatment plan. They also provide preventive and therapeutic programs at work places, schools and similar institutions. Certified Clinical Nutritionists or CCNs, are trained health professionals who also offer dietary advice on the role of nutrition in chronic disease, including possible prevention or remediation by addressing nutritional deficiencies before resorting to drugs. Government regulation especially in terms of licensing, is currently less universal for the CCN than that of RD or RDN. Another advanced Nutrition Professional is a Certified Nutrition Specialist or CNS. These Board Certified Nutritionists typically specialize in obesity and chronic disease. In order to become board certified, potential CNS candidate must pass an examination, much like Registered Dieticians. This exam covers specific domains within the health sphere including; Clinical Intervention and Human Health.

A poor diet may cause health problems, causing deficiency diseases such as blindness, anemia, scurvy, preterm birth, stillbirth and cretinism; health-threatening conditions like obesity and metabolic syndrome; and such common chronic systemic diseases as cardiovascular disease, diabetes, and osteoporosis. A poor diet can cause the wasting of kwashiorkor in acute cases, and the stunting of marasmus in chronic cases of malnutrition.

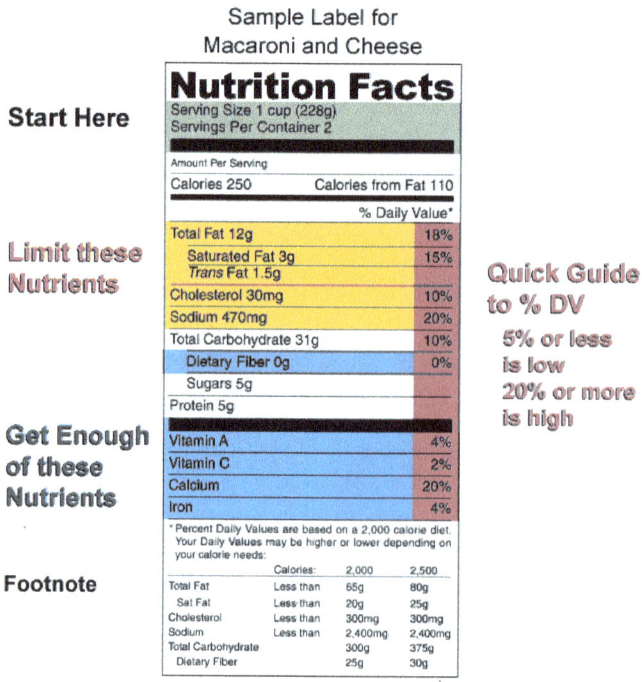

The "Nutrition Facts" table displayed on packaged food labels in the United States indicates the amounts of nutrients recommended by the US Food and Drug Administration to limit or consume according to the Daily Value

HISTORY

Antiquity

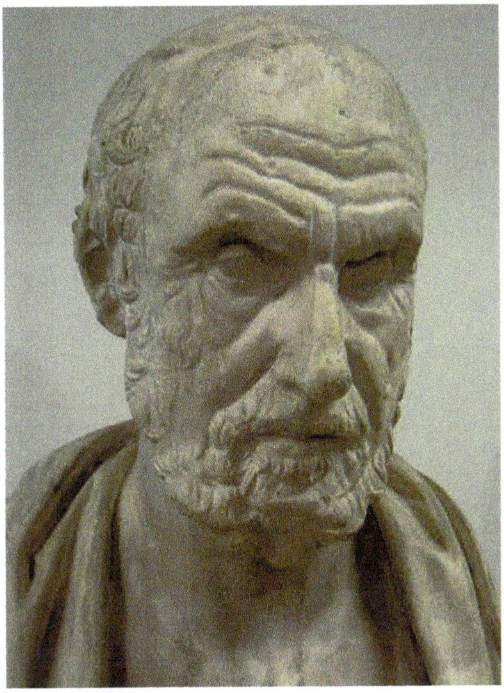

Hippocrates lived about 400 BC, and Galen and the understanding of nutrition followed him for centuries.

The first recorded dietary advice, carved into a Babylonian stone tablet in about 2500 BC, cautioned those with pain inside to avoid eating onions for three days. Scurvy, later found to be a vitamin C deficiency, was first described in 1500 BC in the Ebers Papyrus.

According to Walter Gratzer, the study of nutrition probably began during the 6th century BC. In China, the concept of *Qi* developed, a spirit or "wind" similar to what Western Europeans later called *pneuma*. Food was classified into "hot" (for example, meats, blood, ginger, and hot spices) and "cold" (green vegetables) in China, India, Malaya, and Persia. *Humours* developed perhaps first in China alongside *qi*. Ho the Physician concluded that diseases are caused by deficiencies of elements (Wu Xing: fire, water, earth, wood, and metal), and he classified diseases as well as prescribed diets. About the same time in Italy, Alcmaeon of Croton (a Greek) wrote of the importance of equilibrium between what goes in and what goes out, and warned that imbalance would result in disease marked by obesity or emaciation.

The first recorded nutritional experiment with human subjects is found in the Bible's Book of Daniel. Daniel and his friends were captured by the king of Babylon during an invasion of Israel. Selected as court servants, they were to share in the king's fine foods and wine. But they objected, preferring vegetables (pulses) and water in accordance with their Jewish dietary restrictions. The king's chief steward reluctantly agreed to a trial. Daniel and his friends received their diet for ten days and were then compared to the king's men. Appearing healthier, they were allowed to continue with their diet.

Around 475 BC, Anaxagoras stated that food is absorbed by the human body and, therefore, contains "homeomerics" (generative components), suggesting the existence of nutrients. Around 400 BC, Hippocrates, who recognized and was concerned with obesity, which may have been common in southern Europe at the time, said, "Let food be your medicine and medicine be your food." The works that are still attributed to him, *Corpus Hippocraticum*, called for moderation and emphasized exercise.

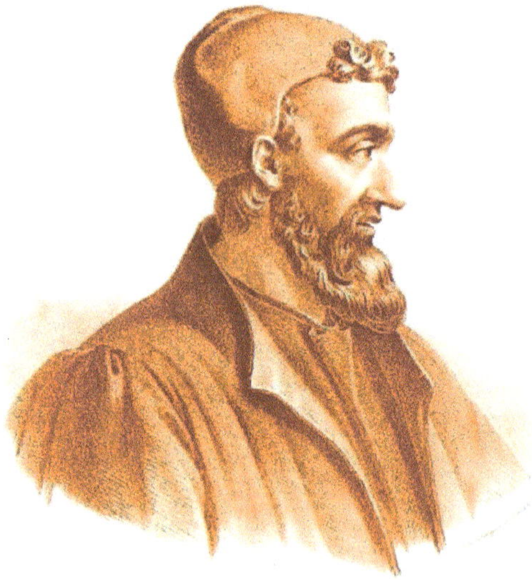

Followed for a millennium and a half, Galen (1st century) created the first coherent (although mistaken) theory of nutrition.

Salt, pepper and other spices were prescribed for various ailments in various preparations for example mixed with vinegar. In the 2nd century BC, Cato the Elder believed that cabbage (or the urine of cabbage-eaters) could cure digestive diseases, ulcers, warts, and intoxication. Living about the turn of the millennium, Aulus Celsus, an ancient Roman doctor, believed in "strong" and "weak" foods (bread for example was strong, as were older animals and vegetables).

Galen to Lind

One mustn't overlook the doctrines of Galen: In use from his life in the 1st century AD until the 17th century, it was heresy to disagree with him for 1500 years. Galen was physician to gladiators in Pergamon, and in Rome, physician to Marcus Aurelius and the three emperors who succeeded him. Most of Galen's teachings were gathered and enhanced in the late 11th century by Benedictine monks at the School of Salerno in

Regimen sanitatis Salernitanum, which still had users in the 17th century. Galen believed in the bodily *humours* of Hippocrates, and he taught that *pneuma* is the source of life. Four elements (earth, air, fire and water) combine into "complexion", which combines into states (the four temperaments: sanguine, phlegmatic, choleric, and melancholic). The states are made up of pairs of attributes (hot and moist, cold and moist, hot and dry, and cold and dry), which are made of four humours: blood, phlegm, green (or yellow) bile, and black bile (the bodily form of the elements). Galen thought that for a person to have gout, kidney stones, or arthritis was scandalous, which Gratzer likens to Samuel Butler›s *Erehwon* (1872) where sickness is a crime.

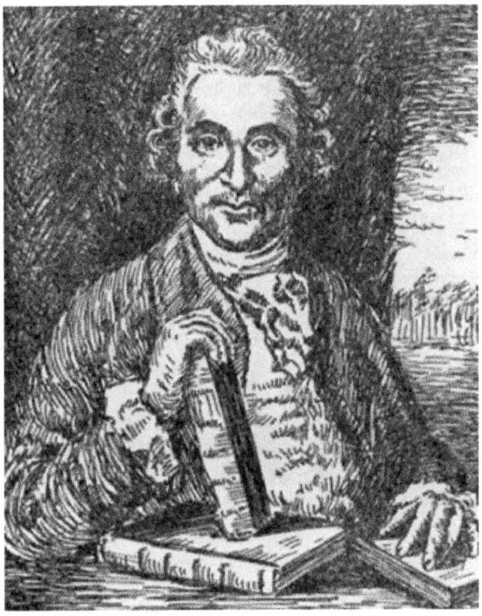

James Lind conducted in 1747 the first controlled clinical trial in modern times, and in 1753 published *Treatise on Scurvy*.

In the 1500s, Paracelsus was probably the first to criticize Galen publicly. Also in the 16th century, scientist and artist Leonardo da Vinci compared metabolism to a burning candle. Leonardo did not publish his works on this subject, but he was not afraid of thinking for himself and he definitely disagreed with Galen. Ultimately, 16th century works of Andreas Vesalius, sometimes called the father of modern medicine, overturned Galen's ideas. He was followed by piercing thought amalgamated with the era's mysticism and religion sometimes fueled by the mechanics of Newton and Galileo. Jan Baptist van Helmont, who discovered several gases such as carbon dioxide, performed the first quantitative experiment. Robert Boyle advanced chemistry. Sanctorius measured body weight. Physician Herman Boerhaave modeled the digestive process. Physiologist Albrecht von Haller worked out the difference between nerves and muscles.

Sometimes overlooked during his life, James Lind, a physician in the British navy, performed the first scientific nutrition experiment in 1747. Lind discovered that lime juice saved sailors that had been at sea for years from scurvy, a deadly and painful bleeding disorder. Between 1500 and 1800, an estimated two million sailors had died of scurvy. The discovery was ignored for forty years, after which British sailors became known as «limeys.» The essential vitamin C within citrus fruits would not be identified by scientists until 1932.

Lavoisier and Modern Science

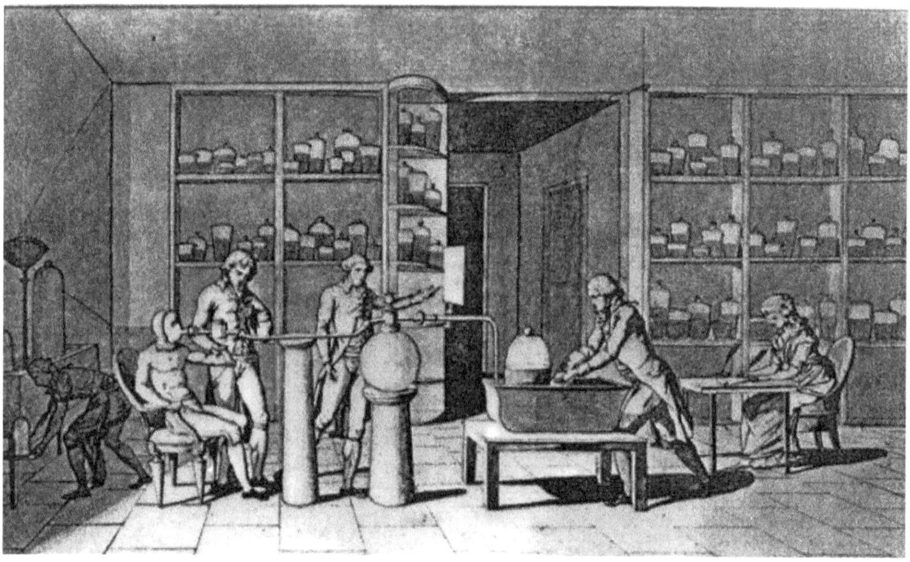

By containing his assistant, Armand Seguin, inside a rubber suit fitted with a tube sealed to his mouth with putty, Antoine Lavoisier first measured basal metabolic rate. Drawing by Madame Lavoisier (seated at right).

Around 1770, Antoine Lavoisier discovered the details of metabolism, demonstrating that the oxidation of food is the source of body heat. Called the most fundamental chemical discovery of the 18th century, Lavoisier discovered the principle of conservation of mass. His ideas made the phlogiston theory of combustion obsolete.

In 1790, George Fordyce recognized calcium as necessary for the survival of fowl. In the early 19th century, the elements carbon, nitrogen, hydrogen, and oxygen were recognized as the primary components of food, and methods to measure their proportions were developed.

In 1816, François Magendie discovered that dogs fed only carbohydrates (sugar), fat (olive oil), and water died evidently of starvation, but dogs also fed protein survived, identifying protein as an essential dietary component. William Prout in 1827 was the first person to divide foods into carbohydrates, fat, and protein. During the 19th century, Jean-Baptiste Dumas and Justus von Liebig quarrelled over their shared belief that animals get their protein directly from plants (animal and plant protein are the same and that humans do not create organic compounds). With a reputation as the leading organic chemist of his day but with no credentials in animal physiology, Liebig grew rich making food extracts like beef bouillon and infant formula that were later found to be of questionable nutritious value. In the 1860s, Claude Bernard discovered that body fat can be synthesized from carbohydrate and protein, showing that the energy in blood glucose can be stored as fat or as glycogen.

In the early 1880s, Kanehiro Takaki observed that Japanese sailors (whose diets consisted almost entirely of white rice) developed beriberi (or endemic neuritis, a disease causing heart problems and paralysis), but British sailors and Japanese naval officers did not. Adding various types of vegetables and meats to the diets of Japanese sailors prevented the disease, (not because of the increased protein as Takaki supposed but because it introduced a few parts per million of thiamine to the diet, later understood as a cure).

In 1896, Eugen Baumann observed iodine in thyroid glands. In 1897, Christiaan Eijkman worked with natives of Java, who also suffered from beriberi. Eijkman observed that chickens fed the native diet of white rice developed the symptoms of beriberi but remained healthy when fed unprocessed brown rice with the outer bran intact. Eijkman cured the natives by feeding them brown rice, discovering that food can cure disease. Over two decades later, nutritionists learned that the outer rice bran contains vitamin B1, also known as thiamine.

From 1900 to the Present

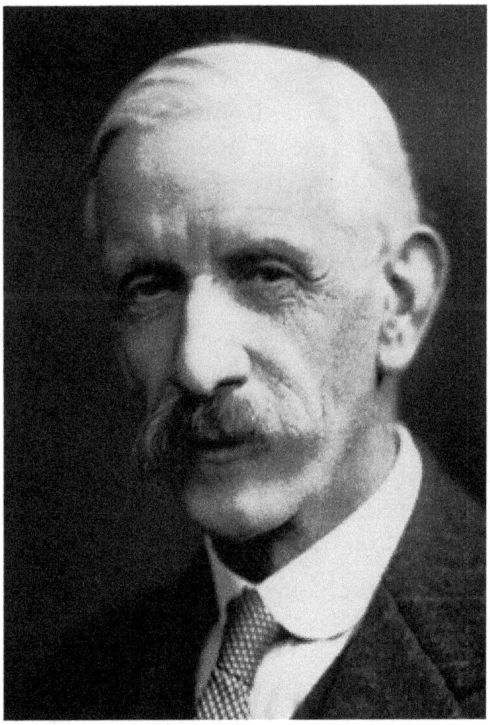

Frederick Hopkins discovered vitamins, for which he shared a Nobel prize with Eijkman.

In the early 20th century, Carl von Voit and Max Rubner independently measured caloric energy expenditure in different species of animals, applying principles of physics in nutrition. In 1906, Edith G. Willcock and Frederick Hopkins showed that the amino acid tryptophan aids the well-being of mice but it did not assure their growth. In the middle of twelve years of attempts to isolate them, Hopkins said in a 1906 lecture that «unsuspected dietetic factors,» other than calories, protein, and minerals, are needed to prevent deficiency diseases. In 1907, Stephen M. Babcock and Edwin B. Hart conducted the single-grain experiment, which took nearly four years to complete.

Vitamin	Year Isolated
Thiamin	1926
Vitamin C	1926
Vitamin A	1939
Vitamin D	1931
Vitamin E	1936
Niacin	1937
Biotin	1939
Vitamin K	1939
Pantothenic acid	1939
Folate	1939
Riboflavin	1933
Vitamin B6	1936

Oxford University closed down its nutrition department after World War II because the subject seemed to have been completed between 1912 and 1944.

In 1912, Casimir Funk coined the term vitamin, a vital factor in the diet, from the words "vital" and "amine," because these unknown substances preventing scurvy, beriberi, and pellagra, were thought then to be derived from ammonia. The vitamins were studied in the first half of the 20th century.

In 1913, Elmer McCollum and Marguerite Davis discovered the first vitamin, fat-soluble vitamin A, then water-soluble vitamin B (in 1915; now known to be a complex of several water-soluble vitamins) and named vitamin C as the then-unknown substance preventing scurvy. Lafayette Mendel and Thomas Osborne also performed pioneering work on vitamins A and B. In 1919, Sir Edward Mellanby incorrectly identified rickets as a vitamin A deficiency because he could cure it in dogs with cod liver oil. In 1922, McCollum destroyed the vitamin A in cod liver oil, but found that it still cured rickets. Also in 1922, H.M. Evans and L.S. Bishop discover vitamin E as essential for rat pregnancy, originally calling it "food factor X" until 1925.

In 1925, Hart discovered that trace amounts of copper are necessary for iron absorption. In 1927, Adolf Otto Reinhold Windaus synthesized vitamin D, and was awarded the Nobel Prize in Chemistry in 1928. In 1928, Albert Szent-Györgyi isolated ascorbic acid, and in 1932 proved that it is vitamin C by preventing scurvy. In 1935, he synthesized it, and in 1937, he won a Nobel Prize for his efforts. Szent-Györgyi concurrently elucidated much of the citric acid cycle.

In the 1930s, William Cumming Rose identified essential amino acids, necessary protein components that the body cannot synthesize. In 1935, Underwood and Marston independently discovered the necessity of cobalt. In 1936, Eugene Floyd DuBois showed that work and school performance are related to caloric intake. In 1938, Erhard Fernholz discovered the chemical structure of vitamin E and then he tragically disappeared. It was synthesised the same year by Paul Karrer.

In 1940, rationing in the United Kingdom during and after World War II took place according to nutritional principles drawn up by Elsie Widdowson and others. In 1941, the first Recommended Dietary Allowances (RDAs) were established by the National Research Council.

In 1992, The U.S. Department of Agriculture introduced the Food Guide Pyramid. In 2002, a Natural Justice study showed a relation between nutrition and violent behavior. In 2005, one inconclusive study found that obesity could be caused by adenovirus in addition to bad nutrition.

World leaders are looking at alternatives like genetically modified foods to tackle the problem of world hunger and food shortages.

NUTRIENTS

The list of nutrients that people are known to require is, in the words of Marion Nestle, "almost certainly incomplete". As of 2014, nutrients are thought to be of two types: macro-nutrients which are needed in relatively large amounts, and micronutrients which are needed in smaller quantities. A type of carbohydrate, dietary fiber, i.e. non-digestible material such as cellulose, is required, for both mechanical and biochemical reasons, although the exact reasons remain unclear. Other micronutrients include antioxidants and phytochemicals, which are said to influence (or protect) some body systems. Their necessity is not as well established as in the case of, for instance, vitamins.

Most foods contain a mix of some or all of the nutrient types, together with other substances, such as toxins of various sorts. Some nutrients can be stored internally (e.g., the fat-soluble vitamins), while others are required more or less continuously. Poor health can be caused by a lack of required nutrients or, in extreme cases, too much of a required nutrient. For example, both salt and water (both absolutely required) will cause illness or even death in excessive amounts.

Macronutrients

The macronutrients are carbohydrates, fiber, fats, protein, and water. The macronutrients (excluding fiber and water) provide structural material (amino acids from which proteins are built, and lipids from which cell membranes and some signaling molecules are built) and energy. Some of the structural material can be used to generate energy internally, and in either case it is measured in Joules or kilocalories (often called "Calories" and written with a capital *C* to distinguish them from little 'c' calories). Carbohydrates and proteins provide 17 kJ approximately (4 kcal) of energy per gram, while fats provide 37 kJ (9 kcal) per gram, though the net energy from either depends on such factors as absorption and digestive effort, which vary substantially from instance to instance. Vitamins, minerals, fiber, and water do not provide energy, but are required for other reasons.

Molecules of carbohydrates and fats consist of carbon, hydrogen, and oxygen atoms. Carbohydrates range from simple monosaccharides (glucose, fructose, galactose) to complex polysaccharides (starch). Fats are triglycerides, made of assorted fatty acid monomers bound to a glycerol backbone. Some fatty acids, but not all, are essential in the diet: they cannot be synthesized in the body. Protein molecules contain nitrogen atoms in addition to carbon, oxygen, and hydrogen. The fundamental components of protein are nitrogen-containing amino acids, some of which are essential in the sense that humans cannot make them internally. Some of the amino acids are convertible (with the expenditure of energy) to glucose and can be used for energy production, just as ordinary glucose, in a process known as gluconeogenesis. By breaking down existing protein, the carbon skeleton of the various amino acids can be metabolized to intermediates in cellular respiration; the remaining ammonia is discarded primarily as urea in urine. This occurs normally only during prolonged starvation.

Carbohydrates

Carbohydrates may be classified as monosaccharides, disaccharides, or polysaccharides depending on the number of monomer (sugar) units they contain. They constitute a large part of foods such as rice, noodles, bread, and other grain-based products. Monosaccharides, disaccharides, and polysaccharides contain one, two, and three or more sugar units, respectively. Polysaccharides are often referred to as *complex* carbohydrates because they are typically long, multiple branched chains of sugar units.

Traditionally, simple carbohydrates are believed to be absorbed quickly, and therefore to raise blood-glucose levels more rapidly than complex carbohydrates. This, however, is not accurate. Some simple carbohydrates (e.g., fructose) follow different metabolic pathways (e.g., fructolysis) that result in only a partial catabolism to glucose, while, in essence, many complex carbohydrates may be digested at the same rate as simple carbohydrates. Glucose stimulates the production of insulin through food entering the bloodstream, which is grasped by the beta cells in the pancreas.

Fiber

Dietary fiber is a carbohydrate that is incompletely absorbed in humans and in some animals. Like all carbohydrates, when it is metabolized it can produce four Calories (kilocalories) of energy per gram. However, in most circumstances it accounts for less than that because of its limited absorption and digestibility. Dietary fiber consists mainly of cellulose, a large carbohydrate polymer which is indigestible as humans do not have the required enzymes to disassemble it. There are two subcategories: soluble and insoluble fiber. Whole grains, fruits (especially plums, prunes, and figs), and vegetables are good sources of dietary fiber. There are many health benefits of a high-fiber diet. Dietary fiber helps reduce the chance of gastrointestinal problems such as constipation and diarrhea by increasing the weight and size of stool and softening it. Insoluble fiber, found in whole wheat flour, nuts and vegetables, especially stimulates peristalsis – the rhythmic muscular contractions of the intestines, which move digesta along the digestive tract. Soluble fiber, found in oats, peas, beans, and many fruits, dissolves in water in the intestinal tract to produce a gel that slows the movement of food through the intestines. This may help lower blood glucose levels because it can slow the absorption of sugar. Additionally, fiber, perhaps especially that from whole grains, is thought to possibly help lessen insulin spikes, and therefore reduce the risk of type 2 diabetes. The link between increased fiber consumption and a decreased risk of colorectal cancer is still uncertain.

Fat

A molecule of dietary fat typically consists of several fatty acids (containing long chains of carbon and hydrogen atoms), bonded to a glycerol. They are typically found as triglycerides (three fatty acids attached to one glycerol backbone). Fats may be classified as saturated or unsaturated depending on the detailed structure of the fatty acids involved. Saturated fats have all of the carbon atoms in their fatty acid chains bonded to hydrogen atoms, whereas unsaturated fats have some of these carbon atoms double-bonded, so their molecules have relatively fewer hydrogen atoms than a saturated fatty acid of the same length. Unsaturated fats may be further classified as monounsaturated (one double-bond) or polyunsaturated (many double-bonds). Furthermore, depending on the location of the double-bond in the fatty acid chain, unsaturated fatty acids are classified as omega-3 or omega-6 fatty acids. Trans fats are a type of unsaturated fat with *trans*-isomer bonds; these are rare in nature and in foods from natural sources; they are typically created in an industrial process called (partial) hydrogenation. There are nine kilocalories in each gram of fat. Fatty acids such as conjugated linoleic acid, catalpic acid, eleostearic acid and punicic acid, in addition to providing energy, represent potent immune modulatory molecules.

Saturated fats (typically from animal sources) have been a staple in many world cultures for millennia. Unsaturated fats (e. g., vegetable oil) are considered healthier, while trans fats are to be avoided. Saturated and some trans fats are typically solid at room temperature (such as butter or lard), while unsaturated fats are typically liquids (such as olive oil or flaxseed oil). Trans fats are very rare in nature, and have been shown to be highly detrimental to human health, but have properties useful in the food processing industry, such as rancidity resistance.

Essential Fatty Acids

Most fatty acids are non-essential, meaning the body can produce them as needed, generally from other fatty acids and always by expending energy to do so. However, in humans, at least two fatty acids are essential and must be included in the diet. An appropriate balance of essential fatty acids—omega-3 and omega-6 fatty acids—seems also important for health, although definitive experimental demonstration has been elusive. Both of these "omega" long-chain polyunsaturated fatty acids are substrates for a class of eicosanoids known as prostaglandins, which have roles throughout the human body. They are hormones, in some respects. The omega-3 eicosapentaenoic acid (EPA), which can be made in the human body from the omega-3 essential fatty acid alpha-linolenic acid (ALA), or taken in through marine food sources, serves as a building block for series 3 prostaglandins (e.g., weakly inflammatory PGE3). The omega-6 dihomo-gamma-linolenic acid (DGLA) serves as a building block for series 1 prostaglandins (e.g. anti-inflammatory PGE1), whereas arachidonic acid (AA) serves as a building block for series 2 prostaglandins (e.g. pro-inflammatory PGE 2). Both DGLA and AA can be made from the omega-6 linoleic acid (LA) in the human body, or can be taken in directly through food. An appropriately balanced intake of omega-3 and omega-6 partly determines the relative production of different prostaglandins, which is one reason why a balance between omega-3 and omega-6 is believed important for cardiovascular health. In industrialized societies, people typically consume large amounts of processed vegetable oils, which have reduced amounts of the essential fatty acids along with too much of omega-6 fatty acids relative to omega-3 fatty acids.

The conversion rate of omega-6 DGLA to AA largely determines the production of the prostaglandins PGE1 and PGE2. Omega-3 EPA prevents AA from being released from membranes, thereby skewing prostaglandin balance away from pro-inflammatory PGE2 (made from AA) toward anti-inflammatory PGE1 (made from DGLA). Moreover, the conversion (desaturation) of DGLA to AA is controlled by the enzyme delta-5-desaturase, which in turn is controlled by hormones such as insulin (up-regulation) and glucagon (down-regulation). The amount and type of carbohydrates consumed, along with some types of amino acid, can influence processes involving insulin, glucagon, and other hormones; therefore, the ratio of omega-3 versus omega-6 has wide effects on general health, and specific effects on immune function and inflammation, and mitosis (i.e., cell division).

Protein

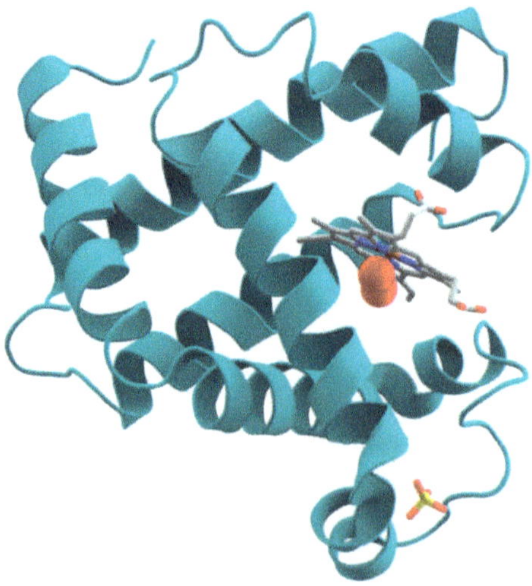

Proteins are chains of amino acids found in most nutritional foods.

Proteins are structural materials in much of the animal body (e.g. muscles, skin, and hair). They also form the enzymes that control chemical reactions throughout the body. Each protein molecule is composed of amino acids, which are characterized by inclusion of nitrogen and sometimes sulphur (these components are responsible for the distinctive smell of burning protein, such as the keratin in hair). The body requires amino acids to produce new proteins (protein retention) and to replace damaged proteins (maintenance). As there is no protein or amino acid storage provision, amino acids must be present in the diet. Excess amino acids are discarded, typically in the urine. For all animals, some amino acids are *essential* (an animal cannot produce them internally) and some are *non-essential* (the animal can produce them from other nitrogen-containing compounds). About twenty amino acids are found in the human body, and about ten of these are essential and, therefore, must be included in the diet. A diet that contains adequate amounts of amino acids (especially those that are essential) is particularly important in some situations: during early development and maturation, pregnancy, lactation, or injury (a burn, for instance). A *complete* protein source contains all the essential amino acids; an *incomplete* protein source lacks one or more of the essential amino acids.

It is possible with protein combinations of two incomplete protein sources (e.g., rice and beans) to make a complete protein source, and characteristic combinations are the basis of distinct cultural cooking traditions. However, complementary sources of protein do not need to be eaten at the same meal to be used together by the body. Excess amino acids from protein can be converted into glucose and used for fuel through a process called gluconeogenesis. The amino acids remaining after such conversion are discarded.

Water

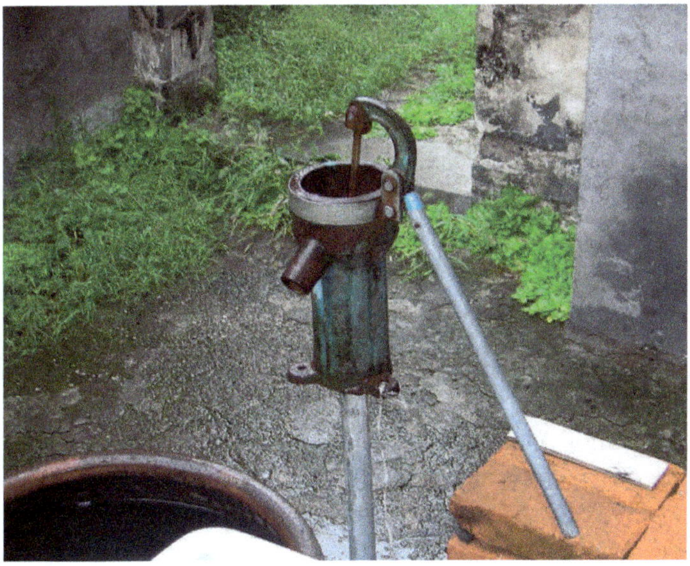

A manual water pump in China

Water is excreted from the body in multiple forms; including urine and feces, sweating, and by water vapour in the exhaled breath. Therefore, it is necessary to adequately rehydrate to replace lost fluids.

Early recommendations for the quantity of water required for maintenance of good health suggested that 6–8 glasses of water daily is the minimum to maintain proper hydration. However the notion that a person should consume eight glasses of water per day cannot be traced to a credible scientific source. The original water intake recommendation in 1945 by the Food and Nutrition Board of the National Research Council read: «An ordinary standard for diverse persons is 1 milliliter for each calorie of food. Most of this quantity is contained in prepared foods.» More recent comparisons of well-known recommendations on fluid intake have revealed large discrepancies in the volumes of water we need to consume for good health. Therefore, to help standardize guidelines, recommendations for water consumption are included in two recent European Food Safety Authority (EFSA) documents (2010): (i) Food-based dietary guidelines and (ii) Dietary reference values for water or adequate daily intakes (ADI). These specifications were provided by calculating adequate intakes from measured intakes in populations of individuals with "desirable osmolarity values of urine and desirable water volumes per energy unit consumed." For healthful hydration, the current EFSA guidelines recommend total water intakes of 2.0 L/day for adult females and 2.5 L/day for adult males. These reference values include water from drinking water, other beverages, and from food. About 80% of our daily water requirement comes from the beverages we drink, with the remaining 20% coming from food. Water content varies depending on the type of food consumed, with fruit and vegetables containing more than cereals, for example. These values are estimated using country-specific food balance sheets published by the Food and Agriculture Organisation of the United Nations. Other guidelines for nutrition also have implications for the beverages we consume for healthy hydration- for example, the World Health Organization (WHO) recommend that added sugars should represent no more than 10% of total energy intake. The EFSA panel also determined intakes for different populations. Recommended intake volumes in the elderly are the same as for adults as despite lower energy consumption, the water requirement of this group is increased due to a reduction in renal concentrating capacity. Pregnant and breastfeeding women require additional fluids to stay hydrated. The EFSA panel proposes that pregnant women should consume the same volume of water as non-pregnant women, plus an increase in proportion to the higher energy requirement, equal to 300 mL/day. To compensate for additional fluid output, breastfeeding women require an additional 700 mL/day above the recommended intake values for non-lactating women.

For those who have healthy kidneys, it is somewhat difficult to drink too much water, but (especially in warm humid weather and while exercising) it is dangerous to drink too little. While overhydration is much less common than dehydration, it is also possible to drink far more water than necessary, which can result in water intoxication, a serious and potentially fatal condition. In particular, large amounts of de-ionized water are dangerous.

Micronutrients

Minerals

Dietary minerals are inorganic chemical elements required by living organisms, other than the four elements carbon, hydrogen, nitrogen, and oxygen that are present in nearly all organic molecules. The term "mineral" is archaic, since the intent is to describe simply the less common elements in the diet. Some are heavier than the four just mentioned, including several metals, which often occur as ions in the body. Some dietitians recommend that these be supplied from foods in which they occur naturally, or at least as complex compounds, or sometimes even from natural inorganic sources (such as calcium carbonate from ground oyster shells). Some minerals are absorbed much more readily in the ionic forms found in such sources. On the other hand, minerals are often artificially added to the diet as supplements; the most famous is likely iodine in iodized salt which prevents goiter.

Macrominerals

Many elements are essential in relative quantity; they are usually called "bulk minerals". Some are structural, but many play a role as electrolytes. Elements with recommended dietary allowance (RDA) greater than 150 mg/day are, in alphabetical order (with informal or folk-medicine perspectives in parentheses):

- Calcium, a common electrolyte, but also needed structurally (for muscle and digestive system health, bone strength, some forms neutralize acidity, may help clear toxins, provides signaling ions for nerve and membrane functions)
- Chlorine as chloride ions; very common electrolyte; see sodium, below
- Magnesium, required for processing ATP and related reactions (builds bone, causes strong peristalsis, increases flexibility, increases alkalinity)
- Phosphorus, required component of bones; essential for energy processing
- Potassium, a very common electrolyte (heart and nerve health)
- Sodium, a very common electrolyte; in general not found in dietary supplements, despite being needed in large quantities, because the ion is very common in food: typically as sodium chloride, or common salt. Excessive sodium consumption can deplete calcium and magnesium leading to high blood pressure and osteoporosis.
- Sulfur, for three essential amino acids and therefore many proteins (skin, hair, nails, liver, and pancreas). Sulfur is not consumed alone, but in the form of sulfur-containing amino acids

Trace Minerals

Many elements are required in trace amounts, usually because they play a catalytic role in enzymes. Some trace mineral elements (RDA < 200 mg/day) are, in alphabetical order:

- Cobalt required for biosynthesis of vitamin B12 family of coenzymes. Animals cannot biosynthesize B12, and must obtain this cobalt-containing vitamin in their diet.
- Copper required component of many redox enzymes, including cytochrome c oxidase
- Chromium required for sugar metabolism

- Iodine required not only for the biosynthesis of thyroxine but also — it is presumed — for other important organs as breast, stomach, salivary glands, thymus, etc. (see Extrathyroidal iodine); for this reason iodine is needed in larger quantities than others in this list, and sometimes classified with the macrominerals
- Iron required for many enzymes, and for hemoglobin and some other proteins
- Manganese (processing of oxygen)
- Molybdenum required for xanthine oxidase and related oxidases
- Selenium required for peroxidase (antioxidant proteins)
- Zinc required for several enzymes such as carboxypeptidase, liver alcohol dehydrogenase, and carbonic anhydrase

Vitamins

As with the minerals discussed above, some vitamins are recognized as organic essential nutrients, necessary in the diet for good health. (Vitamin D is the exception: it can be synthesized in the skin, in the presence of UVB radiation.) Certain vitamin-like compounds that are recommended in the diet, such as carnitine, are thought useful for survival and health, but these are not "essential" dietary nutrients because the human body has some capacity to produce them from other compounds. Moreover, thousands of different phytochemicals have recently been discovered in food (particularly in fresh vegetables), which may have desirable properties including antioxidant activity (see below); however, experimental demonstration has been suggestive but inconclusive. Other essential nutrients that are not classified as vitamins include essential amino acids (see above), choline, essential fatty acids (see above), and the minerals discussed in the preceding section.

Vitamin deficiencies may result in disease conditions, including goitre, scurvy, osteoporosis, impaired immune system, disorders of cell metabolism, certain forms of cancer, symptoms of premature aging, and poor psychological health (including eating disorders), among many others. Excess levels of some vitamins are also dangerous to health (notably vitamin A). Deficient or excess levels of minerals can also have serious health consequences.

HEALTHY DIETS

Whole Plant Food Diet

Heart disease, cancer, obesity, and diabetes are commonly called "Western" diseases because these maladies were once rarely seen in developing countries. An international study in China found some regions had virtually no cancer or heart disease, while in other areas they reflected "up to a 100-fold increase" coincident with shifts from diets that were found to be entirely plant-based to heavily animal-based, respectively. In contrast, diseases of affluence like cancer and heart disease are common throughout the developed world, including the United States. Adjusted for age and exercise, large regional clusters of people in China rarely suffered from these "Western" diseases possibly because their diets are rich in vegetables, fruits, and whole grains, and have little dairy and meat products. Some studies show these to be, in high quantities, possible causes of some cancers. There are arguments for and against this controversial issue.

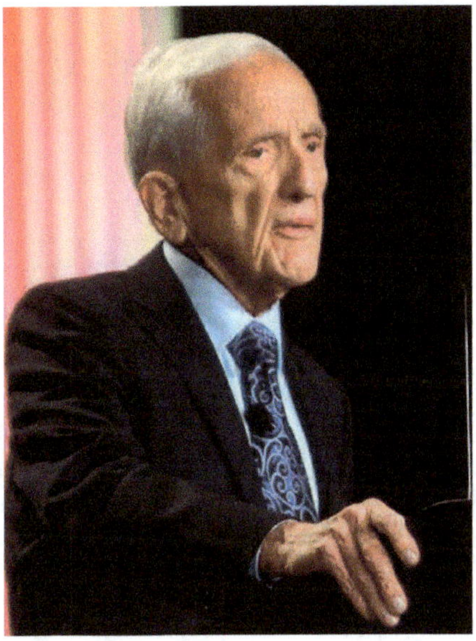

T. Colin Campbell is among the scientists who advocate a plant-based diet

The United Healthcare/Pacificare nutrition guideline recommends a whole plant food diet, and recommends using protein only as a condiment with meals. A *National Geographic* cover article from November 2005, entitled *The Secrets of Living Longer*, also recommends a whole plant food diet. The article is a lifestyle survey of three populations, Sardinians, Okinawans, and Adventists, who generally display longevity and "suffer a fraction of the diseases that commonly kill people in other parts of the developed world, and enjoy more healthy years of life." In common with all three groups is to "Eat fruits, vegetables, and whole grains."

The *National Geographic* article noted that an NIH funded study of 34,000 Seventh-day Adventists between 1976 and 1988 "...found that the Adventists' habit of consuming beans, soy milk, tomatoes, and other fruits lowered their risk of developing certain cancers. It also suggested that eating whole grain bread, drinking five glasses of water a day, and, most surprisingly, consuming four servings of nuts a week reduced their risk of heart disease."

The French «Paradox»

The French paradox is the observation that the French suffer a relatively low incidence of coronary heart disease, despite having a diet relatively rich in saturated fats. A number of explanations have been suggested:

- Saturated fat consumption does not cause heart disease
- Reduced consumption of processed carbohydrate and other junk foods.
- Regular consumption of red wine.
- Higher consumption of artificially produced trans-fats by Americans, which has been shown to have greater lipoprotein effects per gram than saturated fat.

However, statistics collected by the World Health Organization from 1990–2000 show that the incidence of heart disease in France may have been underestimated and, in fact, may be similar to that of neighboring countries.

Phytochemicals

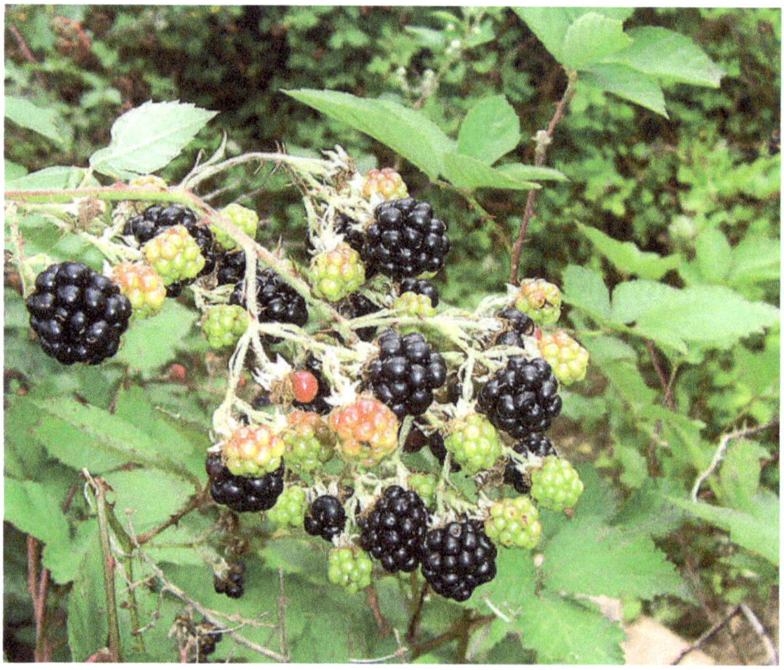

Blackberries are a source of polyphenols

Phytochemicals such as polyphenols are compounds produced naturally in plants (phyto means "plant" in Greek). In general, the term is used to refer to those chemicals under research to assess whether they have biological significance. To date, there is no evidence in humans that polyphenols or other non-nutrient compounds from plants have health effects. Further, dietary supplements containing phytochemicals also have no proven health benefit.

While initial studies sought to reveal if antioxidant or phytochemical supplements might promote health, later large clinical trials did not detect any benefit and showed instead that excess supplementation could be harmful.

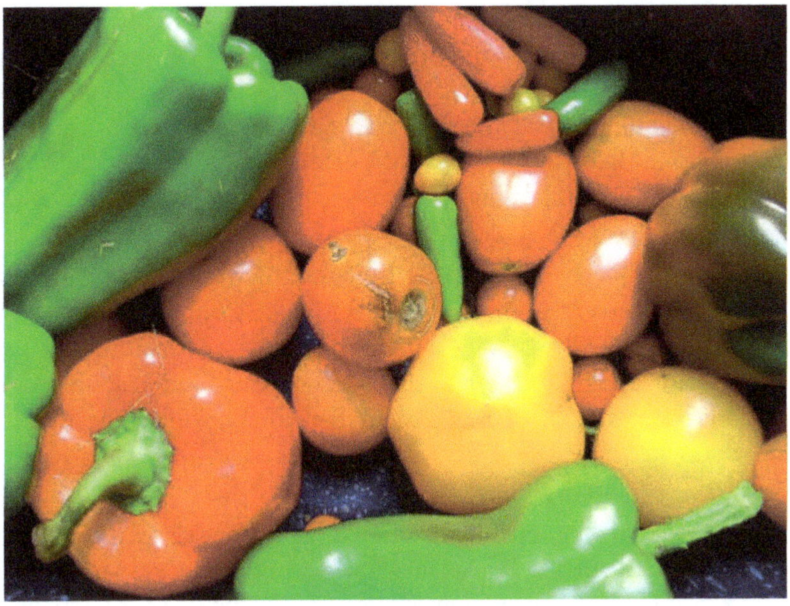

Colorful fruits and vegetables can be components of a healthy diet.

Intestinal Bacterial Flora

Animal intestines contain a large population of gut flora. In humans, the four dominant phyla are Firmicutes, Bacteroidetes, Actinobacteria, and Proteobacteria. They are essential to digestion and are also affected by food that is consumed. Bacteria in the gut perform many important functions for humans, including breaking down and aiding in the absorption of otherwise indigestible food; stimulating cell growth; repressing the growth of harmful bacteria, training the immune system to respond only to pathogens; producing vitamin B_{12}; and defending against some infectious diseases.

Animal Nutrition

Nutritional science investigates the metabolic and physiological responses of the body to diet. With advances in the fields of molecular biology, biochemistry, nutritional immunology, molecular medicine and genetics, the study of nutrition is increasingly concerned with metabolism and metabolic pathways: the sequences of biochemical steps through which substances in living things change from one form to another.

Carnivore and herbivore diets are contrasting, with basic nitrogen and carbon proportions vary for their particular foods. "The nitrogen content of plant tissues averages about 2%, while in fungi, animals, and bacteria it averages about 5% to 10%." Many herbivores rely on bacterial fermentation to create digestible nutrients from indigestible plant cellulose, while obligate carnivores must eat animal meats to obtain certain vitamins or nutrients their bodies cannot otherwise synthesize. All animals' diets must provide sufficient amounts of the basic building blocks they need, up to the point where their particular biology can synthesize the rest. Animal tissue contains chemical compounds, such as water, carbohydrates (sugar, starch, and fiber), amino acids (in proteins), fatty acids (in lipids), and nucleic acids (DNA and RNA). These compounds in turn consist of elements such as carbon, hydrogen, oxygen, nitrogen, phosphorus, calcium, iron, zinc, magnesium, manganese, and so on. All of these chemical compounds and elements occur in various forms and combinations (e.g. hormones, vitamins, phospholipids, hydroxyapatite).

Animal tissue consists of elements and compounds ingested, digested, absorbed, and circulated through the bloodstream to feed the cells of the body. Except in the unborn fetus, the digestive system is the first system involved. Digestive juices break chemical bonds in ingested molecules, and modify their conformations and energy states. Though some molecules are absorbed into the bloodstream unchanged, digestive processes release them from the matrix of foods. Unabsorbed matter, along with some waste products of metabolism, is eliminated from the body in the feces.

Studies of nutritional status must take into account the state of the body before and after experiments, as well as the chemical composition of the whole diet and of all material excreted and eliminated from the body (in urine and feces). Comparing the food to the waste can help determine the specific compounds and elements absorbed and metabolized in the body. The effects of nutrients may only be discernible over an extended period, during which all food and waste must be analyzed. The number of variables involved in such experiments is high, making nutritional studies time-consuming and expensive, which explains why the science of animal nutrition is still slowly evolving.

In particular, the consumption of whole-plant foods slows digestion and allows better absorption, and a more favorable balance of essential nutrients per Calorie, resulting in better management of cell growth, maintenance, and mitosis (cell division), as well as better regulation of appetite and blood sugar. Regularly scheduled meals (every few hours) have also proven more wholesome than infrequent or haphazard ones.

Plant Nutrition

Plant nutrition is the study of the chemical elements that are necessary for plant growth. There are several principles that apply to plant nutrition. Some elements are directly involved in plant metabolism. However, this principle does not account for the so-called beneficial elements, whose presence, while not required, has clear positive effects on plant growth.

A nutrient that is able to limit plant growth according to Liebig's law of the minimum is considered an essential plant nutrient if the plant cannot complete its full life cycle without it. There are 16 essential plant soil nutrients, besides the three major elemental nutrients carbon and oxygen that are obtained by photosynthetic plants from carbon dioxide in air, and hydrogen, which is obtained from water.

Plants uptake essential elements from the soil through their roots and from the air (consisting of mainly nitrogen and oxygen) through their leaves. Green plants obtain their carbohydrate supply from the carbon dioxide in the air by the process of photosynthesis. Carbon and oxygen are absorbed from the air, while other nutrients are absorbed from the soil. Nutrient uptake in the soil is achieved by cation exchange, wherein root hairs pump hydrogen ions (H^+) into the soil through proton pumps. These hydrogen ions displace cations attached to negatively charged soil particles so that the cations are available for uptake by the root. In the leaves, stomata open to take in carbon dioxide and expel oxygen. The carbon dioxide molecules are used as the carbon source in photosynthesis.

Although nitrogen is plentiful in the Earth's atmosphere, very few plants can use this directly. Most plants, therefore, require nitrogen compounds to be present in the soil in which they grow. This is made possible by the fact that largely inert atmospheric nitrogen is changed in a nitrogen fixation process to biologically usable forms in the soil by bacteria.

Plant nutrition is a difficult subject to understand completely, partially because of the variation between different plants and even between different species or individuals of a given clone. Elements present at low levels may cause deficiency symptoms, and toxicity is possible at levels that are too high. Furthermore, deficiency of one element may present as symptoms of toxicity from another element, and vice versa.

ENVIRONMENTAL NUTRITION

Research in the field of nutrition has greatly contributed in finding out the essential facts about how environmental depletion can lead to crucial nutrition-related health problems like contamination, spread of contagious diseases, malnutrition, etc. Moreover, environmental contamination due to discharge of agricultural as well as industrial chemicals like organocholrines, heavy metal, and radionucleotides may adversely affect the human and the ecosystem as a whole. As far as safety of the human health is concerned, then these environmental contaminants can reduce people's nutritional status and health. This could directly or indirectly cause drastic changes in their diet habits. Hence, food-based remedial as well as preventive strategies are essential to address global issues like hunger and malnutrition and to enable the susceptible people to adapt themselves to all these environmental as well as socio-economic alterations.

ADVICE AND GUIDANCE

Government Policies

Canada's Food Guide is another example government-run nutrition program. Produced by Health Canada, the guide advises food quantities, provides education on balanced nutrition, and promotes physical activity in accordance with government-mandated nutrient needs. Like other nutrition programs around the world, Canada's Food Guide divides nutrition into four main food groups: vegetables and fruit, grain products, milk and alternatives, and meat and alternatives. It is interesting to note that, unlike its American counterpart, the Canadian guide references and provides alternative to meat and dairy, which can be attributed to the growing vegan and vegetarian movements.

In the US, dietitians are registered (RD) or licensed (LD) with the Commission for Dietetic Registration and the American Dietetic Association, and are only able to use the title "dietitian," as described by the business and professions codes of each respective state, when they have met specific educational and experiential prerequisites and passed a national registration or licensure examination, respectively. In California, registered dietitians must abide by the *"Business and Professions Code of Section 2585-2586.8"*. Anyone may call themselves a nutritionist, including unqualified dietitians, as this term is unregulated. Some states, such as the State of Florida, have begun to include the title "nutritionist" in state licensure requirements. Most governments provide guidance on nutrition, and some also impose mandatory disclosure/labeling requirements for processed food manufacturers and restaurants to assist consumers in complying with such guidance.

In the US, nutritional standards and recommendations are established jointly by the US Department of Agriculture and US Department of Health and Human Services. Dietary and physical activity guidelines from the USDA are presented in the concept of MyPlate, which superseded the food pyramid, which replaced the Four Food Groups. The Senate committee currently responsible for oversight of the USDA is the *Agriculture, Nutrition and Forestry Committee*. Committee hearings are often televised on C-SPAN. The U.S. Department of Health and Human Services provides a sample week-long menu that fulfills the nutritional recommendations of the government.

Government Programs

Governmental organisations have been working on nutrition literacy interventions in non-primary health care settings to address the nutrition information problem in the U.S. Some programs include:

The Family Nutrition Program (FNP) is a free nutrition education program serving low-income adults around the U.S. This program is funded by the Food Nutrition Service's (FNS) branch of the United States Department of Agriculture (USDA) usually through a local state academic institution that runs the program. The FNP has developed a series of tools to help families participating in the Food Stamp Program stretch their food dollar and form healthful eating habits including nutrition education.

Expanded Food and Nutrition Education Program (ENFEP) is a unique program that currently operates in all 50 states and in American Samoa, Guam, Micronesia, Northern Marianas, Puerto Rico, and the Virgin Islands. It is designed to assist limited-resource audiences in acquiring the knowledge, skills, attitudes, and changed behavior necessary for nutritionally sound diets, and to contribute to their personal development and the improvement of the total family diet and nutritional well-being.

An example of a state initiative to promote nutrition literacy is Smart Bodies, a public-private partnership between the state's largest university system and largest health insurer, Louisiana State Agricultural Center and Blue Cross and Blue Shield of Louisiana Foundation. Launched in 2005, this program promotes lifelong healthful eating patterns and physically active lifestyles for children and their families. It is an interactive educational program designed to help prevent childhood obesity through classroom activities that teach children healthful eating habits and physical exercise.

Education

Nutrition is taught in schools in many countries. In England and Wales, the Personal and Social Education and Food Technology curricula include nutrition, stressing the importance of a balanced diet and teaching how to read nutrition labels on packaging. In many schools, a Nutrition class will fall within the Family and Consumer Science or Health departments. In some American schools, students are required to take a certain number of FCS or Health related classes. Nutrition is offered at many schools, and, if it is not a class of its own, nutrition is included in other FCS or Health classes such as: Life Skills, Independent Living, Single Survival, Freshmen Connection, Health etc. In many Nutrition classes, students learn about the food groups, the food pyramid, Daily Recommended Allowances, calories, vitamins, minerals, malnutrition, physical activity, healthful food choices, portion sizes, and how to live a healthy life.

A 1985, US National Research Council report entitled *Nutrition Education in US Medical Schools* concluded that nutrition education in medical schools was inadequate. Only 20% of the schools surveyed taught nutrition as a separate, required course. A 2006 survey found that this number had risen to 30%. Membership by physicians in leading professional nutrition societies such as the American Society for Nutrition has generally declined from the 1990s.

NUTRITION LITERACY

At the time of this entry, we were not able to identify any specific nutrition literacy studies in the U.S. at a national level. However, the findings of the 2003 National Assessment of Adult Literacy (NAAL) provide a basis upon which to frame the nutrition literacy problem in the U.S. NAAL introduced the first ever measure of "the degree to which individuals have the capacity to obtain, process and understand basic health information and services needed to make appropriate health decisions" – an objective of Healthy People 2010 and of which nutrition literacy might be considered an important subset. On a scale of below basic, basic, intermediate and proficient, NAAL found 13 percent of adult Americans have proficient health literacy, 44% have intermediate literacy, 29 percent have basic literacy and 14 percent have below basic health literacy. The study found that health literacy increases with education and people living below the level of poverty have lower health literacy than those above it.

Another study examining the health and nutrition literacy status of residents of the lower Mississippi Delta found that 52 percent of participants had a high likelihood of limited literacy skills. While a precise comparison between the NAAL and Delta studies is difficult, primarily because of methodological differences, Zoellner et al. suggest that health literacy rates in the Mississippi Delta region are different from the U.S. general population and that they help establish the scope of the problem of health literacy among adults in the Delta region. For example, only 12 percent of study participants identified the My Pyramid graphic two years after it had been launched by the USDA. The study also found significant relationships between nutrition literacy and income level and nutrition literacy and educational attainment further delineating priorities for the region.

These statistics point to the complexities surrounding the lack of health/nutrition literacy and reveal the degree to which they are embedded in the social structure and interconnected with other problems. Among these problems are the lack of information about food choices, a lack of understanding of nutritional information and its application to individual circumstances, limited or difficult access to healthful foods, and a range of cultural influences and socioeconomic constraints such as low levels of education and high levels of poverty that decrease opportunities for healthful eating and living.

The links between low health literacy and poor health outcomes has been widely documented and there is evidence that some interventions to improve health literacy have produced successful results in the primary care setting. More must be done to further our understanding of nutrition literacy specific interventions in non-primary care settings in order to achieve better health outcomes.

MALNUTRITION

Malnutrition refers to insufficient, excessive, or imbalanced consumption of nutrients by an organism. In developed countries, the diseases of malnutrition are most often associated with nutritional imbalances or excessive consumption. In developing countries, malnutrition is more likely to be caused by poor access to a range of nutritious foods or inadequate knowledge. In Mali the International Crops Research Institute for the Semi-Arid Tropics (ICRISAT) and the Aga Khan Foundation, trained women's groups to make *equinut*, a healthy and nutritional version of the traditional recipe *di-dègué* (comprising peanut paste, honey and millet or rice flour). The aim was to boost nutrition and livelihoods by producing a product that women could make and sell, and which would be accepted by the local community because of its local heritage.

Although there are more organisms in the world who are malnourished due to insufficient consumption, increasingly more organisms suffer from excessive over-nutrition; a problem caused by an over abundance of sustenance coupled with the instinctual desire (by animals in particular) to consume all that it can.

Nutritionism is the view that excessive reliance on food science and the study of nutrition can lead to poor nutrition and to ill health. It was originally credited to Gyorgy Scrinis, and was popularized by Michael Pollan. Since nutrients are invisible, policy makers rely on nutrition experts to advise on food choices. Because science has an incomplete understanding of how food affects the human body, Pollan argues, nutritionism can be blamed for many of the health problems relating to diet in the Western World today.

Insufficient

In general, *under-consumption* refers to the long-term consumption of insufficient sustenance in relation to the energy that an organism expends or expels, leading to poor health.

Excessive

In general, *over-consumption* refers to the long-term consumption of excess sustenance in relation to the energy that an organism expends or expels, leading to poor health and, in animals, obesity. It can cause excessive hair loss, brittle nails, and irregular premenstrual cycles for females.

Unbalanced

When too much of one or more nutrients is present in the diet to the exclusion of the proper amount of other nutrients, the diet is said to be unbalanced.

Illnesses Caused by Improper Nutrient Consumption

Nutrients	Deficiency	Excess
Macronutrients		
Calories	Starvation, marasmus	Obesity, diabetes mellitus, cardiovascular disease
Simple carbohydrates	Low energy levels.	Obesity, diabetes mellitus, cardiovascular disease
Complex carbohydrates	Micronutrient deficiency	Obesity, cardiovascular disease (high glycemic index foods)
Protein	Kwashiorkor	Rabbit starvation
Saturated fat	Low testosterone levels, vitamin deficiencies.	Obesity, cardiovascular disease
Trans fat	None	Obesity, cardiovascular disease
Unsaturated fat	Fat-soluble vitamin deficiency	Obesity, cardiovascular disease
Micronutrients		
Vitamin A	Xerophthalmia and night blindness	Hypervitaminosis A (cirrhosis, hair loss)
Vitamin B_1	Beri-Beri	?
Vitamin B_2	Skin and corneal lesions	?
Niacin	Pellagra	Dyspepsia, cardiac arrhythmias, birth defects
Vitamin B_{12}	Pernicious anemia	?
Vitamin C	Scurvy	Diarrhea causing dehydration
Vitamin D	Rickets	Hypervitaminosis D (dehydration, vomiting, constipation)
Vitamin E	Neurological disease	Hypervitaminosis E (anticoagulant: excessive bleeding)
Vitamin K	Hemorrhage	Liver damage
Omega-3 fats	Cardiovascular Disease	Bleeding, Hemorrhages, Hemorrhagic stroke, reduced glycemic control among diabetics
Omega-6 fats	None	Cardiovascular Disease, Cancer
Cholesterol	None	Cardiovascular Disease
Macrominerals		
Calcium	Osteoporosis, tetany, carpopedal spasm, laryngospasm, cardiac arrhythmias	Fatigue, depression, confusion, nausea, vomiting, constipation, pancreatitis, increased urination, kidney stones
Magnesium	Hypertension	Weakness, nausea, vomiting, impaired breathing, and hypotension
Potassium	Hypokalemia, cardiac arrhythmias	Hyperkalemia, palpitations
Sodium	Hyponatremia	Hypernatremia, hypertension
Trace minerals		

Iron	Anemia	Cirrhosis, Hereditary hemochromatosis, heart disease
Iodine	Goiter, hypothyroidism	Iodine toxicity (goiter, hypothyroidism)

Mental Agility

Research indicates that improving the awareness of nutritious meal choices and establishing long-term habits of healthy eating have a positive effect on cognitive and spatial memory capacity, with potential to increase a student's ability to process and retain academic information.

Some organizations have begun working with teachers, policymakers, and managed foodservice contractors to mandate improved nutritional content and increased nutritional resources in school cafeterias from primary to university level institutions. Health and nutrition have been proven to have close links with overall educational success. Currently, less than 10% of American college students report that they eat the recommended five servings of fruit and vegetables daily. Better nutrition has been shown to affect both cognitive and spatial memory performance; a study showed those with higher blood sugar levels performed better on certain memory tests. In another study, those who consumed yogurt performed better on thinking tasks when compared to those that consumed caffeine-free diet soda or confections. Nutritional deficiencies have been shown to have a negative effect on learning behavior in mice as far back as 1951.

"Better learning performance is associated with diet-induced effects on learning and memory ability".

The "nutrition-learning nexus" demonstrates the correlation between diet and learning and has application in a higher education setting.

"We find that better-nourished children perform significantly better in school, partly because they enter school earlier and thus have more time to learn but mostly because of greater learning productivity per year of schooling."

91% of college students feel that they are in good health, whereas only 7% eat their recommended daily allowance of fruits and vegetables.

Nutritional education is an effective and workable model in a higher education setting.

More "engaged" learning models that encompass nutrition is an idea that is picking up steam at all levels of the learning cycle.

There is limited research available that directly links a student's Grade Point Average (G.P.A.) to their overall nutritional health. Additional substantive data is needed to prove that overall intellectual health is closely linked to a person's diet, rather than just another correlation fallacy.

Mental Disorders

Nutritional supplement treatment may be appropriate for major depression, bipolar disorder, schizophrenia, and obsessive compulsive disorder, the four most common mental disorders in developed countries. Supplements that have been studied most for mood elevation and stabilization include eicosapentaenoic acid and docosahexaenoic acid (each of which an omega-3 fatty acid contained in fish oil but not in flaxseed oil), vitamin B12, folic acid, and inositol.

Cancer

Cancer is now common in developing countries. According to a study by the International Agency for Research on Cancer, "In the developing world, cancers of the liver, stomach and esophagus were more common, often linked to consumption of carcinogenic preserved foods, such as smoked or salted food, and parasitic infections that attack organs." Lung cancer rates are rising rapidly in poorer nations because of increased use of tobacco. Developed countries "tended to have cancers linked to affluence or a 'Western lifestyle' — cancers of the colon, rectum, breast and prostate — that can be caused by obesity, lack of exercise, diet and age."

Metabolic Syndrome

Several lines of evidence indicate lifestyle-induced hyperinsulinemia and reduced insulin function (i.e., insulin resistance) as a decisive factor in many disease states. For example, hyperinsulinemia and insulin resistance are strongly linked to chronic inflammation, which in turn is strongly linked to a variety of adverse developments such as arterial microinjuries and clot formation (i.e., heart disease) and exaggerated cell division (i.e., cancer). Hyperinsulinemia and insulin resistance (the so-called metabolic syndrome) are characterized by a combination of abdominal obesity, elevated blood sugar, elevated blood pressure, elevated blood triglycerides, and reduced HDL cholesterol. The negative effect of hyperinsulinemia on prostaglandin PGE1/PGE2 balance may be significant.

The state of obesity clearly contributes to insulin resistance, which in turn can cause type 2 diabetes. Virtually all obese and most type 2 diabetic individuals have marked insulin resistance. Although the association between overweight and insulin resistance is clear, the exact (likely multifarious) causes of insulin resistance remain less clear. It is important to note that it has been demonstrated that appropriate exercise, more regular food intake, and reducing glycemic load (see below) all can reverse insulin resistance in overweight individuals (and thereby lower blood sugar levels in those with type 2 diabetes).

Obesity can unfavourably alter hormonal and metabolic status via resistance to the hormone leptin, and a vicious cycle may occur in which insulin/leptin resistance and obesity aggravate one another. The vicious cycle is putatively fuelled by continuously high insulin/leptin stimulation and fat storage, as a result of high intake of strongly insulin/leptin stimulating foods and energy. Both insulin and leptin normally function as satiety signals to the hypothalamus in the brain; however, insulin/leptin resistance may reduce this signal and therefore allow continued overfeeding despite large body fat stores. In addition, reduced leptin signalling to the brain may reduce leptin's normal effect to maintain an appropriately high metabolic rate.

There is a debate about how and to what extent different dietary factors— such as intake of processed carbohydrates, total protein, fat, and carbohydrate intake, intake of saturated and trans fatty acids, and low intake of vitamins/minerals—contribute to the development of insulin and leptin resistance. In any case, analogous to the way modern man-made pollution may possess the potential to overwhelm the environment's ability to maintain homeostasis, the recent explosive introduction of high glycemic index and processed foods into the human diet may possess the potential to overwhelm the body's ability to maintain homeostasis and health (as evidenced by the metabolic syndrome epidemic).

Hyponatremia

Excess water intake, without replenishment of sodium and potassium salts, leads to hyponatremia, which can further lead to water intoxication at more dangerous levels. A well-publicized case occurred in 2007, when Jennifer Strange died while participating in a water-drinking contest. More usually, the condition occurs in long-distance endurance events (such as marathon or triathlon competition and training) and causes gradual mental dulling, headache, drowsiness, weakness, and confusion; extreme cases may result in coma, convulsions, and death. The primary damage comes from swelling of the brain, caused by increased osmosis as blood salinity decreases. Effective fluid replacement techniques include water aid stations during running/cycling races, trainers providing water during team games, such as soccer, and devices such as Camel Baks, which can provide water for a person without making it too hard to drink the water.

Antinutrient

Antinutrients are natural or synthetic compounds that interfere with the absorption of nutrients. Nutrition studies focus on antinutrients commonly found in food sources and beverages.

Sugar Consumption in the United States

The relatively recent increased consumption of sugar has been linked to the rise of some afflictions such as diabetes, obesity, and more recently heart disease. Increased consumption of sugar has been tied to these three, among others. Obesity levels have more than doubled in the last 30 years among adults, going from 15% to 35% in the United States. Obesity and diet also happen to be high risk factors for diabetes. In the same time span that obesity doubled, diabetes numbers quadrupled in America. Increased weight, especially in the form of belly fat, and high sugar intake are also high risk factors for heart disease. Both sugar intake and fatty tissue increase the probability of elevated LDL cholesterol in the bloodstream. Elevated amounts of Low-density lipoprotein (LDL) cholesterol, is the primary factor in heart disease. In order to avoid all the dangers of sugar, moderate consumption is paramount.

Processed Foods

Since the Industrial Revolution some two hundred years ago, the food processing industry has invented many technologies that both help keep foods fresh longer and alter the fresh state of food as they appear in nature. Cooling is the primary technology used to maintain freshness, whereas many more technologies have been invented to allow foods to last longer without becoming spoiled. These latter technologies include pasteurisation, autoclavation, drying, salting, and separation of various components, all of which appearing to alter the original nutritional contents of food. Pasteurisation and autoclavation (heating techniques) have no doubt improved the safety of many common foods, preventing epidemics of bacterial infection. But some of the (new) food processing technologies have downfalls as well.

Modern separation techniques such as milling, centrifugation, and pressing have enabled concentration of particular components of food, yielding flour, oils, juices, and so on, and even separate fatty acids, amino acids, vitamins, and minerals. Inevitably, such large-scale concentration changes the nutritional content of food, saving certain nutrients while removing others. Heating techniques may also reduce food's content of many heat-labile nutrients such as certain vitamins and phytochemicals, and possibly other yet-to-be-discovered substances.Because of reduced nutritional value, processed foods are often 'enriched' or 'fortified' with some of the most critical nutrients (usually certain vitamins) that were lost during processing. Nonetheless, processed foods tend to have an inferior nutritional profile compared to whole, fresh foods, regarding content of both sugar and high GI starches, potassium/sodium, vitamins, fiber, and of intact, unoxidized (essential) fatty acids. In addition, processed foods often contain potentially harmful substances such as oxidized fats and trans fatty acids.

A dramatic example of the effect of food processing on a population's health is the history of epidemics of beri-beri in people subsisting on polished rice. Removing the outer layer of rice by polishing it removes with it the essential vitamin thiamine, causing beri-beri. Another example is the development of scurvy among infants in the late 19th century in the United States. It turned out that the vast majority of sufferers were being fed milk that had been heat-treated (as suggested by Pasteur) to control bacterial disease. Pasteurisation was effective against bacteria, but it destroyed the vitamin C.

As mentioned, lifestyle- and obesity-related diseases are becoming increasingly prevalent all around the world. There is little doubt that the increasingly widespread application of some modern food processing technologies has contributed to this development. The food processing industry is a major part of modern economy, and as such it is influential in political decisions (e.g., nutritional recommendations, agricultural subsidising). In any known profit-driven economy, health considerations are hardly a priority; effective production of cheap foods with a long shelf-life is more the trend. In general, whole, fresh foods have a relatively short shelf-life and are less profitable to produce and sell than are more processed foods. Thus, the consumer is left with the choice between more expensive, but nutritionally superior, whole, fresh foods, and cheap, usually nutritionally inferior, processed foods. Because processed foods are often cheaper, more convenient (in both purchasing, storage, and preparation), and more available, the consumption of nutritionally inferior foods has been increasing throughout the world along with many nutrition-related health complications.

REFERENCES

1. "Joint Collection Development Policy: Human Nutrition and Food". US National Library of Medicine, National Institutes of Health. 14 October 2014. Retrieved 13 December 2014.
2. "What is an RDN and DTR?". Academy of Nutrition and Dietetics. Retrieved May 9, 2015.
3. http://www.iaacn.org/ The International & American Associations of Clinical Nutritionist, 2014, Retrieved 2014-12-14
4. "FAQs about CNS Certification – Certification Board for Nutrition Specialists". Retrieved 2015-09-24.
5. Whitney, Ellie; Rolfes, Sharon Rady (2013). Understanding Nutrition (13 ed.). Wadsworth, Cengage Learning. pp. 667, 670. ISBN 978-1133587521.
6. Obesity, Weight Linked to Prostate Cancer Deaths – National Cancer Institute. Cancer.gov. Retrieved on 2011-10-17.
7. Obesity and Overweight for Professionals: Causes | DNPAO | CDC. Cdc.gov (2011-05-16). Retrieved on 2011-10-17.
8. Metabolic syndrome – PubMed Health. Ncbi.nlm.nih.gov. Retrieved on 2011-10-17.
9. Omega-3 fatty acids. Umm.edu (2011-10-05). Retrieved on 2011-10-17.
10. What I need to know about Eating and Diabetes – National Diabetes Information Clearinghouse. Diabetes.niddk.nih.gov. Retrieved on 2011-10-17.
11. Diabetes Diet and Food Tips: Eating to Prevent and Control Diabetes. Helpguide.org. Retrieved on 2011-10-17.
12. Osteoporosis & Vitamin D: Deficiency, How Much, Benefits, and More. Webmd.com (2005-07-07). Retrieved on 2011-10-17.
13. Dietary Supplement Fact Sheet: Vitamin D. Ods.od.nih.gov. Retrieved on 2011-10-17.
14. Brody, Jane E. (March 19, 1998). "Osteoporosis Linked to Vitamin D Deficiency". The New York Times. Archived from the original on 2008-03-09.
15. Payne-Palacio, June R.; Canter, Deborah D. (2014). The Profession of Dietetics. Jones & Bartlett Learning. pp. 3, 4. ISBN 978-1-284-02608-5.
16. Gratzer 2005, p. 40.
17. Gratzer 2005, p. 41.
18. Gratzer 2005, p. 36.
19. Daniel 1:5–16. Biblegateway.com. Retrieved on 2011-10-17.
20. McCollum, Elmer V. (1957). A History of Nutrition. Cambridge, Mass.: The Riverside Press (Houghton Mifflin). pp. 8–9.
21. History of the Study of Nutrition in Western Culture (Rai University lecture notes for General Nutrition course, 2004)

22. Smith, Richard (24 January 2004). "Let food by thy medicine...". BMJ. 328 (7433): 0–g. doi:10.1136/bmj.328.7433.0-g.
23. Gratzer 2005, p. 37.
24. Gratzer 2005, pp. 38, 39, 41.
25. Gratzer 2005, p. 38.
26. Gratzer 2005, p. 39.
27. Bhatt, Arun (January–March 2010). "Evolution of Clinical Research: A History Before and Beyond James Lind". Perspectives in Clinical Research. Indian Society for Clinical Research via US National Center for Biotechnology Information. 1 (1): 6–10. PMC 3149409 . PMID 21829774.
28. Gratzer 2005, p. 48.
29. Gratzer 2005, pp. 48, 49, 50, 52, 53, 54.
30. Willett, Walter C. with Skerrett, Patrick J. (2005) . Eat, Drink, and be Healthy: The Harvard Medical School Guide To Healthy Eating. Free Press (Simon & Schuster). p. 183. ISBN 0-684-86337-5.
31. Gratzer 2005, pp. 21–24, 32.
32. Gratzer 2005, p. 60.
33. Silberberg, Martin S. (2009). Chemistry: The Molecular Nature of Matter and Change (5 ed.). McGraw-Hill. p. 44. ISBN 978-0-07-304859-8.
34. Gratzer 2005, p. 56.
35. Muljadi, Paul. Health. Paul Muljadi. p. 42.
36. Gratzer 2005, pp. 73–74.
37. Ahrens, Richard (January 1, 1977). "William Prout (1785–1850): A Biographical Sketch" (PDF). The Journal of Nutrition. 107 (1): 15.
38. Gratzer 2005, p. 82.
39. Carpenter 1994, p. 224.
40. Gratzer 2005, pp. 86, 92, 95, 115.
41. Gratzer 2005, pp. 98–99.
42. Carpenter 1994, p. 220.
43. Willcock, Edith G.; F. Gowland Hopkins (1906). "The importance of individual amino-acids in metabolism: Observations on the effect of adding tryptophane to a dietary in which zein is the sole nitrogenous constituent." (PDF). The Journal of Physiology. 35 (1–2): 88–102. doi:10.1113/jphysiol.1906.sp001181. PMC 1465819 . PMID 16992872.
44. Semenza, G., ed. (2012). Comprehensive Biochemistry: Selected Topics in the History of Biochemistry: Personal Recollections, Part 1. 35. Elsevier via Google Books. p. 117. ISBN 0444598200. Retrieved March 15, 2016.
45. Hopkins, F. Gowland (1912). "Feeding Experiments Illustrating the Importance of Accessory Factors in Normal Dietaries" (PDF). The Journal of Physiology.

44 (5–6): 425–460. doi:10.1113/jphysiol.1912.sp001524. PMC 1512834 . PMID 16993143. Retrieved March 15, 2016.

46. Carpenter's table gives the year each vitamin was proposed, the year isolated (shown here), the year the structure was determined, and the year that synthesis was achieved. Carpenter, Kenneth J. (October 1, 2003). "A Short History of Nutritional Science: Part 3 (1912–1944)". The Journal of Nutrition. 133 (10): 3023–3032. PMID 14519779. from Combs, G. F., Jr (1992). The Vitamins: Fundamental Aspects in Nutrition and Health. Academic Press. ISBN 0123819806.
47. Carpenter, Kenneth J. (November 1, 2003). "A Short History of Nutritional Science: Part 4 (1945–1985)". The Journal of Nutrition. 133 (11): 3331–3342. PMID 14608041.
48. Conlan, Roberta; Elizabeth Sherman (October 2000). "Unraveling the Enigma of Vitamin D" (PDF). National Academy of Sciences. Retrieved June 13, 2016.
49. Subcommittee on Vitamin Tolerance, Committee on Animal Nutrition, National Research Council (1987). "Vitamin E, in Vitamin Tolerance of Animals". National Academy of Sciences. Retrieved December 22, 2013.
50. "F.B.I. Joins Hunt for Young German Chemist". San Bernardino Daily Sun. December 18, 1940. Retrieved December 22, 2013.
51. "USDA's Food Guide Pyramid Booklet, 1992" (PDF). United States Department Of Agriculture. Archived from the original (PDF) on August 24, 2014.
52. Contagious obesity? Identifying the human adenoviruses that may make us fat. Science Blog
53. Montouri, Paulo; Triassi, Maria; Sarnacchiaro, Pasquale (2012). "The consumption of genetically modified foods in Italian high school students". Food Quality and preference. 26 (2): 246–251. doi:10.1016/j.foodqual.2012.05.004.
54. Nestle, Marion (2013) . Food Politics: How the Food Industry Influences Nutrition and Health. University of California Press. p. 413. ISBN 978-0-520-27596-6.
55. Fuhrman, Joel (2014). The End of Dieting. Harper One (Harper Collins). pp. 101–102. ISBN 978-0-06-224932-6.
56. "Get the Facts on Fiber". webmd.com.
57. "Strange but True: Drinking Too Much Water Can Kill". Scientific American. June 21, 2007.
58. "Can shipwrecked men survive if they drink sea water?". Natural History Magazine.
59. Berg J, Tymoczko JL, Stryer L (2002). Biochemistry (5th ed.). San Francisco: W.H. Freeman. p. 603. ISBN 0-7167-4684-0.
60. Otto, H (1973). Diabetik Bei Diabetus Mellitus. Bern: Verlag Hans Huber.
61. Crapo, P; Reaven, Olefsky (1977). "Postprandial plasma-glucose and -insulin responses to different complex carbohydrates". Diabetes. 26 (12): 1178–1183. doi:10.2337/diabetes.26.12.1178. PMID 590639.

62. Crapo, P; Kolterman, Waldeck; Reaven, Olefsky (1980). "Postprandial hormonal responses to different types of complex carbohydrate in individuals with impaired glucose tolerance". Am J Clin Nutr. 33 (8): 1723–1728. PMID 6996472.

63. Jenkins, David; Jenkins, Alexandra L.; Wolever, Thomas M.S.; Thompson, Lilian H. and Rao, A. Venkat (February 1986). "Simple and complex carbohydrates". Nutritional Reviews. 44 (2): 44–49. doi:10.1111/j.1753-4887.1986.tb07585.x.

64. "The Nutrition Source: Carbohydrates". Harvard School of Public Health. Retrieved 2011-07-07.

65. American Dietetic Association; Dietitians Of, Canada (2003). "Position of the American Dietetic Association and Dietitians of Canada: Vegetarian diets". JADA. 103 (6): 748–765. doi:10.1053/jada.2003.50142. PMID 12778049.

66. "Healthy Water Living". BBC. Retrieved 2007-02-01. Archived from the original on 2007-01-01.

67. ""Drink at least eight glasses of water a day." Really? Is thcre scientific evidence for "8 × 8"?". physiology.org.

68. Food and Nutrition Board, National Academy of Sciences. Recommended Dietary Allowances, revised 1945. National Research Council, Reprint and Circular Series, No. 122, 1945 (Aug), pp. 3–18.

69. Le Bellego L, Jean C, Jiménez L, Magnani C, Tang W, Boutrolle I (2010). "Understanding fluid consumption patterns to improve healthy hydration". Nutr Today. 45 (6): S22–S26. doi:10.1097/NT.0b013e3181fe4314.

70. EFSA Panel on Dietetic Products, Nutrition and Allergies (NDA) (2010). "Scientific Opinion on Dietary Reference Values for Water". EFSA Journal. 8 (3): 1459. doi:10.2903/j.efsa.2010.1459.

71. Armstrong LE, Pumerantz AC, Roti MW, Judelson DA, Watson G, Dias JC, Sokmen B, Casa DJ, Maresh CM, et al. (2005). "Fluid, electrolyte, and renal indices of hydration during 11 days of controlled caffeine consumption". Int J Sport Nutr Exerc Metab. 15 (3): 252–65. PMID 16131696.

72. "FAO Corporate Document Repository. Food Balance Sheets- A Handbook." Retrieved 2011-03-07

73. "WHO Technical Report Series. Diet, nutrition and the prevention of chronic diseases." Report of a Joint WHO/FAO Expert Consultation; Geneva 2003. Retrieved 2011-03-07

74. Farrell DJ, Bower L (October 2003). "Fatal water intoxication". J. Clin. Pathol. Journal of Clinical Pathology. 56 (10): 803–4. doi:10.1136/jcp.56.10.803-a. PMC 1770067 . PMID 14514793.

75. Mitchell, Dakota; Haroun, Lee (2012). Introduction to Health Care (3 ed.). Delmar Cengage. p. 279. ISBN 978-1-435-48755-0.

76. Nelson, D. L.; Cox, M. M. (2000). Lehninger Principles of Biochemistry (3rd ed.). New York: Worth Publishing. ISBN 1-57259-153-6.

77. Corbridge, D. E. C. (1995). Phosphorus: An Outline of its Chemistry, Biochemistry, and Technology (5th ed.). Amsterdam: Elsevier. ISBN 0-444-89307-5.

78. Lippard, S. J.; Berg, J. M. (1994). Principles of Bioinorganic Chemistry. Mill Valley, CA: University Science Books. ISBN 0935702725.

79. Shils, M. S.; et al., eds. (2005). Modern Nutrition in Health and Disease. Lippincott Williams and Wilkins. ISBN 0-7817-4133-5.

80. Campbell T.; Campbell T. (2005). The China Study. Dallas: Benella Books. ISBN 1-932100-38-5.

81. Andrew Mente; Lawrence de Koning; Harry S. Shannon; Sonia S. Anand (2009). "A Systematic Review of the Evidence Supporting a Causal Link Between Dietary Factors and Coronary Heart Disease". Arch Intern Med. 169 (7): 659–669. doi:10.1001/archinternmed.2009.38. PMID 19364995.

82. Eckel RH, Borra S, Lichtenstein AH, Yin-Piazza SY (April 2007). "Understanding the complexity of trans fatty acid reduction in the American diet: American Heart Association Trans Fat Conference 2006: report of the Trans Fat Conference Planning Group". Circulation. 115 (16): 2231–46. doi:10.1161/CIRCULATIONAHA.106.181947. PMID 17426064.

83. Ducimetière P, Lang T, Amouyel P, Arveiler D, Ferrières J (January 2000). "Why mortality from heart disease is low in France. Rates of coronary events are similar in France and Southern Europe". BMJ. 320 (7229): 249–50. doi:10.1136/bmj.320.7229.249/a. PMC 1117444 . PMID 10642245.

84. "Phytochemical". American Cancer Society. 17 January 2013. Retrieved 1 October 2013.

85. Woodside JV, McCall D, McGartland C, Young IS (2005). "Micronutrients: dietary intake v. supplement use". The Proceedings of the Nutrition Society. 64 (4): 543–53. doi:10.1079/PNS2005464. PMID 16313697.

86. Bjelakovic G; Nikolova, D; Gluud, LL; Simonetti, RG; Gluud, C (2007). "Mortality in randomized trials of antioxidant supplements for primary and secondary prevention: systematic review and meta-analysis". JAMA. 297 (8): 842–57. doi:10.1001/jama.297.8.842. PMID 17327526.

87. Sepkowitz, Kent (3 August 2011). "The Doctor and the Pomegranate". Slate.

88. Khanna S, Tosh PK (January 2014). "A clinician's primer on the role of the microbiome in human health and disease". Mayo Clin. Proc. 89 (1): 107–14. doi:10.1016/j.mayocp.2013.10.011. PMID 24388028.

89. Guarner, F; Malagelada, J (2003). "Gut flora in health and disease". The Lancet. 361 (9356): 512–9. doi:10.1016/S0140-6736(03)12489-0. PMID 12583961.

90. Chapter 6 Energy and Nutrient Relations, Ecology course text at SCNU.edu

91. Researchers Look at How Frequency of Meals May Affect Health. USDA Agricultural Research Service. Ars.usda.gov (February 15, 2008). Retrieved on 2011-10-17.

92. Allen V. Barker; David J. Pilbeam. Handbook of Plant Nutrition. CRC Press, 2010. p. Preface.

93. Lindemann, W.C. and Glover C.R. (2003) Nitrogen Fixation by Legumes. New Mexico State University/

94. Nutrition and the Environment, Retrieved 20 June 2014.
95. Sample Menus for a 2000 Calorie Food Pattern. mypyramid.gov
96. Commission on Life Sciences. (1985). Nutrition Education in US Medical Schools, p. 4. National Academies Press.
97. Adams KM, Lindell KC, Kohlmeier M, Zeisel SH (2006). "Status of nutrition education in medical schools". Am. J. Clin. Nutr. 83 (4): 941S–4S. PMC 2430660 . PMID 16600952.
98. McClave, Stephen A.; Mechanick, Jeffrey I.; Bistrian, Bruce; Graham, Toby; Hegazi, Refaat; Jensen, Gordon L.; Kushner, Robert F.; Merritt, Russell (2016-12-01). "What is the significance of a physician shortage in nutrition medicine?". JPEN. Journal of parenteral and enteral nutrition. 34 (6 Suppl): 7S–20S. doi:10.1177/0148607110375429. PMID 21149831.
99. Baldi, S. (ED.) et al. (2009). Technical Report and Data File User's Manual for the 2003 National Assessment of Adult Literacy (NCES 2009–47). U.S. Department of Education, National Center for Education Statistics. Washington, D.C.: U.S. Government Printing Office.
100. Zoellner, J., Connell, C., Bounds, W., Crook, L., Yadrick, K. (2009). "Nutrition Literacy Status and Preferred Nutrition Communications Channels Among Adults in the Lower Mississippi Delta". Preventing Chronic Disease. 6 (4): A128. PMC 2774642 . PMID 19755004.
101. Berkman N. D., Sheridan, S.L., Donahue, K. E., Halpern, D.J., Viera, A., Crotty, K., ... Viswanathan, M. (2011). Health and Literacy Intervention Outcomes: an Updated Systematic Review. Evidence Report/Technology Assessment no. 199. Prepared by RTI International – University of North Carolina Evidence-based Practice Center. Publication Number 11-E006. Rockville, MD. Agency for Healthcare Research and Quality.
102. Nourishing communities through holistic farming, Impatient optimists, Bill & Melinda Gates Foundation. April 30th 2013.
103. "Gyorgy Scrinis' Web Page". Retrieved 2009-01-14.
104. Pollan, Michael (2007-01-28). "Unhappy Meals". The New York Times.
105. Pollan, Michael (2008). In Defense of Food: An Eater's Manifesto. New York, USA: Penguin Press. ISBN 978-1594201455.
106. Jere R. Behrman (1996). "The impact of health and nutrition on education". World Bank Research Observer. 11 (1): 23–37. doi:10.1093/wbro/11.1.23.
107. American College Health Association (2007). "American College Health Association National College Health Assessment Spring 2006 Reference Group data report (abridged)". J Am Coll Health. 55 (4): 195–206. doi:10.3200/JACH.55.4.195-206. PMID 17319325.
108. Benton D, Sargent J (July 1992). "Breakfast, blood glucose and memory". Biol Psychol. 33 (2–3): 207–10. doi:10.1016/0301-0511(92)90032-P. PMID 1525295.
109. Kanarek RB, Swinney D (February 1990). "Effects of food snacks on cognitive performance in male college students". Appetite. 14 (1): 15–27. doi:10.1016/0195-

6663(90)90051-9. PMID 2310175.

110. Whitley JR, O'Dell BL, Hogan AG (September 1951). "Effect of diet on maze learning in second generation rats; folic acid deficiency". J. Nutr. 45 (1): 153–60. PMID 14880969.
111. Umezawa M, Kogishi K, Tojo H, et al. (February 1999). "High-linoleate and high-alpha-linolenate diets affect learning ability and natural behavior in SAMR1 mice". J. Nutr. 129 (2): 431–7. PMID 10024623.
112. Glewwe P, Jacoby H, King E (2001). "Early childhood nutrition and academic achievement: A longitudinal analysis". Journal of Public Economics. 81 (3): 345–68. doi:10.1016/S0047-2727(00)00118-3.
113. Glewwe, Paul; Jacoby, Hanan G; King, Elizabeth M (2001). "Managed food service contractors react quickly to the demands of their clients achievement: A longitudinal analysis". Journal of Public Economics. 81 (3): 345–368. doi:10.1016/S0047-2727(00)00118-3.
114. Guernsey L (1993). "Many colleges clear their tables of steak, substitute fruit and pasta". Chronicle of Higher Education. 39 (26): A30.
115. Duster T, Waters A (2006). "Engaged learning across the curriculum: The vertical integration of food for thought". Liberal Education. 92 (2): 42.
116. Lakhan SE, Vieira KF (2008). "Nutritional therapies for mental disorders". Nutr J. 7 (1): 2. doi:10.1186/1475-2891-7-2. PMC 2248201 . PMID 18208598.
117. Coren, Michael (2005-03-10). "Study: Cancer no longer rare in poorer countries". CNN. Retrieved 2007-01-01.
118. "Why is too much water dangerous?". BBC News. 2007-01-15. Retrieved 2008-11-09.
119. Number (in Millions) of Civilian, Non-Institutionalized Persons with Diagnosed Diabetes, United States, 1980–2014. U.S. Centers for Disease Control and Prevention. (3 March 2013)
120. A portfolio of content dedicated to the Cardiovascular and Stroke Professional. American Heart Association.
121. Morris, Audrey; Audia Barnett; Olive-Jean Burrows (2004). "Effect of Processing on Nutrient Content of Foods" (PDF). Cajanus. 37 (3): 160–164. Retrieved 2006-10-26.

CHAPTER 2

Process of Metabolism

Chapter Contents

- **Introduction**
- **Key Biochemicals**
- **Catabolism**
- **Energy Transformations**
- **Investigation and Manipulation**

The term metabolism, derived from the Greek language, simply means change or transformation. It relates to various processes within the body that convert food and other substances into energy and other metabolic byproducts used by the body. It is a necessary function that allows our bodies to use food and other resources to maintain the working parts, repair damage, heal injury and rid the body of toxins. In other words, metabolism is a necessary process, without which living organisms would die. Metabolism aids in digestive function as well as absorption of nutrients. It is most affected by nutrition, hydration and physical activity. Each of these items is an imperative aspect of optimum metabolic health. When any one of these is lacking, the metabolic rate decreases. Consequently, weight loss and weight maintenance are directly related to healthy metabolism.

INTRODUCTION

Metabolism is the set of life-sustaining chemical transformations within the cells of living organisms. The three main purposes of metabolism are the conversion of food/fuel to energy to run cellular processes, the conversion of food/fuel to building blocks for proteins, lipids, nucleic acids, and some carbohydrates, and the elimination of nitrogenous wastes. These enzyme-catalyzed reactions allow organisms to grow and reproduce, maintain their structures, and respond to their environments. The word metabolism can also refer to the sum of all chemical reactions that occur in living organisms, including digestion and the transport of substances into and between different cells, in which case the set of reactions within the cells is called intermediary metabolism or intermediate metabolism.

Metabolism is usually divided into two categories: catabolism, the *breaking down* of organic matter, for example, by cellular respiration, and anabolism, the *building up* of components of cells such as proteins and nucleic acids. Usually, breaking down releases energy and building up consumes energy.

The chemical reactions of metabolism are organized into metabolic pathways, in which one chemical is transformed through a series of steps into another chemical, by a sequence of enzymes. Enzymes are crucial to metabolism because they allow organisms to drive desirable reactions that require energy that will not occur by themselves, by coupling them to spontaneous reactions that release energy. Enzymes act as catalysts that allow the reactions to proceed more rapidly. Enzymes also allow the regulation of metabolic pathways in response to changes in the cell's environment or to signals from other cells.

The metabolic system of a particular organism determines which substances it will find nutritious and which poisonous. For example, some prokaryotes use hydrogen sulfide as a nutrient, yet this gas is poisonous to animals. The speed of metabolism, the metabolic rate, influences how much food an organism will require, and also affects how it is able to obtain that food.

A striking feature of metabolism is the similarity of the basic metabolic pathways and components between even vastly different species. For example, the set of carboxylic acids that are best known as the intermediates in the citric acid cycle are present in all known organisms, being found in species as diverse as the unicellular bacterium *Escherichia coli* and huge multicellular organisms like elephants. These striking similarities in metabolic pathways are likely due to their early appearance in evolutionary history, and their retention because of their efficacy.

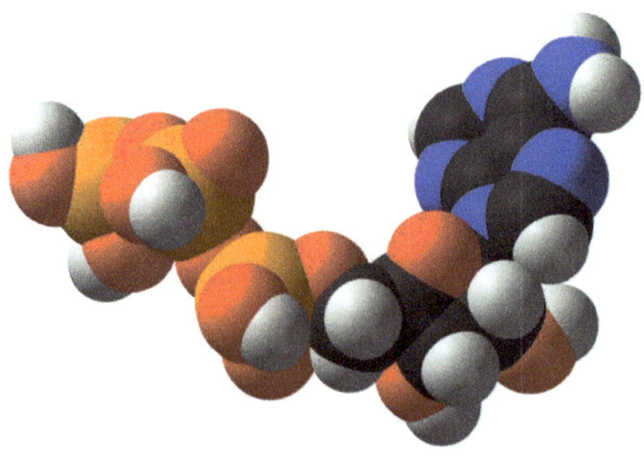

Structure of adenosine triphosphate (ATP), a central intermediate in energy metabolism

KEY BIOCHEMICALS

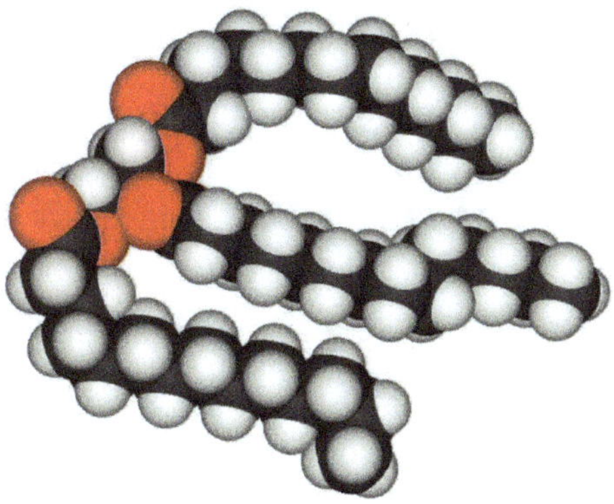

Structure of a triacylglycerol lipid

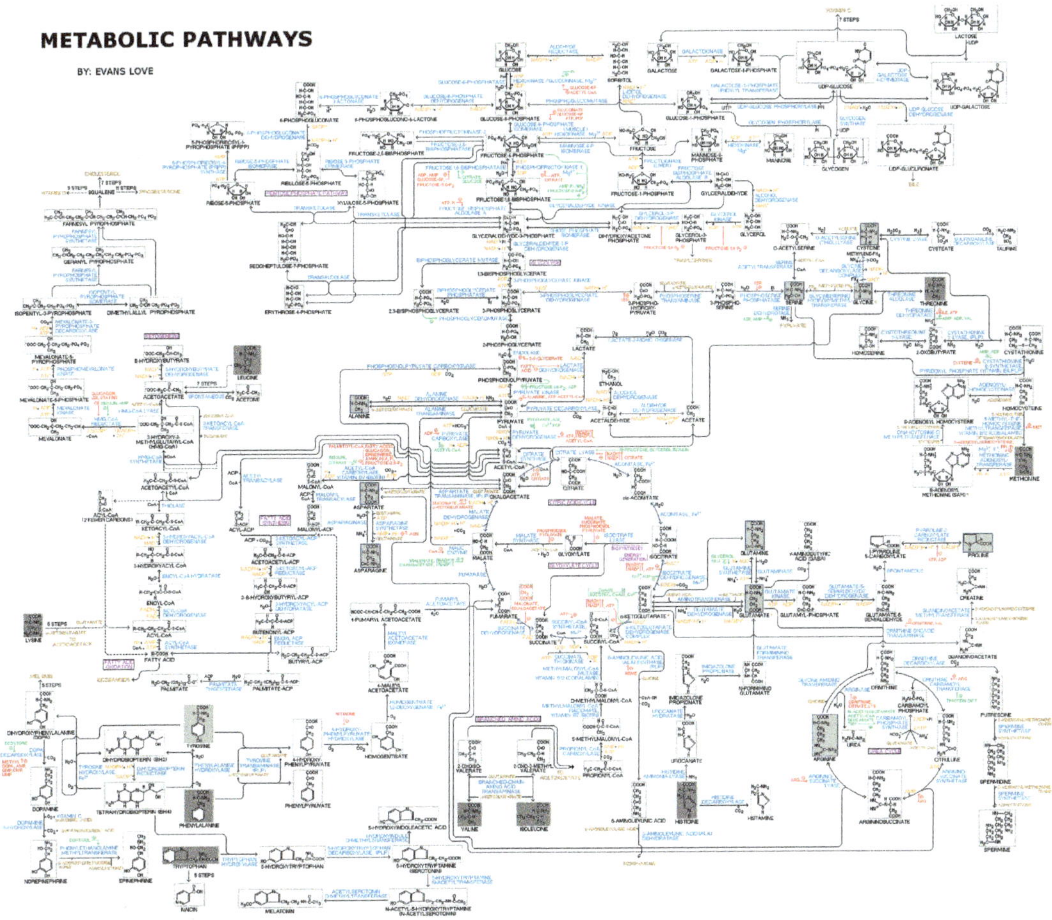

This is a diagram depicting a large set of human metabolic pathways.

Most of the structures that make up animals, plants and microbes are made from three basic classes of molecule: amino acids, carbohydrates and lipids (often called fats). As these molecules are vital for life, metabolic reactions either focus on making these molecules during the construction of cells and tissues, or by breaking them down and using them as a source of energy, by their digestion. These biochemicals can be joined together to make polymers such as DNA and proteins, essential macromolecules of life.

Type of molecule	Name of monomer forms	Name of polymer forms	Examples of polymer forms
Amino acids	Amino acids	Proteins (made of polypeptides)	Fibrous proteins and globular proteins
Carbohydrates	Monosaccharides	Polysaccharides	Starch, glycogen and cellulose
Nucleic acids	Nucleotides	Polynucleotides	DNA and RNA

Amino Acids and Proteins

Proteins are made of amino acids arranged in a linear chain joined together by peptide bonds. Many proteins are enzymes that catalyze the chemical reactions in metabolism. Other proteins have structural or mechanical functions, such as those that form the cytoskeleton, a system of scaffolding that maintains the cell shape. Proteins are also important in cell signaling, immune responses, cell adhesion, active transport across membranes, and the cell cycle. Amino acids also contribute to cellular energy metabolism by providing a carbon source for entry into the citric acid cycle (tricarboxylic acid cycle), especially when a primary source of energy, such as glucose, is scarce, or when cells undergo metabolic stress.

Lipids

Lipids are the most diverse group of biochemicals. Their main structural uses are as part of biological membranes both internal and external, such as the cell membrane, or as a source of energy. Lipids are usually defined as hydrophobic or amphipathic biological molecules but will dissolve in organic solvents such as benzene or chloroform. The fats are a large group of compounds that contain fatty acids and glycerol; a glycerol molecule attached to three fatty acid esters is called a triacylglyceride. Several variations on this basic structure exist, including alternate backbones such as sphingosine in the sphingolipids, and hydrophilic groups such as phosphate as in phospholipids. Steroids such as cholesterol are another major class of lipids.

Carbohydrates

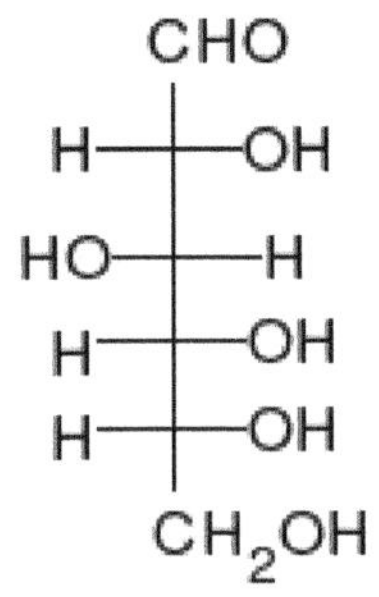

Glucose can exist in both a straight-chain and ring form.

Carbohydrates are aldehydes or ketones, with many hydroxyl groups attached, that can exist as straight chains or rings. Carbohydrates are the most abundant biological molecules, and fill numerous roles, such as the storage and transport of energy (starch, glycogen) and structural components (cellulose in plants, chitin in animals). The basic carbohydrate units are called monosaccharides and include galactose, fructose, and most importantly glucose. Monosaccharides can be linked together to form polysaccharides in almost limitless ways.

Nucleotides

The two nucleic acids, DNA and RNA, are polymers of nucleotides. Each nucleotide is composed of a phosphate attached to a ribose or deoxyribose sugar group which is attached to a nitrogenous base. Nucleic acids are critical for the storage and use of genetic information, and its interpretation through the processes of transcription and protein biosynthesis. This information is protected by DNA repair mechanisms and propagated through DNA replication. Many viruses have an RNA genome, such as HIV, which uses reverse transcription to create a DNA template from its viral RNA genome. RNA in ribozymes such as spliceosomes and ribosomes is similar to enzymes as it can catalyze chemical reactions. Individual nucleosides are made by attaching a nucleobase to a ribose sugar. These bases are heterocyclic rings containing nitrogen, classified as purines or pyrimidines. Nucleotides also act as coenzymes in metabolic-group-transfer reactions.

Coenzymes

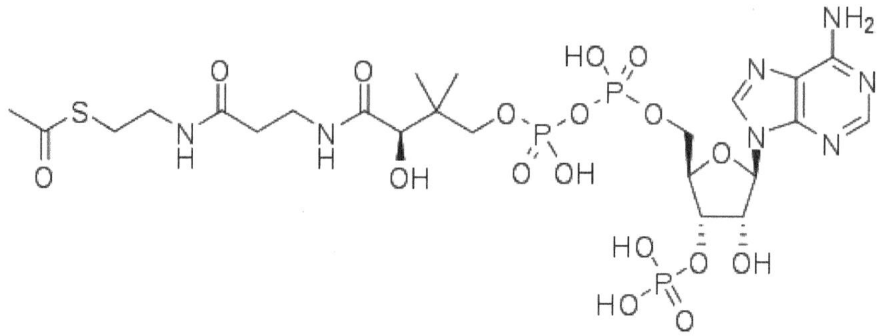

Structure of the coenzyme acetyl-CoA.The transferable acetyl group is bonded to the sulfur atom at the extreme left.

Metabolism involves a vast array of chemical reactions, but most fall under a few basic types of reactions that involve the transfer of functional groups of atoms and their bonds within molecules. This common chemistry allows cells to use a small set of metabolic intermediates to carry chemical groups between different reactions. These group-transfer intermediates are called coenzymes. Each class of group-transfer reactions is carried out by a particular coenzyme, which is the substrate for a set of enzymes that produce it, and a set of enzymes that consume it. These coenzymes are therefore continuously made, consumed and then recycled.

One central coenzyme is adenosine triphosphate (ATP), the universal energy currency of cells. This nucleotide is used to transfer chemical energy between different chemical reactions. There is only a small amount of ATP in cells, but as it is continuously regenerated, the human body can use about its own weight in ATP per day. ATP acts as a bridge between catabolism and anabolism. Catabolism breaks down molecules, and anabolism puts them together. Catabolic reactions generate ATP, and anabolic reactions consume it. It also serves as a carrier of phosphate groups in phosphorylation reactions.

A vitamin is an organic compound needed in small quantities that cannot be made in cells. In human nutrition, most vitamins function as coenzymes after modification; for example, all water-soluble vitamins are phosphorylated or are coupled to nucleotides when they are used in cells. Nicotinamide adenine dinucleotide (NAD^+), a derivative of vitamin B_3 (niacin), is an important coenzyme that acts as a hydrogen acceptor. Hundreds of separate types of dehydrogenases remove electrons from their substrates and reduce NAD^+ into NADH. This reduced form of the coenzyme is then a substrate for any of the reductases in the cell that need to reduce their substrates. Nicotinamide adenine dinucleotide exists in two related forms in the cell, NADH and NADPH. The NAD^+/NADH form is more important in catabolic reactions, while $NADP^+$/NADPH is used in anabolic reactions.

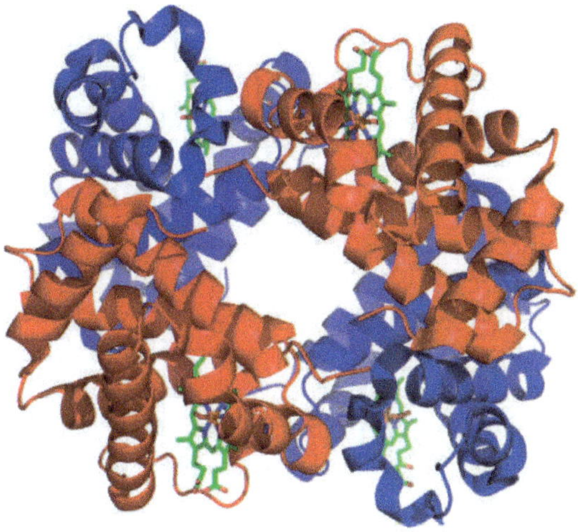

Structure of hemoglobin. The protein subunits are in red and blue, and the iron-containing heme groups in green. From PDB: 1GZX.

Minerals and Cofactors

Inorganic elements play critical roles in metabolism; some are abundant (e.g. sodium and potassium) while others function at minute concentrations. About 99% of a mammal's mass is made up of the elements carbon, nitrogen, calcium, sodium, chlorine, potassium, hydrogen, phosphorus, oxygen and sulfur. Organic compounds (proteins, lipids and carbohydrates) contain the majority of the carbon and nitrogen; most of the oxygen and hydrogen is present as water.

The abundant inorganic elements act as ionic electrolytes. The most important ions are sodium, potassium, calcium, magnesium, chloride, phosphate and the organic ion bicarbonate. The maintenance of precise ion gradients across cell membranes maintains osmotic pressure and pH. Ions are also critical for nerve and muscle function, as action potentials in these tissues are produced by the exchange of electrolytes between the extracellular fluid and the cell's fluid, the cytosol. Electrolytes enter and leave cells through proteins in the cell membrane called ion channels. For example, muscle contraction depends upon the movement of calcium, sodium and potassium through ion channels in the cell membrane and T-tubules.

Transition metals are usually present as trace elements in organisms, with zinc and iron being most abundant of those. These metals are used in some proteins as cofactors and are essential for the activity of enzymes such as catalase and oxygen-carrier proteins such as hemoglobin. Metal cofactors are bound tightly to specific sites in proteins; although enzyme cofactors can be modified during catalysis, they always return to their original state by the end of the reaction catalyzed. Metal micronutrients are taken up into organisms by specific transporters and bind to storage proteins such as ferritin or metallothionein when not in use.

CATABOLISM

Catabolism is the set of metabolic processes that break down large molecules. These include breaking down and oxidizing food molecules. The purpose of the catabolic reactions is to provide the energy and components needed by anabolic reactions. The exact nature of these catabolic reactions differ from organism to organism and organisms can be classified based on their sources of energy and carbon (their primary nutritional groups), as shown in the table below. Organic molecules are used as a source of energy by organotrophs, while lithotrophs use inorganic substrates and phototrophs capture sunlight as chemical energy. However, all these different forms of metabolism depend on redox reactions that involve the transfer of electrons from reduced donor molecules such as organic molecules, water, ammonia, hydrogen sulfide or ferrous ions to acceptor molecules such as oxygen, nitrate or sulfate. In animals these reactions involve complex organic molecules that are broken down to simpler molecules, such as carbon dioxide and water. In photosynthetic organisms such as plants and cyanobacteria, these electron-transfer reactions do not release energy, but are used as a way of storing energy absorbed from sunlight.

<table>
<tr><th colspan="6">Classification of organisms based on their metabolism</th></tr>
<tr><td rowspan="2">Energy source</td><td>sunlight</td><td>photo-</td><td colspan="2" rowspan="2"></td><td rowspan="6">-troph</td></tr>
<tr><td>Preformed molecules</td><td>chemo-</td></tr>
<tr><td rowspan="2">Electron donor</td><td>organic compound</td><td rowspan="2"></td><td>organo-</td><td rowspan="2"></td></tr>
<tr><td>inorganic compound</td><td>litho-</td></tr>
<tr><td rowspan="2">Carbon source</td><td>organic compound</td><td colspan="2"></td><td>hetero-</td></tr>
<tr><td>inorganic compound</td><td colspan="2">auto-</td><td></td></tr>
</table>

The most common set of catabolic reactions in animals can be separated into three main stages. In the first, large organic molecules such as proteins, polysaccharides or lipids are digested into their smaller components outside cells. Next, these smaller molecules are taken up by cells and converted to yet smaller molecules, usually acetyl coenzyme A (acetyl-CoA), which releases some energy. Finally, the acetyl group on the CoA is oxidised to water and carbon dioxide in the citric acid cycle and electron transport chain, releasing the energy that is stored by reducing the coenzyme nicotinamide adenine dinucleotide (NAD^+) into NADH.

Digestion

Macromolecules such as starch, cellulose or proteins cannot be rapidly taken up by cells and must be broken into their smaller units before they can be used in cell metabolism. Several common classes of enzymes digest these polymers. These digestive enzymes include proteases that digest proteins into amino acids, as well as glycoside hydrolases that digest polysaccharides into simple sugars known as monosaccharides.

Microbes simply secrete digestive enzymes into their surroundings, while animals only secrete these enzymes from specialized cells in their guts. The amino acids or sugars released by these extracellular enzymes are then pumped into cells by active transport proteins.

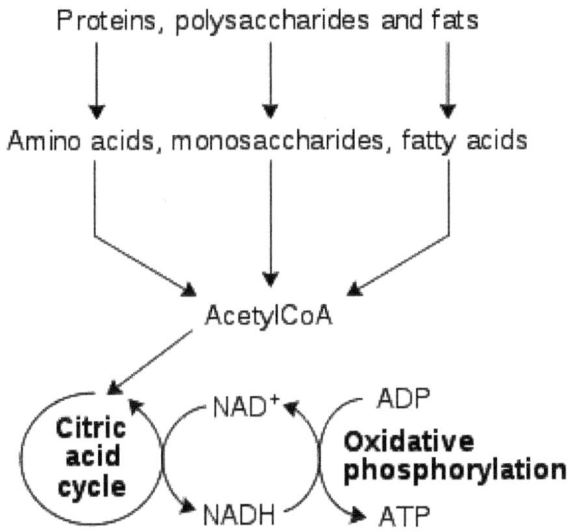

A simplified outline of the catabolism of proteins, carbohydrates and fats

Energy from Organic Compounds

Carbohydrate catabolism is the breakdown of carbohydrates into smaller units. Carbohydrates are usually taken into cells once they have been digested into monosaccharides. Once inside, the major route of breakdown is glycolysis, where sugars such as glucose and fructose are converted into pyruvate and some ATP is generated. Pyruvate is an intermediate in several metabolic pathways, but the majority is converted to acetyl-CoA and fed into the citric acid cycle. Although some more ATP is generated in the citric acid cycle, the most important product is NADH, which is made from NAD^+ as the acetyl-CoA is oxidized. This oxidation releases carbon dioxide as a waste product. In anaerobic conditions, glycolysis produces lactate, through the enzyme lactate dehydrogenase re-oxidizing NADH to NAD+ for re-use in glycolysis. An alternative route for glucose breakdown is the pentose phosphate pathway, which reduces the coenzyme NADPH and produces pentose sugars such as ribose, the sugar component of nucleic acids.

Fats are catabolised by hydrolysis to free fatty acids and glycerol. The glycerol enters glycolysis and the fatty acids are broken down by beta oxidation to release acetyl-CoA, which then is fed into the citric acid cycle. Fatty acids release more energy upon oxidation than carbohydrates because carbohydrates contain more oxygen in their structures. Steroids are also broken down by some bacteria in a process similar to beta oxidation, and this breakdown process involves the release of significant amounts of acetyl-CoA, propionyl-CoA, and pyruvate, which can all be used by the cell for energy. *M. tuberculosis* can also grow on the lipid cholesterol as a sole source of carbon, and genes involved in the cholesterol use pathway(s) have been validated as important during various stages of the infection lifecycle of *M. tuberculosis*.

Amino acids are either used to synthesize proteins and other biomolecules, or oxidized to urea and carbon dioxide as a source of energy. The oxidation pathway starts with the removal of the amino group by a transaminase. The amino group is fed into the urea cycle, leaving a deaminated carbon skeleton in the form of a keto acid. Several of these keto acids are intermediates in the citric acid cycle, for example the deamination of glutamate forms α-ketoglutarate. The glucogenic amino acids can also be converted into glucose, through gluconeogenesis (discussed below).

ENERGY TRANSFORMATIONS

Oxidative Phosphorylation

In oxidative phosphorylation, the electrons removed from organic molecules in areas such as the protagon acid cycle are transferred to oxygen and the energy released is used to make ATP. This is done in eukaryotes by a series of proteins in the membranes of mitochondria called the electron transport chain. In prokaryotes, these proteins are found in the cell's inner membrane. These proteins use the energy released from passing electrons from reduced molecules like NADH onto oxygen to pump protons across a membrane.

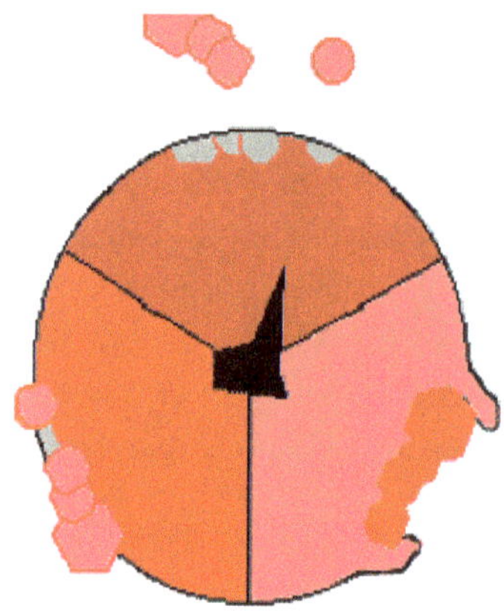

Mechanism of ATP synthase. ATP is shown in red, ADP and phosphate in pink and the rotating stalk subunit in black.

Pumping protons out of the mitochondria creates a proton concentration difference across the membrane and generates an electrochemical gradient. This force drives protons back into the mitochondrion through the base of an enzyme called ATP synthase. The flow of protons makes the stalk subunit rotate, causing the active site of the synthase domain to change shape and phosphorylate adenosine diphosphate – turning it into ATP.

Energy from Inorganic Compounds

Chemolithotrophy is a type of metabolism found in prokaryotes where energy is obtained from the oxidation of inorganic compounds. These organisms can use hydrogen, reduced sulfur compounds (such as sulfide, hydrogen sulfide and thiosulfate), ferrous iron (FeII) or ammonia as sources of reducing power and they gain energy from the oxidation of these compounds with electron acceptors such as oxygen or nitrite. These microbial processes are important in global biogeochemical cycles such as acetogenesis, nitrification and denitrification and are critical for soil fertility.

Energy from Light

The energy in sunlight is captured by plants, cyanobacteria, purple bacteria, green sulfur bacteria and some protists. This process is often coupled to the conversion of carbon dioxide into organic compounds, as part of photosynthesis, which is discussed below. The energy capture and carbon fixation systems can however operate separately in prokaryotes, as purple bacteria and green sulfur bacteria can use sunlight as a source of energy, while switching between carbon fixation and the fermentation of organic compounds.

In many organisms the capture of solar energy is similar in principle to oxidative phosphorylation, as it involves the storage of energy as a proton concentration gradient. This proton motive force then drives ATP synthesis. The electrons needed to drive this electron transport chain come from light-gathering proteins called photosynthetic reaction centres or rhodopsins. Reaction centers are classed into two types depending on the type of photosynthetic pigment present, with most photosynthetic bacteria only having one type, while plants and cyanobacteria have two.

In plants, algae, and cyanobacteria, photosystem II uses light energy to remove electrons from water, releasing oxygen as a waste product. The electrons then flow to the cytochrome b6f complex, which uses their energy to pump protons across the thylakoid membrane in the chloroplast. These protons move back through the membrane as they drive the ATP synthase, as before. The electrons then flow through photosystem I and can then either be used to reduce the coenzyme $NADP^+$, for use in the Calvin cycle, which is discussed below, or recycled for further ATP generation.

Anabolism

Anabolism is the set of constructive metabolic processes where the energy released by catabolism is used to synthesize complex molecules. In general, the complex molecules that make up cellular structures are constructed step-by-step from small and simple precursors. Anabolism involves three basic stages. First, the production of precursors such as amino acids, monosaccharides, isoprenoids and nucleotides, secondly, their activation into reactive forms using energy from ATP, and thirdly, the assembly of these precursors into complex molecules such as proteins, polysaccharides, lipids and nucleic acids.

Organisms differ in how many of the molecules in their cells they can construct for themselves. Autotrophs such as plants can construct the complex organic molecules in cells such as polysaccharides and proteins from simple molecules like carbon dioxide and water. Heterotrophs, on the other hand, require a source of more complex substances, such as monosaccharides and amino acids, to produce these complex molecules. Organisms can be further classified by ultimate source of their energy: photoautotrophs and photoheterotrophs obtain energy from light, whereas chemoautotrophs and chemoheterotrophs obtain energy from inorganic oxidation reactions.

Carbon Fixation

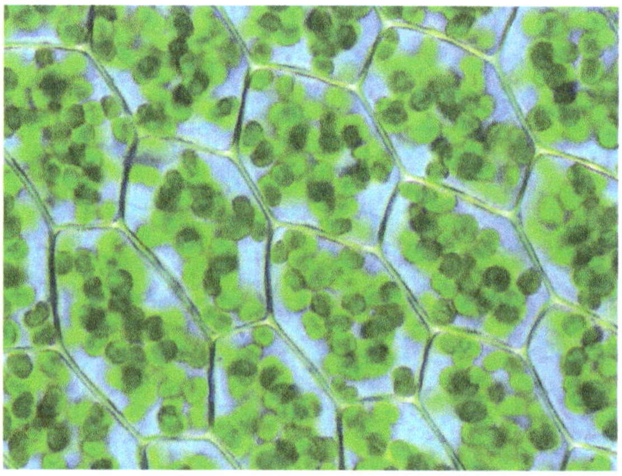

Plant cells (bounded by purple walls) filled with chloroplasts (green), which are the site of photosynthesis

Photosynthesis is the synthesis of carbohydrates from sunlight and carbon dioxide (CO_2). In plants, cyanobacteria and algae, oxygenic photosynthesis splits water, with oxygen produced as a waste product. This process uses the ATP and NADPH produced by the photosynthetic reaction centres, as described above, to convert CO_2 into glycerate 3-phosphate, which can then be converted into glucose. This carbon-fixation reaction is carried out by the enzyme RuBisCO as part of the Calvin – Benson cycle. Three types of photosynthesis occur in plants, C3 carbon fixation, C4 carbon fixation and CAM photosynthesis. These differ by the route that carbon dioxide takes to the Calvin cycle, with C3 plants fixing CO_2 directly, while C4 and CAM photosynthesis incorporate the CO_2 into other compounds first, as adaptations to deal with intense sunlight and dry conditions.

In photosynthetic prokaryotes the mechanisms of carbon fixation are more diverse. Here, carbon dioxide can be fixed by the Calvin – Benson cycle, a reversed citric acid cycle, or the carboxylation of acetyl-CoA. Prokaryotic chemoautotrophs also fix CO_2 through the Calvin – Benson cycle, but use energy from inorganic compounds to drive the reaction.

Carbohydrates and Glycans

In carbohydrate anabolism, simple organic acids can be converted into monosaccharides such as glucose and then used to assemble polysaccharides such as starch. The generation of glucose from compounds like pyruvate, lactate, glycerol, glycerate 3-phosphate and amino acids is called gluconeogenesis. Gluconeogenesis converts pyruvate to glucose-6-phosphate through a series of intermediates, many of which are shared with glycolysis. However, this pathway is not simply glycolysis run in reverse, as several steps are catalyzed by non-glycolytic enzymes. This is important as it allows the formation and breakdown of glucose to be regulated separately, and prevents both pathways from running simultaneously in a futile cycle.

Although fat is a common way of storing energy, in vertebrates such as humans the fatty acids in these stores cannot be converted to glucose through gluconeogenesis as these organisms cannot convert acetyl-CoA into pyruvate; plants do, but animals do not, have the necessary enzymatic machinery. As a result, after long-term starvation, vertebrates need to produce ketone bodies from fatty acids to replace glucose in tissues such as the brain that cannot metabolize fatty acids. In other organisms such as plants and bacteria, this metabolic problem is solved using the glyoxylate cycle, which bypasses the decarboxylation step in the citric acid cycle and allows the transformation of acetyl-CoA to oxaloacetate, where it can be used for the production of glucose.

Polysaccharides and glycans are made by the sequential addition of monosaccharides by glycosyltransferase from a reactive sugar-phosphate donor such as uridine diphosphate glucose (UDP-glucose) to an acceptor hydroxyl group on the growing polysaccharide. As any of the hydroxyl groups on the ring of the substrate can be acceptors, the polysaccharides produced can have straight or branched structures. The polysaccharides produced can have structural or metabolic functions themselves, or be transferred to lipids and proteins by enzymes called oligosaccharyltransferases.

Fatty Acids, Isoprenoids and Steroids

Fatty acids are made by fatty acid synthases that polymerize and then reduce acetyl-CoA units. The acyl chains in the fatty acids are extended by a cycle of reactions that add the acyl group, reduce it to an alcohol, dehydrate it to an alkene group and then reduce it again to an alkane group. The enzymes of fatty acid biosynthesis are divided into two groups: in animals and fungi, all these fatty acid synthase reactions are carried out by a single multifunctional type I protein, while in plant plastids and bacteria separate type II enzymes perform each step in the pathway.

Terpenes and isoprenoids are a large class of lipids that include the carotenoids and form the largest class of plant natural products. These compounds are made by the assembly and modification of isoprene units donated from the reactive precursors isopentenyl pyrophosphate and dimethylallyl pyrophosphate. These precursors can be made in different ways. In animals and archaea, the mevalonate pathway produces these compounds from acetyl-CoA, while in plants and bacteria the non-mevalonate pathway uses pyruvate and glyceraldehyde 3-phosphate as substrates. One important reaction that uses these activated isoprene donors is steroid biosynthesis. Here, the isoprene units are joined together to make squalene and then folded up and formed into a set of rings to make lanosterol. Lanosterol can then be converted into other steroids such as cholesterol and ergosterol.

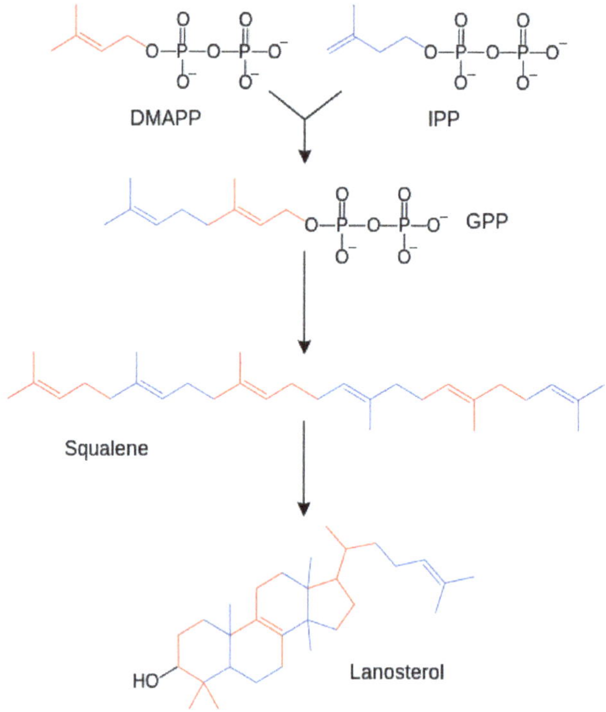

Simplified version of the steroid synthesis pathway with the intermediates isopentenyl pyrophosphate (IPP), dimethylallyl pyrophosphate (DMAPP), geranyl pyrophosphate (GPP) and squalene shown. Some intermediates are omitted for clarity.

Proteins

Organisms vary in their ability to synthesize the 20 common amino acids. Most bacteria and plants can synthesize all twenty, but mammals can only synthesize eleven nonessential amino acids, so nine essential amino acids must be obtained from food. Some simple parasites, such as the bacteria *Mycoplasma pneumoniae*, lack all amino acid synthesis and take their amino acids directly from their hosts. All amino acids are synthesized from intermediates in glycolysis, the citric acid cycle, or the pentose phosphate pathway. Nitrogen is provided by glutamate and glutamine. Amino acid synthesis depends on the formation of the appropriate alpha-keto acid, which is then transaminated to form an amino acid.

Amino acids are made into proteins by being joined together in a chain of peptide bonds. Each different protein has a unique sequence of amino acid residues: this is its primary structure. Just as the letters of the alphabet can be combined to form an almost endless variety of words, amino acids can be linked in varying sequences to form a huge variety of proteins. Proteins are made from amino acids that have been activated by attachment to a transfer RNA molecule through an ester bond. This aminoacyl-tRNA precursor is produced in an ATP-dependent reaction carried out by an aminoacyl tRNA synthetase. This aminoacyl-tRNA is then a substrate for the ribosome, which joins the amino acid onto the elongating protein chain, using the sequence information in a messenger RNA.

Nucleotide Synthesis and Salvage

Nucleotides are made from amino acids, carbon dioxide and formic acid in pathways that require large amounts of metabolic energy. Consequently, most organisms have efficient systems to salvage preformed nucleotides. Purines are synthesized as nucleosides (bases attached to ribose). Both adenine and guanine are made from the precursor nucleoside inosine monophosphate, which is synthesized using atoms from the amino acids glycine, glutamine, and aspartic acid, as well as formate transferred from the coenzyme tetrahydrofolate. Pyrimidines, on the other hand, are synthesized from the base orotate, which is formed from glutamine and aspartate.

Xenobiotics and Redox Metabolism

All organisms are constantly exposed to compounds that they cannot use as foods and would be harmful if they accumulated in cells, as they have no metabolic function. These potentially damaging compounds are called xenobiotics. Xenobiotics such as synthetic drugs, natural poisons and antibiotics are detoxified by a set of xenobiotic-metabolizing enzymes. In humans, these include cytochrome P450 oxidases, UDP-glucuronosyltransferases, and glutathione *S*-transferases. This system of enzymes acts in three stages to firstly oxidize the xenobiotic (phase I) and then conjugate water-soluble groups onto the molecule (phase II). The modified water-soluble xenobiotic can then be pumped out of cells and in multicellular organisms may be further metabolized before being excreted (phase III). In ecology, these reactions are particularly important in microbial biodegradation of pollutants and the bioremediation of contaminated land and oil spills. Many of these microbial reactions are shared with multicellular organisms, but due to the incredible diversity of types of microbes these organisms are able to deal with a far wider range of xenobiotics than multicellular organisms, and can degrade even persistent organic pollutants such as organochloride compounds.

A related problem for aerobic organisms is oxidative stress. Here, processes including oxidative phosphorylation and the formation of disulfide bonds during protein folding produce reactive oxygen species such as hydrogen peroxide. These damaging oxidants are removed by antioxidant metabolites such as glutathione and enzymes such as catalases and peroxidases.

Thermodynamics of Living Organisms

Living organisms must obey the laws of thermodynamics, which describe the transfer of heat and work. The second law of thermodynamics states that in any closed system, the amount of entropy (disorder) cannot decrease. Although living organisms' amazing complexity appears to contradict this law, life is possible as all organisms are open systems that exchange matter and energy with their surroundings. Thus living systems are not in equilibrium, but instead are dissipative systems that maintain their state of high complexity by causing a larger increase in the entropy of their environments. The metabolism of a cell achieves this by coupling the spontaneous processes of catabolism to the non-spontaneous processes of anabolism. In thermodynamic terms, metabolism maintains order by creating disorder.

Regulation and Control

As the environments of most organisms are constantly changing, the reactions of metabolism must be finely regulated to maintain a constant set of conditions within cells, a condition called homeostasis. Metabolic regulation also allows organisms to respond to signals and interact actively with their environments. Two closely linked concepts are important for understanding how metabolic pathways are controlled. Firstly, the *regulation* of an enzyme in a pathway is how its activity is increased and decreased in response to signals. Secondly, the *control* exerted by this enzyme is the effect that these changes in its activity have on the overall rate of the pathway (the flux through the pathway). For example, an enzyme may show large changes in activity (*i.e.* it is highly regulated) but if these changes have little effect on the flux of a metabolic pathway, then this enzyme is not involved in the control of the pathway.

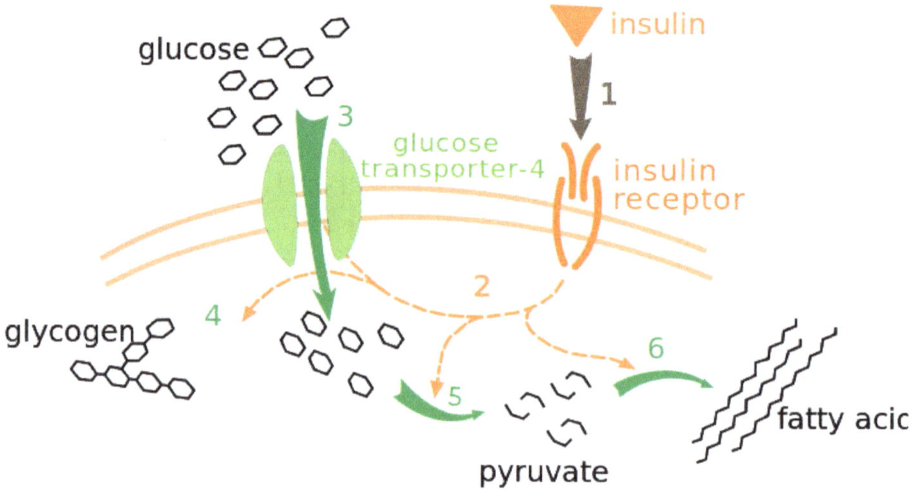

Effect of insulin on glucose uptake and metabolism. Insulin binds to its receptor (1), which in turn starts many protein activation cascades (2). These include: translocation of Glut-4 transporter to the plasma membrane and influx of glucose (3), glycogen synthesis (4), glycolysis (5) and fatty acid synthesis (6).

There are multiple levels of metabolic regulation. In intrinsic regulation, the metabolic pathway self-regulates to respond to changes in the levels of substrates or products; for example, a decrease in the amount of product can increase the flux through the pathway to compensate. This type of regulation often involves allosteric regulation of the activities of multiple enzymes in the pathway.Extrinsic control involves a cell in a multicellular organism changing its metabolism in response to signals from other cells. These signals are usually in the form of soluble messengers such as hormones and growth factors and are detected by specific receptors on the cell surface. These signals are then transmitted inside the cell by second messenger systems that often involved the phosphorylation of proteins.

A very well understood example of extrinsic control is the regulation of glucose metabolism by the hormone insulin. Insulin is produced in response to rises in blood glucose levels. Binding of the hormone to insulin receptors on cells then activates a cascade of protein kinases that cause the cells to take up glucose and convert it into storage molecules such as fatty acids and glycogen. The metabolism of glycogen is controlled by activity of phosphorylase, the enzyme that breaks down glycogen, and glycogen synthase, the enzyme that makes it. These enzymes are regulated in a reciprocal fashion, with phosphorylation inhibiting glycogen synthase, but activating phosphorylase. Insulin causes glycogen synthesis by activating protein phosphatases and producing a decrease in the phosphorylation of these enzymes.

Evolution

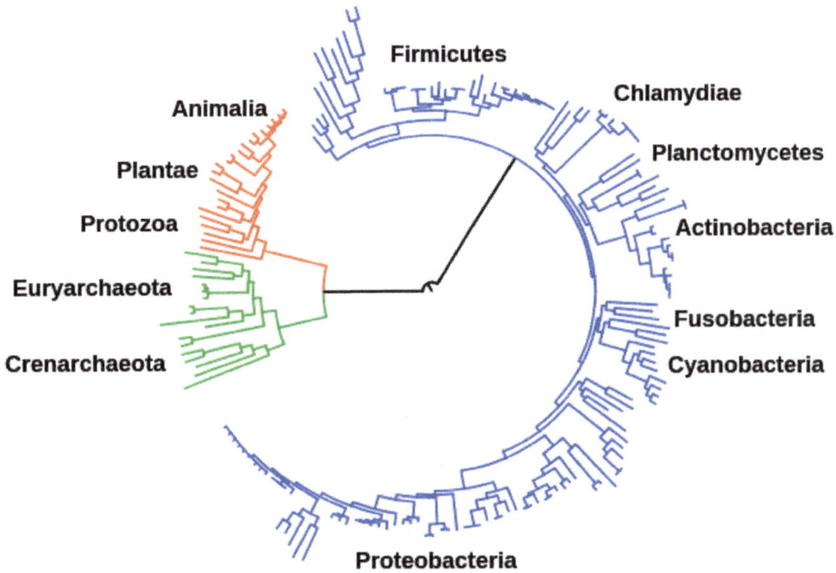

Evolutionary tree showing the common ancestry of organisms from all three domains of life. Bacteria are colored blue, eukaryotes red, and archaea green. Relative positions of some of the phyla included are shown around the tree.

The central pathways of metabolism described above, such as glycolysis and the citric acid cycle, are present in all three domains of living things and were present in the last universal common ancestor. This universal ancestral cell was prokaryotic and probably a methanogen that had extensive amino acid, nucleotide, carbohydrate and lipid metabolism. The retention of these ancient pathways during later evolution may be the result of these reactions having been an optimal solution to their particular metabolic problems, with pathways such as glycolysis and the citric acid cycle producing their end products highly efficiently and in a minimal number of steps. The first pathways of enzyme-based metabolism may have been parts of purine nucleotide metabolism, while previous metabolic pathways were a part of the ancient RNA world.

Many models have been proposed to describe the mechanisms by which novel metabolic pathways evolve. These include the sequential addition of novel enzymes to a short ancestral pathway, the duplication and then divergence of entire pathways as well as the recruitment of pre-existing enzymes and their assembly into a novel reaction pathway. The relative importance of these mechanisms is unclear, but genomic studies have shown that enzymes in a pathway are likely to have a shared ancestry, suggesting that many pathways have evolved in a step-by-step fashion with novel functions created from pre-existing steps in the pathway. An alternative model comes from studies that trace the evolution of proteins' structures in metabolic networks, this has suggested that enzymes are pervasively recruited, borrowing enzymes to perform similar functions in different metabolic pathways (evident in the MANET database) These recruitment processes result in an evolutionary enzymatic mosaic. A third possibility is that some parts of metabolism might exist as "modules" that can be reused in different pathways and perform similar functions on different molecules.

As well as the evolution of new metabolic pathways, evolution can also cause the loss of metabolic functions. For example, in some parasites metabolic processes that are not essential for survival are lost and preformed amino acids, nucleotides and carbohydrates may instead be scavenged from the host. Similar reduced metabolic capabilities are seen in endosymbiotic organisms.

INVESTIGATION AND MANIPULATION

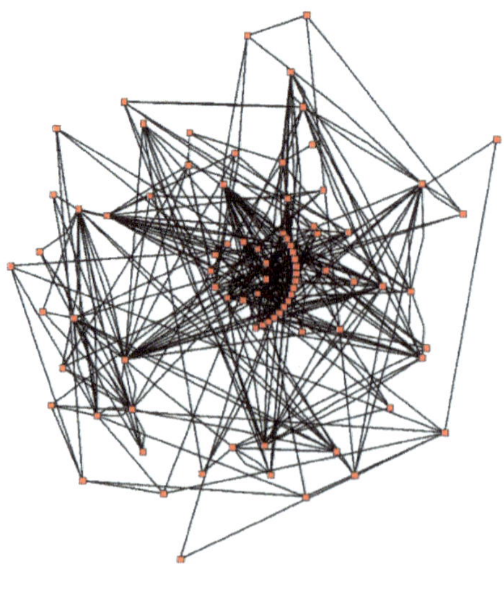

Metabolic network of the *Arabidopsis thaliana* citric acid cycle. Enzymes and metabolites are shown as red squares and the interactions between them as black lines.

Classically, metabolism is studied by a reductionist approach that focuses on a single metabolic pathway. Particularly valuable is the use of radioactive tracers at the whole-organism, tissue and cellular levels, which define the paths from precursors to final products by identifying radioactively labelled intermediates and products. The enzymes that catalyze these chemical reactions can then be purified and their kinetics and responses to inhibitors investigated. A parallel approach is to identify the small molecules in a cell or tissue; the complete set of these molecules is called the metabolome. Overall, these studies give a good view of the structure and function of simple metabolic pathways, but are inadequate when applied to more complex systems such as the metabolism of a complete cell.

An idea of the complexity of the metabolic networks in cells that contain thousands of different enzymes is given by the figure showing the interactions between just 43 proteins and 40 metabolites to the right: the sequences of genomes provide lists containing anything up to 45,000 genes. However, it is now possible to use this genomic data to reconstruct complete networks of biochemical reactions and produce more holistic mathematical models that may explain and predict their behavior. These models are especially powerful when used to integrate the pathway and metabolite data obtained through classical methods with data on gene expression from proteomic and DNA microarray studies. Using these techniques, a model of human metabolism has now been produced, which will guide future drug discovery and biochemical research. These models are now used in network analysis, to classify human diseases into groups that share common proteins or metabolites.

Bacterial metabolic networks are a striking example of bow-tie organization, an architecture able to input a wide range of nutrients and produce a large variety of products and complex macromolecules using a relatively few intermediate common currencies.

A major technological application of this information is metabolic engineering. Here, organisms such as yeast, plants or bacteria are genetically modified to make them more useful in biotechnology and aid the production of drugs such as antibiotics or industrial chemicals such as 1,3-propanediol and shikimic acid. These genetic modifications usually aim to reduce the amount of energy used to produce the product, increase yields and reduce the production of wastes.

The term *metabolism* is derived from the Greek Μεταβολισμός – "Metabolismos" for "change", or "overthrow". The first documented references of metabolism were made by Ibn al-Nafis in his 1260 AD work titled Al-Risalah al-Kamiliyyah fil Siera al-Nabawiyyah (The Treatise of Kamil on the Prophet's Biography) which included the following phrase "Both the body and its parts are in a continuous state of dissolution and nourishment, so they are inevitably undergoing permanent change." The history of the scientific study of metabolism spans several centuries and has moved from examining whole animals in early studies, to examining individual metabolic reactions in modern biochemistry. The first controlled experiments in human metabolism were published by Santorio Santorio in 1614 in his book *Ars de statica medicina*. He described how he weighed himself before and after eating, sleep, working, sex, fasting, drinking, and excreting. He found that most of the food he took in was lost through what he called "insensible perspiration".

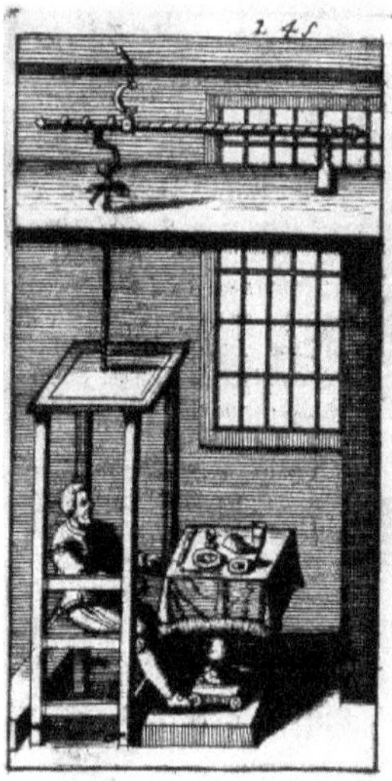

Santorio Santorio in his steelyard balance, from *Ars de statica medicina*, first published 1614

In these early studies, the mechanisms of these metabolic processes had not been identified and a vital force was thought to animate living tissue. In the 19th century, when studying the fermentation of sugar to alcohol by yeast, Louis Pasteur concluded that fermentation was catalyzed by substances within the yeast cells he called "ferments". He wrote that "alcoholic fermentation is an act correlated with the life and organization of the yeast cells, not with the death or putrefaction of the cells." This discovery, along with the publication by Friedrich Wöhler in 1828 of a paper on the chemical synthesis of urea, and is notable for being the first organic compound prepared from wholly inorganic precursors. This proved that the organic compounds and chemical reactions found in cells were no different in principle than any other part of chemistry.

It was the discovery of enzymes at the beginning of the 20th century by Eduard Buchner that separated the study of the chemical reactions of metabolism from the biological study of cells, and marked the beginnings of biochemistry. The mass of biochemical knowledge grew rapidly throughout the early 20th century. One of the most prolific of these modern biochemists was Hans Krebs who made huge contributions to the study of metabolism. He discovered the urea cycle and later, working with Hans Kornberg, the citric acid cycle and the glyoxylate cycle. Modern biochemical research has been greatly aided by the development of new techniques such as chromatography, X-ray diffraction, NMR spectroscopy, radioisotopic labelling, electron microscopy and molecular dynamics simulations. These techniques have allowed the discovery and detailed analysis of the many molecules and metabolic pathways in cells.

REFERENCES

1. Friedrich C (1998). "Physiology and genetics of sulfur-oxidizing bacteria". Adv Microb Physiol. Advances in Microbial Physiology. 39: 235–89. doi:10.1016/

S0065-2911(08)60018-1. ISBN 978-0-12-027739-1. PMID 9328649.

2. Pace NR (January 2001). "The universal nature of biochemistry". Proc. Natl. Acad. Sci. U.S.A. 98 (3): 805–8. Bibcode:2001PNAS...98..805P. doi:10.1073/pnas.98.3.805. PMC 33372 . PMID 11158550.
3. Smith E, Morowitz H (2004). "Universality in intermediary metabolism". Proc Natl Acad Sci USA. 101 (36): 13168–73. Bibcode:2004PNAS..10113168S. doi:10.1073/pnas.0404922101. PMC 516543 . PMID 15340153.
4. Ebenhöh O, Heinrich R (2001). "Evolutionary optimization of metabolic pathways. Theoretical reconstruction of the stoichiometry of ATP and NADH producing systems". Bull Math Biol. 63 (1): 21–55. doi:10.1006/bulm.2000.0197. PMID 11146883.
5. Meléndez-Hevia E, Waddell T, Cascante M (1996). "The puzzle of the Krebs citric acid cycle: assembling the pieces of chemically feasible reactions, and opportunism in the design of metabolic pathways during evolution". J Mol Evol. 43 (3): 293–303. doi:10.1007/BF02338838. PMID 8703096.
6. Michie K, Löwe J (2006). "Dynamic filaments of the bacterial cytoskeleton". Annu Rev Biochem. 75: 467–92. doi:10.1146/annurev.biochem.75.103004.142452. PMID 16756499.
7. Nelson, David L.; Michael M. Cox (2005). Lehninger Principles of Biochemistry. New York: W. H. Freeman and company. p. 841. ISBN 0-7167-4339-6.
8. Kelleher J, Bryan 3rd, B, Mallet R, Holleran A, Murphy A, and Fiskum G (1987). "Analysis of tricarboxylic acid-cycle metabolism of hepatoma cells by comparison of 14CO2ratios". Biochem J. 246 (3): 633–639. doi:10.1042/bj2460633. PMC 1148327 . PMID 3120698.
9. Hothersall, J & Ahmed, A (2013). "Metabolic fate of the increased yeast amino acid uptake subsequent to catabolite derepression". J Amino Acids. 2013: e461901. doi:10.1155/2013/461901. PMC 3575661 . PMID 23431419.
10. Fahy E, Subramaniam S, Brown H, Glass C, Merrill A, Murphy R, Raetz C, Russell D, Seyama Y, Shaw W, Shimizu T, Spener F, van Meer G, VanNieuwenhze M, White S, Witztum J, Dennis E (2005). "A comprehensive classification system for lipids". J Lipid Res. 46 (5): 839–61. doi:10.1194/jlr.E400004-JLR200. PMID 15722563.
11. "Nomenclature of Lipids". IUPAC-IUB Commission on Biochemical Nomenclature (CBN). Retrieved 2007-03-08.
12. Hegardt F (1999). "Mitochondrial 3-hydroxy-3-methylglutaryl-CoA synthase: a control enzyme in ketogenesis". Biochem J. 338 (Pt 3): 569–82. doi:10.1042/0264-6021:3380569. PMC 1220089 . PMID 10051425.
13. Raman R, Raguram S, Venkataraman G, Paulson J, Sasisekharan R (2005). "Glycomics: an integrated systems approach to structure-function relationships of glycans". Nat Methods. 2 (11): 817–24. doi:10.1038/nmeth807. PMID 16278650.
14. Sierra S, Kupfer B, Kaiser R (2005). "Basics of the virology of HIV-1 and its replication". J Clin Virol. 34 (4): 233–44. doi:10.1016/j.jcv.2005.09.004. PMID

16198625.

15. Wimmer M, Rose I (1978). "Mechanisms of enzyme-catalyzed group transfer reactions". Annu Rev Biochem. 47: 1031–78. doi:10.1146/annurev.bi.47.070178.005123. PMID 354490.
16. Mitchell P (1979). "The Ninth Sir Hans Krebs Lecture. Compartmentation and communication in living systems. Ligand conduction: a general catalytic principle in chemical, osmotic and chemiosmotic reaction systems". Eur J Biochem. 95 (1): 1–20. doi:10.1111/j.1432-1033.1979.tb12934.x. PMID 378655.
17. Dimroth P, von Ballmoos C, Meier T (March 2006). "Catalytic and mechanical cycles in F-ATP synthases: Fourth in the Cycles Review Series". EMBO Rep. 7 (3): 276–82. doi:10.1038/sj.embor.7400646. PMC 1456893 . PMID 16607397.
18. Coulston, Ann; Kerner, John; Hattner, JoAnn; Srivastava, Ashini (2006). "Nutrition Principles and Clinical Nutrition". Stanford School of Medicine Nutrition Courses. SUMMIT.
19. Pollak N, Dölle C, Ziegler M (2007). "The power to reduce: pyridine nucleotides – small molecules with a multitude of functions". Biochem J. 402 (2): 205–18. doi:10.1042/BJ20061638. PMC 1798440 . PMID 17295611.
20. Heymsfield S, Waki M, Kehayias J, Lichtman S, Dilmanian F, Kamen Y, Wang J, Pierson R (1991). "Chemical and elemental analysis of humans in vivo using improved body composition models". Am J Physiol. 261 (2 Pt 1): E190–8. PMID 1872381.
21. Sychrová H (2004). "Yeast as a model organism to study transport and homeostasis of alkali metal cations" (PDF). Physiol Res. 53 Suppl 1: S91–8. PMID 15119939.
22. Levitan I (1988). "Modulation of ion channels in neurons and other cells". Annu Rev Neurosci. 11: 119–36. doi:10.1146/annurev.ne.11.030188.001003. PMID 2452594.
23. Dulhunty A (2006). "Excitation-contraction coupling from the 1950s into the new millennium". Clin Exp Pharmacol Physiol. 33 (9): 763–72. doi:10.1111/j.1440-1681.2006.04441.x. PMID 16922804.
24. Mahan D, Shields R (1998). "Macro- and micromineral composition of pigs from birth to 145 kilograms of body weight" (PDF). J Anim Sci. 76 (2): 506–12. PMID 9498359.
25. Husted S, Mikkelsen B, Jensen J, Nielsen N (2004). "Elemental fingerprint analysis of barley (Hordeum vulgare) using inductively coupled plasma mass spectrometry, isotope-ratio mass spectrometry, and multivariate statistics". Anal Bioanal Chem. 378 (1): 171–82. doi:10.1007/s00216-003-2219-0. PMID 14551660.
26. Finney L, O'Halloran T (2003). "Transition metal speciation in the cell: insights from the chemistry of metal ion receptors". Science. 300 (5621): 931–6. Bibcode:2003Sci...300..931F. doi:10.1126/science.1085049. PMID 12738850.

27. Cousins R, Liuzzi J, Lichten L (2006). "Mammalian zinc transport, trafficking, and signals". J Biol Chem. 281 (34): 24085–9. doi:10.1074/jbc.R600011200. PMID 16793761.

28. Dunn L, Rahmanto Y, Richardson D (2007). "Iron uptake and metabolism in the new millennium". Trends Cell Biol. 17 (2): 93–100. doi:10.1016/j.tcb.2006.12.003. PMID 17194590.

29. Nealson K, Conrad P (1999). "Life: past, present and future". Philos Trans R Soc Lond B Biol Sci. 354 (1392): 1923–39. doi:10.1098/rstb.1999.0532. PMC 1692713 . PMID 10670014.

30. Nelson N, Ben-Shem A (2004). "The complex architecture of oxygenic photosynthesis". Nat Rev Mol Cell Biol. 5 (12): 971–82. doi:10.1038/nrm1525. PMID 15573135.

31. Häse C, Finkelstein R (December 1993). "Bacterial extracellular zinc-containing metalloproteases". Microbiol Rev. 57 (4): 823–37. PMC 372940 . PMID 8302217.

32. Gupta R, Gupta N, Rathi P (2004). "Bacterial lipases: an overview of production, purification and biochemical properties". Appl Microbiol Biotechnol. 64 (6): 763–81. doi:10.1007/s00253-004-1568-8. PMID 14966663.

33. Hoyle T (1997). "The digestive system: linking theory and practice". Br J Nurs. 6 (22): 1285–91. PMID 9470654.

34. Souba W, Pacitti A (1992). "How amino acids get into cells: mechanisms, models, menus, and mediators". JPEN J Parenter Enteral Nutr. 16 (6): 569–78. doi:10.1177/0148607192016006569. PMID 1494216.

35. Barrett M, Walmsley A, Gould G (1999). "Structure and function of facilitative sugar transporters". Curr Opin Cell Biol. 11 (4): 496–502. doi:10.1016/S0955-0674(99)80072-6. PMID 10449337.

36. Bell G, Burant C, Takeda J, Gould G (1993). "Structure and function of mammalian facilitative sugar transporters". J Biol Chem. 268 (26): 19161–4. PMID 8366068.

37. Bouché C, Serdy S, Kahn C, Goldfine A (2004). "The cellular fate of glucose and its relevance in type 2 diabetes". Endocr Rev. 25 (5): 807–30. doi:10.1210/er.2003-0026. PMID 15466941.

38. Wipperman, Matthew, F.; Thomas, Suzanne, T.; Sampson, Nicole, S. (2014). "Pathogen roid rage: Cholesterol utilization by Mycobacterium tuberculosis". Crit. Rev. Biochem. Mol. Biol. 49 (4): 269–93. doi:10.3109/10409238.2014.895700. PMID 24611808.

39. Sakami W, Harrington H (1963). "Amino acid metabolism". Annu Rev Biochem. 32: 355–98. doi:10.1146/annurev.bi.32.070163.002035. PMID 14144484.

40. Brosnan J (2000). "Glutamate, at the interface between amino acid and carbohydrate metabolism". J Nutr. 130 (4S Suppl): 988S–90S. PMID 10736367.

41. Young V, Ajami A (2001). "Glutamine: the emperor or his clothes?". J Nutr. 131 (9 Suppl): 2449S–59S; discussion 2486S–7S. PMID 11533293.

42. Hosler J, Ferguson-Miller S, Mills D (2006). "Energy Transduction: Proton Transfer Through the Respiratory Complexes". Annu Rev Biochem. 75: 165–87. doi:10.1146/annurev.biochem.75.062003.101730. PMC 2659341 . PMID 16756489.

43. Schultz B, Chan S (2001). "Structures and proton-pumping strategies of mitochondrial respiratory enzymes". Annu Rev Biophys Biomol Struct. 30: 23–65. doi:10.1146/annurev.biophys.30.1.23. PMID 11340051.

44. Capaldi R, Aggeler R (2002). "Mechanism of the F(1)F(0)-type ATP synthase, a biological rotary motor". Trends Biochem Sci. 27 (3): 154–60. doi:10.1016/S0968-0004(01)02051-5. PMID 11893513.

45. Friedrich B, Schwartz E (1993). "Molecular biology of hydrogen utilization in aerobic chemolithotrophs". Annu Rev Microbiol. 47: 351–83. doi:10.1146/annurev.mi.47.100193.002031. PMID 8257102.

46. Weber K, Achenbach L, Coates J (2006). "Microorganisms pumping iron: anaerobic microbial iron oxidation and reduction". Nat Rev Microbiol. 4 (10): 752–64. doi:10.1038/nrmicro1490. PMID 16980937.

47. Jetten M, Strous M, van de Pas-Schoonen K, Schalk J, van Dongen U, van de Graaf A, Logemann S, Muyzer G, van Loosdrecht M, Kuenen J (1998). "The anaerobic oxidation of ammonium". FEMS Microbiol Rev. 22 (5): 421–37. doi:10.1111/j.1574-6976.1998.tb00379.x. PMID 9990725.

48. Simon J (2002). "Enzymology and bioenergetics of respiratory nitrite ammonification". FEMS Microbiol Rev. 26 (3): 285–309. doi:10.1111/j.1574-6976.2002.tb00616.x. PMID 12165429.

49. Conrad R (1996). "Soil microorganisms as controllers of atmospheric trace gases (H2, CO, CH4, OCS, N2O, and NO)". Microbiol Rev. 60 (4): 609–40. PMC 239458 . PMID 8987358.

50. Barea J, Pozo M, Azcón R, Azcón-Aguilar C (2005). "Microbial co-operation in the rhizosphere". J Exp Bot. 56 (417): 1761–78. doi:10.1093/jxb/eri197. PMID 15911555.

51. van der Meer M, Schouten S, Bateson M, Nübel U, Wieland A, Kühl M, de Leeuw J, Sinninghe Damsté J, Ward D (July 2005). "Diel Variations in Carbon Metabolism by Green Nonsulfur-Like Bacteria in Alkaline Siliceous Hot Spring Microbial Mats from Yellowstone National Park". Appl Environ Microbiol. 71 (7): 3978–86. doi:10.1128/AEM.71.7.3978-3986.2005. PMC 1168979 . PMID 16000812.

52. Tichi M, Tabita F (2001). "Interactive Control of Rhodobacter capsulatus Redox-Balancing Systems during Phototrophic Metabolism". J Bacteriol. 183 (21): 6344–54. doi:10.1128/JB.183.21.6344-6354.2001. PMC 100130 . PMID 11591679.

53. Allen J, Williams J (1998). "Photosynthetic reaction centers". FEBS Lett. 438 (1–2): 5–9. doi:10.1016/S0014-5793(98)01245-9. PMID 9821949.

54. Munekage Y, Hashimoto M, Miyake C, Tomizawa K, Endo T, Tasaka M, Shikanai T (2004). "Cyclic electron flow around photosystem I is essential for

photosynthesis". Nature. 429 (6991): 579–82. Bibcode:2004Natur.429..579M. doi:10.1038/nature02598. PMID 15175756.

55. Miziorko H, Lorimer G (1983). "Ribulose-1,5-bisphosphate carboxylase-oxygenase". Annu Rev Biochem. 52: 507–35. doi:10.1146/annurev.bi.52.070183.002451. PMID 6351728.
56. Dodd A, Borland A, Haslam R, Griffiths H, Maxwell K (2002). "Crassulacean acid metabolism: plastic, fantastic". J Exp Bot. 53 (369): 569–80. doi:10.1093/jexbot/53.369.569. PMID 11886877.
57. Hügler M, Wirsen C, Fuchs G, Taylor C, Sievert S (May 2005). "Evidence for Autotrophic CO2 Fixation via the Reductive Tricarboxylic Acid Cycle by Members of the Subdivision of Proteobacteria". J Bacteriol. 187 (9): 3020–7. doi:10.1128/JB.187.9.3020-3027.2005. PMC 1082812 . PMID 15838028.
58. Strauss G, Fuchs G (1993). "Enzymes of a novel autotrophic CO2 fixation pathway in the phototrophic bacterium Chloroflexus aurantiacus, the 3-hydroxypropionate cycle". Eur J Biochem. 215 (3): 633–43. doi:10.1111/j.1432-1033.1993.tb18074.x. PMID 8354269.
59. Wood H (1991). "Life with CO or CO2 and H2 as a source of carbon and energy". FASEB J. 5 (2): 156–63. PMID 1900793.
60. Shively J, van Keulen G, Meijer W (1998). "Something from almost nothing: carbon dioxide fixation in chemoautotrophs". Annu Rev Microbiol. 52: 191–230. doi:10.1146/annurev.micro.52.1.191. PMID 9891798.
61. Boiteux A, Hess B (1981). "Design of glycolysis". Philos Trans R Soc Lond B Biol Sci. 293 (1063): 5–22. Bibcode:1981RSPTB.293....5B. doi:10.1098/rstb.1981.0056. PMID 6115423.
62. Pilkis S, el-Maghrabi M, Claus T (1990). "Fructose-2,6-bisphosphate in control of hepatic gluconeogenesis. From metabolites to molecular genetics". Diabetes Care. 13 (6): 582–99. doi:10.2337/diacare.13.6.582. PMID 2162755.
63. Ensign S (2006). "Revisiting the glyoxylate cycle: alternate pathways for microbial acetate assimilation". Mol Microbiol. 61 (2): 274–6. doi:10.1111/j.1365-2958.2006.05247.x. PMID 16856935.
64. Finn P, Dice J (2006). "Proteolytic and lipolytic responses to starvation". Nutrition. 22 (7–8): 830–44. doi:10.1016/j.nut.2006.04.008. PMID 16815497.
65. Kornberg H, Krebs H (1957). "Synthesis of cell constituents from C2-units by a modified tricarboxylic acid cycle". Nature. 179 (4568): 988–91. Bibcode:1957Natur.179..988K. doi:10.1038/179988a0. PMID 13430766.
66. Rademacher T, Parekh R, Dwek R (1988). "Glycobiology". Annu Rev Biochem. 57: 785–838. doi:10.1146/annurev.bi.57.070188.004033. PMID 3052290.
67. Opdenakker G, Rudd P, Ponting C, Dwek R (1993). "Concepts and principles of glycobiology". FASEB J. 7 (14): 1330–7. PMID 8224606.
68. McConville M, Menon A (2000). "Recent developments in the cell biology and biochemistry of glycosylphosphatidylinositol lipids (review)". Mol Membr Biol. 17 (1): 1–16. doi:10.1080/096876800294443. PMID 10824734.

69. Chirala S, Wakil S (2004). "Structure and function of animal fatty acid synthase". Lipids. 39 (11): 1045–53. doi:10.1007/s11745-004-1329-9. PMID 15726818.

70. White S, Zheng J, Zhang Y (2005). "The structural biology of type II fatty acid biosynthesis". Annu Rev Biochem. 74: 791–831. doi:10.1146/annurev.biochem.74.082803.133524. PMID 15952903.

71. Ohlrogge J, Jaworski J (1997). "Regulation of fatty acid synthesis". Annu Rev Plant Physiol Plant Mol Biol. 48: 109–136. doi:10.1146/annurev.arplant.48.1.109. PMID 15012259.

72. Dubey V, Bhalla R, Luthra R (2003). "An overview of the non-mevalonate pathway for terpenoid biosynthesis in plants" (PDF). J Biosci. 28 (5): 637–46. doi:10.1007/BF02703339. PMID 14517367.

73. Kuzuyama T, Seto H (2003). "Diversity of the biosynthesis of the isoprene units". Nat Prod Rep. 20 (2): 171–83. doi:10.1039/b109860h. PMID 12735695.

74. Grochowski L, Xu H, White R (May 2006). "Methanocaldococcus jannaschii Uses a Modified Mevalonate Pathway for Biosynthesis of Isopentenyl Diphosphate". J Bacteriol. 188 (9): 3192–8. doi:10.1128/JB.188.9.3192-3198.2006. PMC 1447442 . PMID 16621811.

75. Lichtenthaler H (1999). "The 1-Ddeoxy-D-xylulose-5-phosphate pathway of isoprenoid biosynthesis in plants". Annu Rev Plant Physiol Plant Mol Biol. 50: 47–65. doi:10.1146/annurev.arplant.50.1.47. PMID 15012203.

76. Schroepfer G (1981). "Sterol biosynthesis". Annu Rev Biochem. 50: 585–621. doi:10.1146/annurev.bi.50.070181.003101. PMID 7023367.

77. Lees N, Skaggs B, Kirsch D, Bard M (1995). "Cloning of the late genes in the ergosterol biosynthetic pathway of Saccharomyces cerevisiae—a review". Lipids. 30 (3): 221–6. doi:10.1007/BF02537824. PMID 7791529.

78. Himmelreich R, Hilbert H, Plagens H, Pirkl E, Li BC, Herrmann R (November 1996). "Complete sequence analysis of the genome of the bacterium Mycoplasma pneumoniae". Nucleic Acids Res. 24 (22): 4420–49. doi:10.1093/nar/24.22.4420. PMC 146264 . PMID 8948633.

79. Guyton, Arthur C.; John E. Hall (2006). Textbook of Medical Physiology. Philadelphia: Elsevier. pp. 855–6. ISBN 0-7216-0240-1.

80. Ibba M, Söll D (2001). "The renaissance of aminoacyl-tRNA synthesis". EMBO Rep. 2 (5): 382–7. doi:10.1093/embo-reports/kve095. PMC 1083889 . PMID 11375928.

81. Lengyel P, Söll D (1969). "Mechanism of protein biosynthesis". Bacteriol Rev. 33 (2): 264–301. PMC 378322 . PMID 4896351.

82. Rudolph F (1994). "The biochemistry and physiology of nucleotides". J Nutr. 124 (1 Suppl): 124S–127S. PMID 8283301. Zrenner R, Stitt M, Sonnewald U, Boldt R (2006). "Pyrimidine and purine biosynthesis and degradation in plants". Annu Rev Plant Biol. 57: 805–36. doi:10.1146/annurev.arplant.57.032905.105421. PMID 16669783.

83. Stasolla C, Katahira R, Thorpe T, Ashihara H (2003). "Purine and pyrimidine

nucleotide metabolism in higher plants". J Plant Physiol. 160 (11): 1271–95. doi:10.1078/0176-1617-01169. PMID 14658380.

84. Davies O, Mendes P, Smallbone K, Malys N (2012). "Characterisation of multiple substrate-specific (d)ITP/(d)XTPase and modelling of deaminated purine nucleotide metabolism". BMB Reports. 45 (4): 259–64. doi:10.5483/BMBRep.2012.45.4.259. PMID 22531138.

85. Smith J (1995). "Enzymes of nucleotide synthesis". Curr Opin Struct Biol. 5 (6): 752–7. doi:10.1016/0959-440X(95)80007-7. PMID 8749362.

86. Testa B, Krämer S (2006). "The biochemistry of drug metabolism—an introduction: part 1. Principles and overview". Chem Biodivers. 3 (10): 1053–101. doi:10.1002/cbdv.200690111. PMID 17193224.

87. Danielson P (2002). "The cytochrome P450 superfamily: biochemistry, evolution and drug metabolism in humans". Curr Drug Metab. 3 (6): 561–97. doi:10.2174/1389200023337054. PMID 12369887.

88. King C, Rios G, Green M, Tephly T (2000). "UDP-glucuronosyltransferases". Curr Drug Metab. 1 (2): 143–61. doi:10.2174/1389200003339171. PMID 11465080.

89. Sheehan D, Meade G, Foley V, Dowd C (November 2001). "Structure, function and evolution of glutathione transferases: implications for classification of non-mammalian members of an ancient enzyme superfamily". Biochem J. 360 (Pt 1): 1–16. doi:10.1042/0264-6021:3600001. PMC 1222196 . PMID 11695986.

90. Galvão T, Mohn W, de Lorenzo V (2005). "Exploring the microbial biodegradation and biotransformation gene pool". Trends Biotechnol. 23 (10): 497–506. doi:10.1016/j.tibtech.2005.08.002. PMID 16125262.

91. Janssen D, Dinkla I, Poelarends G, Terpstra P (2005). "Bacterial degradation of xenobiotic compounds: evolution and distribution of novel enzyme activities". Environ Microbiol. 7 (12): 1868–82. doi:10.1111/j.1462-2920.2005.00966.x. PMID 16309386.

92. Davies K (1995). "Oxidative stress: the paradox of aerobic life". Biochem Soc Symp. 61: 1–31. doi:10.1042/bss0610001. PMID 8660387.

93. Tu B, Weissman J (2004). "Oxidative protein folding in eukaryotes: mechanisms and consequences". J Cell Biol. 164 (3): 341–6. doi:10.1083/jcb.200311055. PMC 2172237 . PMID 14757749.

94. Sies H (1997). "Oxidative stress: oxidants and antioxidants" (PDF). Exp Physiol. 82 (2): 291–5. doi:10.1113/expphysiol.1997.sp004024. PMID 9129943.

95. Vertuani S, Angusti A, Manfredini S (2004). "The antioxidants and pro-antioxidants network: an overview". Curr Pharm Des. 10 (14): 1677–94. doi:10.2174/1381612043384655. PMID 15134565.

96. von Stockar U, Liu J (1999). "Does microbial life always feed on negative entropy? Thermodynamic analysis of microbial growth". Biochim Biophys Acta. 1412 (3): 191–211. doi:10.1016/S0005-2728(99)00065-1. PMID 10482783.

97. Demirel Y, Sandler S (2002). "Thermodynamics and bioenergetics". Biophys Chem. 97 (2–3): 87–111. doi:10.1016/S0301-4622(02)00069-8. PMID 12050002.

98. Albert R (2005). "Scale-free networks in cell biology". J Cell Sci. 118 (Pt 21): 4947–57. doi:10.1242/jcs.02714. PMID 16254242.

99. Brand M (1997). "Regulation analysis of energy metabolism". J Exp Biol. 200 (Pt 2): 193–202. PMID 9050227.

100. Soyer O, Salathé M, Bonhoeffer S (2006). "Signal transduction networks: topology, response and biochemical processes". J Theor Biol. 238 (2): 416–25. doi:10.1016/j.jtbi.2005.05.030. PMID 16045939.

101. Salter M, Knowles R, Pogson C (1994). "Metabolic control". Essays Biochem. 28: 1–12. PMID 7925313.

102. Westerhoff H, Groen A, Wanders R (1984). "Modern theories of metabolic control and their applications (review)". Biosci Rep. 4 (1): 1–22. doi:10.1007/BF01120819. PMID 6365197.

103. Fell D, Thomas S (1995). "Physiological control of metabolic flux: the requirement for multisite modulation". Biochem J. 311 (Pt 1): 35–9. PMC 1136115 . PMID 7575476.

104. Hendrickson W (2005). "Transduction of biochemical signals across cell membranes". Q Rev Biophys. 38 (4): 321–30. doi:10.1017/S0033583506004136. PMID 16600054.

105. Cohen P (2000). "The regulation of protein function by multisite phosphorylation—a 25 year update". Trends Biochem Sci. 25 (12): 596–601. doi:10.1016/S0968-0004(00)01712-6. PMID 11116185.

106. Lienhard G, Slot J, James D, Mueckler M (1992). "How cells absorb glucose". Sci Am. 266 (1): 86–91. doi:10.1038/scientificamerican0192-86. PMID 1734513.

107. Roach P (2002). "Glycogen and its metabolism". Curr Mol Med. 2 (2): 101–20. doi:10.2174/1566524024605761. PMID 11949930.

108. Newgard C, Brady M, O'Doherty R, Saltiel A (2000). "Organizing glucose disposal: emerging roles of the glycogen targeting subunits of protein phosphatase-1" (PDF). Diabetes. 49 (12): 1967–77. doi:10.2337/diabetes.49.12.1967. PMID 11117996.

109. Romano A, Conway T (1996). "Evolution of carbohydrate metabolic pathways". Res Microbiol. 147 (6–7): 448–55. doi:10.1016/0923-2508(96)83998-2. PMID 9084754.

110. Koch A (1998). "How did bacteria come to be?". Adv Microb Physiol. Advances in Microbial Physiology. 40: 353–99. doi:10.1016/S0065-2911(08)60135-6. ISBN 978-0-12-027740-7. PMID 9889982.

111. Ouzounis C, Kyrpides N (1996). "The emergence of major cellular processes in evolution". FEBS Lett. 390 (2): 119–23. doi:10.1016/0014-5793(96)00631-X. PMID 8706840.

112. Caetano-Anolles G, Kim HS, Mittenthal JE (2007). "The origin of modern metabolic networks inferred from phylogenomic analysis of protein architecture". Proc Natl Acad Sci USA. 104 (22): 9358–63. Bibcode:2007PNAS..104.9358C. doi:10.1073/pnas.0701214104. PMC 1890499 . PMID 17517598.

113. Schmidt S, Sunyaev S, Bork P, Dandekar T (2003). "Metabolites: a helping hand

for pathway evolution?". Trends Biochem Sci. 28 (6): 336–41. doi:10.1016/S0968-0004(03)00114-2. PMID 12826406.

114. Light S, Kraulis P (2004). "Network analysis of metabolic enzyme evolution in Escherichia coli". BMC Bioinformatics. 5: 15. doi:10.1186/1471-2105-5-15. PMC 394313 . PMID 15113413. Alves R, Chaleil R, Sternberg M (2002). "Evolution of enzymes in metabolism: a network perspective". J Mol Biol. 320 (4): 751–70. doi:10.1016/S0022-2836(02)00546-6. PMID 12095253.

115. Kim HS, Mittenthal JE, Caetano-Anolles G (2006). "MANET: tracing evolution of protein architecture in metabolic networks". BMC Bioinformatics. 7: 351. doi:10.1186/1471-2105-7-351. PMC 1559654 . PMID 16854231.

116. Teichmann SA, Rison SC, Thornton JM, Riley M, Gough J, Chothia C (2001). "Small-molecule metabolsim: an enzyme mosaic". Trends Biotechnol. 19 (12): 482–6. doi:10.1016/S0167-7799(01)01813-3. PMID 11711174.

117. Spirin V, Gelfand M, Mironov A, Mirny L (June 2006). "A metabolic network in the evolutionary context: Multiscale structure and modularity". Proc Natl Acad Sci USA. 103 (23): 8774–9. Bibcode:2006PNAS..103.8774S. doi:10.1073/pnas.0510258103. PMC 1482654 . PMID 16731630.

118. Lawrence J (2005). "Common themes in the genome strategies of pathogens". Curr Opin Genet Dev. 15 (6): 584–8. doi:10.1016/j.gde.2005.09.007. PMID 16188434.Wernegreen J (2005). "For better or worse: genomic consequences of intracellular mutualism and parasitism". Curr Opin Genet Dev. 15 (6): 572–83. doi:10.1016/j.gde.2005.09.013. PMID 16230003.

119. Pál C, Papp B, Lercher M, Csermely P, Oliver S, Hurst L (2006). "Chance and necessity in the evolution of minimal metabolic networks". Nature. 440 (7084): 667–70. Bibcode:2006Natur.440..667P. doi:10.1038/nature04568. PMID 16572170.

120. Rennie M (1999). "An introduction to the use of tracers in nutrition and metabolism". Proc Nutr Soc. 58 (4): 935–44. doi:10.1017/S002966519900124X. PMID 10817161.

121. Phair R (1997). "Development of kinetic models in the nonlinear world of molecular cell biology". Metabolism. 46 (12): 1489–95. doi:10.1016/S0026-0495(97)90154-2. PMID 9439549.

122. Sterck L, Rombauts S, Vandepoele K, Rouzé P, Van de Peer Y (2007). "How many genes are there in plants (... and why are they there)?". Curr Opin Plant Biol. 10 (2): 199–203. doi:10.1016/j.pbi.2007.01.004. PMID 17289424.

123. Borodina I, Nielsen J (2005). "From genomes to in silico cells via metabolic networks". Curr Opin Biotechnol. 16 (3): 350–5. doi:10.1016/j.copbio.2005.04.008. PMID 15961036.

124. Gianchandani E, Brautigan D, Papin J (2006). "Systems analyses characterize integrated functions of biochemical networks". Trends Biochem Sci. 31 (5): 284–91. doi:10.1016/j.tibs.2006.03.007. PMID 16616498.

125. Duarte NC, Becker SA, Jamshidi N, et al. (February 2007). "Global reconstruction

of the human metabolic network based on genomic and bibliomic data". Proc. Natl. Acad. Sci. U.S.A. 104 (6): 1777–82. Bibcode:2007PNAS..104.1777D. doi:10.1073/pnas.0610772104. PMC 1794290 . PMID 17267599.

126. Goh KI, Cusick ME, Valle D, Childs B, Vidal M, Barabási AL (May 2007). "The human disease network". Proc. Natl. Acad. Sci. U.S.A. 104 (21): 8685–90. Bibcode:2007PNAS..104.8685G. doi:10.1073/pnas.0701361104. PMC 1885563 . PMID 17502601.
127. Lee DS, Park J, Kay KA, Christakis NA, Oltvai ZN, Barabási AL (July 2008). "The implications of human metabolic network topology for disease comorbidity". Proc. Natl. Acad. Sci. U.S.A. 105 (29): 9880–9885. Bibcode:2008PNAS..105.9880L. doi:10.1073/pnas.0802208105. PMC 2481357 . PMID 18599447.
128. Csete M, Doyle J (2004). "Bow ties, metabolism and disease". Trends Biotechnol. 22 (9): 446–50. doi:10.1016/j.tibtech.2004.07.007. PMID 15331224.
129. Ma HW, Zeng AP (2003). "The connectivity structure, giant strong component and centrality of metabolic networks". Bioinformatics. 19 (11): 1423–30. doi:10.1093/bioinformatics/btg177. PMID 12874056.
130. Zhao J, Yu H, Luo JH, Cao ZW, Li YX (2006). "Hierarchical modularity of nested bow-ties in metabolic networks". BMC Bioinformatics. 7: 386. doi:10.1186/1471-2105-7-386. PMC 1560398 . PMID 16916470.
131. Thykaer J, Nielsen J (2003). "Metabolic engineering of beta-lactam production". Metab Eng. 5 (1): 56–69. doi:10.1016/S1096-7176(03)00003-X. PMID 12749845. González-Pajuelo M, Meynial-Salles I, Mendes F, Andrade J, Vasconcelos I, Soucaille P (2005). "Metabolic engineering of Clostridium acetobutylicum for the industrial production of 1,3-propanediol from glycerol". Metab Eng. 7 (5–6): 329–36. doi:10.1016/j.ymben.2005.06.001. PMID 16095939.Krämer M, Bongaerts J, Bovenberg R, Kremer S, Müller U, Orf S, Wubbolts M, Raeven L (2003). "Metabolic engineering for microbial production of shikimic acid". Metab Eng. 5 (4): 277–83. doi:10.1016/j.ymben.2003.09.001. PMID 14642355.
132. Koffas M, Roberge C, Lee K, Stephanopoulos G (1999). "Metabolic engineering". Annu Rev Biomed Eng. 1: 535–57. doi:10.1146/annurev.bioeng.1.1.535. PMID 11701499.
133. "Metabolism". The Online Etymology Dictionary. Retrieved 2007-02-20.
134. Dr. Abu Shadi Al-Roubi (1982), "Ibn Al-Nafis as a philosopher", Symposium on Ibn al-Nafis, Second International Conference on Islamic Medicine: Islamic Medical Organization, Kuwait (cf. Ibn al-Nafis As a Philosopher, Encyclopedia of Islamic World)
135. Eknoyan G (1999). "Santorio Sanctorius (1561–1636) – founding father of metabolic balance studies". Am J Nephrol. 19 (2): 226–33. doi:10.1159/000013455. PMID 10213823.
136. Williams, H. S. (1904) A History of Science: in Five Volumes. Volume IV: Modern Development of the Chemical and Biological Sciences Harper and Brothers (New York) Retrieved on 2007-03-26

137. Dubos J. (1951). "Louis Pasteur: Free Lance of Science, Gollancz. Quoted in Manchester K. L. (1995) Louis Pasteur (1822–1895)—chance and the prepared mind". Trends Biotechnol. 13 (12): 511–515. doi:10.1016/S0167-7799(00)89014-9. PMID 8595136.

138. Kinne-Saffran E, Kinne R (1999). "Vitalism and synthesis of urea. From Friedrich Wöhler to Hans A. Krebs". Am J Nephrol. 19 (2): 290–4. doi:10.1159/000013463. PMID 10213830.

139. Eduard Buchner's 1907 Nobel lecture at http://nobelprize.org Accessed 2007-03-20

140. Kornberg H (2000). "Krebs and his trinity of cycles". Nat Rev Mol Cell Biol. 1 (3): 225–8. doi:10.1038/35043073. PMID 11252898.

141. Krebs HA, Henseleit K (1932). "Untersuchungen über die Harnstoffbildung im tierkorper". Z. Physiol. Chem. 210: 33–66. doi:10.1515/bchm2.1932.210.1-2.33.

142. Krebs H, Johnson W (April 1937). "Metabolism of ketonic acids in animal tissues". Biochem J. 31 (4): 645–60. doi:10.1042/bj0310645. PMC 1266984 . PMID 16746382.

CHAPTER 3

Metabolic Pathways

Chapter Contents

The term 'metabolism' comes from the Greek word, metabole, which means change. It refers to the total of an organism's chemical reactions. A metabolic pathway is a series of steps found in biochemical reactions that help convert molecules or substrates, such as sugar, into different, more readily usable materials. These reactions occur inside of a cell, where enzymes, or protein molecules, break down or build up molecules. These enzymes are similar to traffic lights in that they can slow, speed up, and stop metabolic processes.

INTRODUCTION

In biochemistry, a metabolic pathway is a linked series of chemical reactions occurring within a cell. The reactants, products, and intermediates of an enzymatic reaction are known as metabolites, which are modified by a sequence of chemical reactions catalyzed by enzymes. In a metabolic pathway, the product of one enzyme acts as the substrate for the next. These enzymes often require dietary minerals, vitamins, and other cofactors to function.

Different metabolic pathways function based on the position within a eukaryotic cell and the significance of the pathway in the given compartment of the cell. For instance, the citric acid cycle, electron transport chain, and oxidative phosphorylation all take place in the mitochondrial membrane. In contrast, glycolysis, pentose phosphate pathway, and fatty acid biosynthesis all occur in the cytosol of a cell.

There are two types of metabolic pathways that are characterized by their ability to either synthesize molecules with the utilization of energy (anabolic pathway) or break down of complex molecules by releasing energy in the process (catabolic pathway). The two pathways complement each other in that the energy released from one is used up by the other. The degradative process of a catabolic pathway provides the energy required to conduct a biosynthesis of an anabolic pathway. In addition to the two distinct metabolic pathways is the amphibolic pathway, which can be either catabolic or anabolic based on the need for or the availability of energy.

Pathways are required for the maintenance of homeostasis within an organism and the flux of metabolites through a pathway is regulated depending on the needs of the cell and the availability of the substrate. The end product of a pathway may be used immediately, initiate another metabolic pathway or be stored for later use. The metabolism of a cell consists of an elaborate network of interconnected pathways that enable the synthesis and breakdown of molecules (anabolism and catabolism)

OVERVIEW

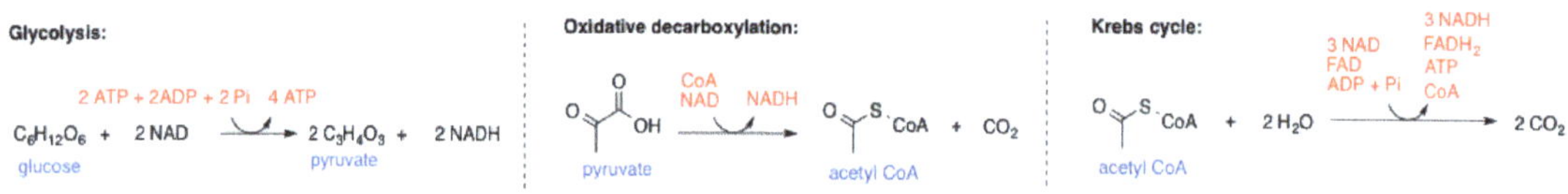

Net reactions of common metabolic pathways

Each metabolic pathway consists of a series of biochemical reactions that are connected by their intermediates: the products of one reaction are the substrates for subsequent reactions, and so on. Metabolic pathways are often considered to flow in one direction. Although all chemical reactions are technically reversible, conditions in the cell are often such that it is thermodynamically more favorable for flux to flow in one direction of a reaction. For example, one pathway may be responsible for the synthesis of a particular amino acid, but the breakdown of that amino acid may occur via a separate and distinct pathway. One example of an exception to this "rule" is the metabolism of glucose. Glycolysis results in the breakdown of glucose, but several reactions in the glycolysis pathway are reversible and participate in the re-synthesis of glucose (gluconeogenesis).

- Glycolysis was the first metabolic pathway discovered:
- As glucose enters a cell, it is immediately phosphorylated by ATP to glucose 6-phosphate in the irreversible first step.
- In times of excess lipid or protein energy sources, certain reactions in the glycolysis pathway may run in reverse in order to produce glucose 6-phosphate which is then used for storage as glycogen or starch.

- Metabolic pathways are often regulated by feedback inhibition.
- Some metabolic pathways flow in a 'cycle' wherein each component of the cycle is a substrate for the subsequent reaction in the cycle, such as in the Krebs Cycle (see below).
- Anabolic and catabolic pathways in eukaryotes often occur independently of each other, separated either physically by compartmentalization within organelles or separated biochemically by the requirement of different enzymes and co-factors.

Major Metabolic Pathways

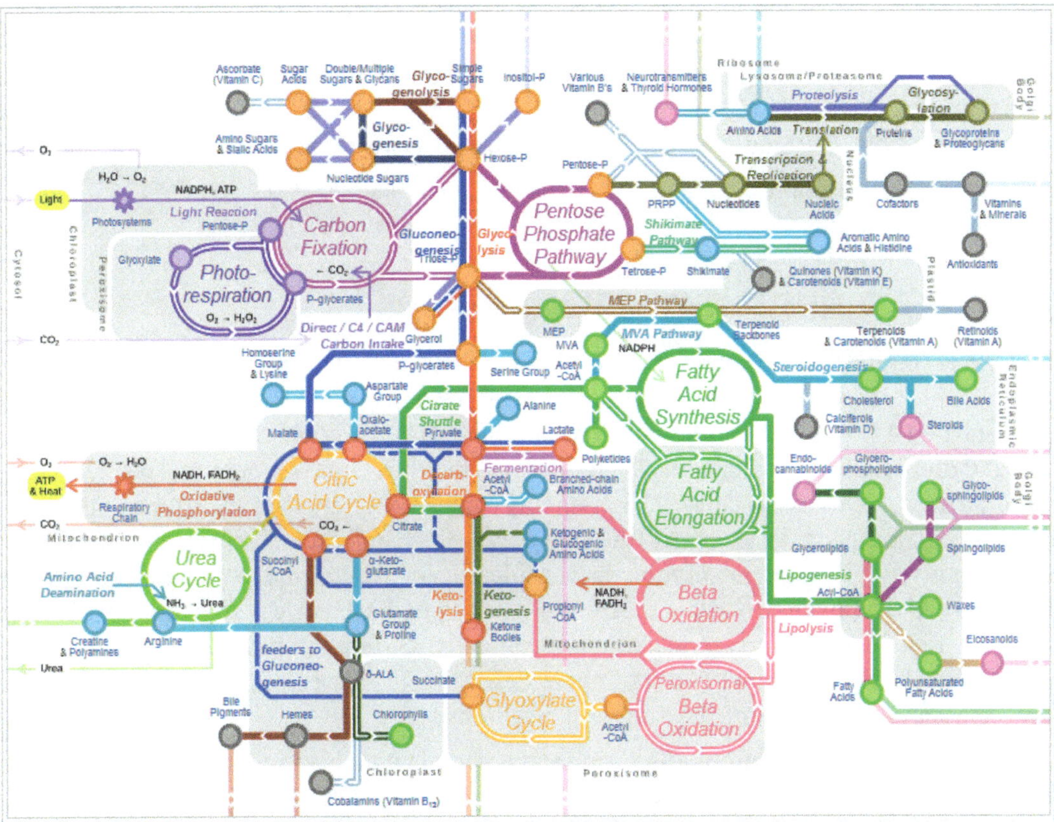

Major metabolic pathways in metro-style map. Click any text (name of pathway or metabolites) to link to the corresponding article.
Single lines: pathways common to most lifeforms. Double lines: pathways not in humans (occurs in e.g. plants, fungi, prokaryotes).
Orange nodes: carbohydrate metabolism. Violet nodes: photosynthesis. Red nodes: cellular respiration. Pink nodes: cell signaling.
Blue nodes: amino acid metabolism. Grey nodes: vitamin and cofactor metabolism. Brown nodes: nucleotide and protein metabolism.
Green nodes: lipid metabolism.

Catabolic Pathway (Catabolism)

A **catabolic pathway** is a series of reactions that bring about a net release of energy in the form of a high energy phosphate bond formed with the energy carriers Adenosine Diphosphate (ADP) and Guanosine Diphosphate (GDP) to produce Adenosine Triphosphate (ATP) and Guanosine Triphosphate (GTP), respectively. The net reaction is, therefore, thermodynamically favorable, for it results in a lower free energy for the final products. A catabolic pathway is an exergonic system that produces chemical energy in the form of ATP, GTP, NADH, NADPH, FADH2, etc. from energy containing sources such as carbohydrates, fats, and proteins. The end products are often carbon dioxide, water, and ammonia. Coupled with an endergonic reaction of anabolism, the cell can synthesize new macromolecules using the original precursors of the anabolic pathway. An example of a coupled reaction is the phosphorylation of fructose-6-phosphate to form the intermediate fructose-1,6-bisphosphate by the enzyme phsophofructokinase accompanied by the hydrolysis of ATP in the pathway of glycolysis. The resulting chemical reaction within the metabolic pathway is highly thermodynamically favorable and, as a result, irreversible in the cell.

$$Fructose - 6 - Phosphate + ATP \longrightarrow Fructose - 1,6 - Bisphosphate + ADP$$

CELLULAR RESPIRATION

Cellular respiration is a set of metabolic reactions and processes that take place in the cells of organisms to convert biochemical energy from nutrients into adenosine triphosphate (ATP), and then release waste products. The reactions involved in respiration are catabolic reactions, which break large molecules into smaller ones, releasing energy in the process, as weak so-called "high-energy" bonds are replaced by stronger bonds in the products. Respiration is one of the key ways a cell releases chemical energy to fuel cellular activity. Cellular respiration is considered an exothermic redox reaction which releases heat. The overall reaction occurs in a series of biochemical steps, most of which are redox reactions themselves. Although technically, cellular respiration is a combustion reaction, it clearly does not resemble one when it occurs in a living cell because of the slow release of energy from the series of reactions.

Nutrients that are commonly used by animal and plant cells in respiration include sugar, amino acids and fatty acids, and the most common oxidizing agent (electron acceptor) is molecular oxygen (O2). The chemical energy stored in ATP (its third phosphate group is weakly bonded to the rest of the molecule and is cheaply broken allowing stronger bonds to form, thereby transferring energy for use by the cell) can then be used to drive processes requiring energy, including biosynthesis, locomotion or transportation of molecules across cell membranes.

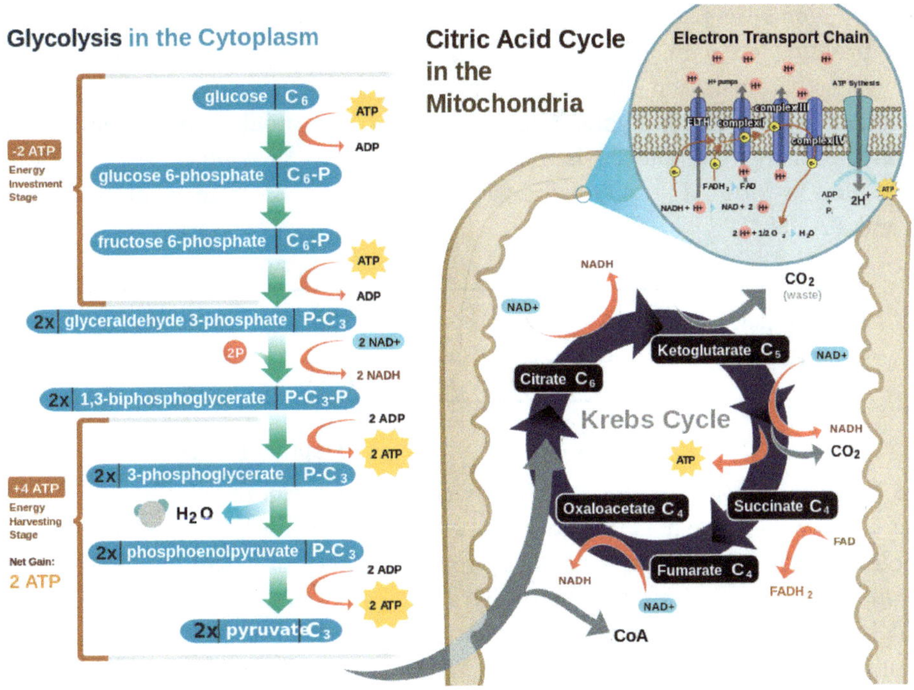

Typical eukaryotic cell

Aerobic Respiration

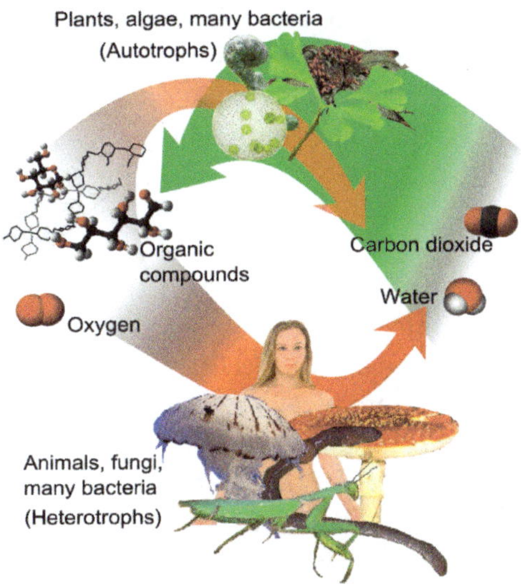

Aerobic respiration (red arrows) is the main means by which both fungi and animals utilize chemical energy in the form of organic compounds that were previously created through photosynthesis (green arrow).

Aerobic respiration requires oxygen (O_2) in order to create ATP. Although carbohydrates, fats, and proteins are consumed as reactants, it is the preferred method of pyruvate breakdown in glycolysis and requires that pyruvate enter the mitochondria in order to be fully oxidized by the Krebs cycle. The products of this process are carbon dioxide and water, but the energy transferred is used to break bonds in ADP as the third phosphate group is added to form ATP (adenosine triphosphate), by substrate-level phosphorylation, NADH and $FADH_2$

Simplified reaction:	$C_6H_{12}O_6$ (s) + 6 O_2 (g) → 6 CO_2 (g) + 6 H_2O (l) + heat
	$\Delta G = -2880$ kJ per mol of $C_6H_{12}O_6$

The negative ΔG indicates that the reaction can occur spontaneously.

The potential of NADH and $FADH_2$ is converted to more ATP through an electron transport chain with oxygen as the "terminal electron acceptor". Most of the ATP produced by aerobic cellular respiration is made by oxidative phosphorylation. This works by the energy released in the consumption of pyruvate being used to create a chemiosmotic potential by pumping protons across a membrane. This potential is then used to drive ATP synthase and produce ATP from ADP and a phosphate group. Biology textbooks often state that 38 ATP molecules can be made per oxidised glucose molecule during cellular respiration (2 from glycolysis, 2 from the Krebs cycle, and about 34 from the electron transport system). However, this maximum yield is never quite reached because of losses due to leaky membranes as well as the cost of moving pyruvate and ADP into the mitochondrial matrix, and current estimates range around 29 to 30 ATP per glucose.

Aerobic metabolism is up to 15 times more efficient than anaerobic metabolism (which yields 2 molecules ATP per 1 molecule glucose). However some anaerobic organisms, such as methanogens are able to continue with anaerobic respiration, yielding more ATP by using other inorganic molecules (not oxygen) as final electron acceptors in the electron transport chain. They share the initial pathway of glycolysis but aerobic metabolism continues with the Krebs cycle and oxidative phosphorylation. The post-glycolytic reactions take place in the mitochondria in eukaryotic cells, and in the cytoplasm in prokaryotic cells.

Glycolysis

Out of the cytoplasm it goes into the Krebs cycle with the acetyl CoA. It then mixes with CO_2 and makes 2 ATP, NADH, and FADH. From there the NADH and FADH go into the NADH reductase, which produces the enzyme. The NADH pulls the enzyme's electrons to send through the electron transport chain. The electron transport chain pulls H^+ ions through the chain. From the electron transport chain, the released hydrogen ions make ADP for an end result of 32 ATP. O_2 attracts itself to the left over electron to make water. Lastly, ATP leaves through the ATP channel and out of the mitochondria.

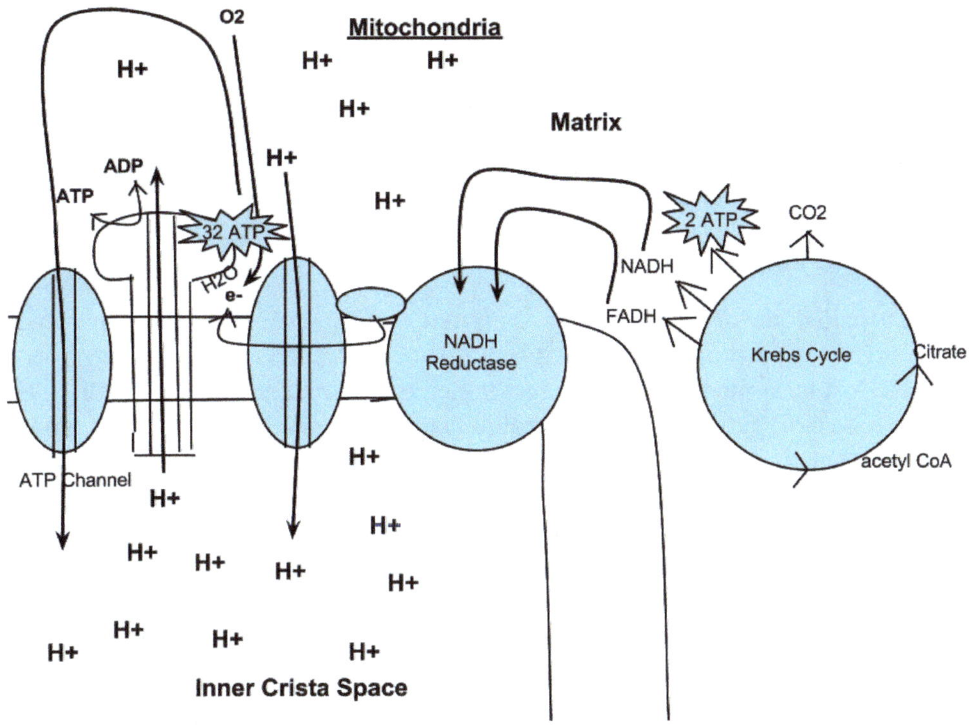

Glycolysis is a metabolic pathway that takes place in the cytosol of cells in all living organisms. This pathway can function with or without the presence of oxygen. In humans, aerobic conditions produce pyruvate and anaerobic conditions produce lactate. In aerobic conditions, the process converts one molecule of glucose into two molecules of pyruvate (pyruvic acid), generating energy in the form of two net molecules of ATP. Four molecules of ATP per glucose are actually produced, however, two are consumed as part of the preparatory phase. The initial phosphorylation of glucose is required to increase the reactivity (decrease its stability) in order for the molecule to be cleaved into two pyruvate molecules by the enzyme aldolase. During the pay-off phase of glycolysis, four phosphate groups are transferred to ADP by substrate-level phosphorylation to make four ATP, and two NADH are produced when the pyruvate are oxidized. The overall reaction can be expressed this way:

Glucose + 2 NAD^+ + 2 P_i + 2 ADP → 2 pyruvate + 2 NADH + 2 ATP + 2 H^+ + 2 H_2O + heat

Starting with glucose, 1 ATP is used to donate a phosphate to glucose to produce glucose 6-phosphate. Glycogen can be converted into glucose 6-phosphate as well with the help of glycogen phosphorylase. During energy metabolism, glucose 6-phosphate becomes fructose 6-phosphate. An additional ATP is used to phosphorylate fructose 6-phosphate into fructose 1,6-disphosphate by the help of phosphofructokinase. Fructose 1,6-diphosphate then splits into two phosphorylated molecules with three carbon chains which later degrades into pyruvate.

Glycolysis can be literally translated as “sugar splitting”.

Oxidative Decarboxylation of Pyruvate

Pyruvate is oxidized to acetyl-CoA and CO_2 by the pyruvate dehydrogenase complex (PDC). The PDC contains multiple copies of three enzymes and is located in the mitochondria of eukaryotic cells and in the cytosol of prokaryotes. In the conversion of pyruvate to acetyl-CoA, one molecule of NADH and one molecule of CO_2 is formed.

Citric Acid Cycle

This is also called the *Krebs cycle* or the *tricarboxylic acid cycle*. When oxygen is present, acetyl-CoA is produced from the pyruvate molecules created from glycolysis. Once acetyl-CoA is formed, aerobic or anaerobic respiration can occur. When oxygen is present, the mitochondria will undergo aerobic respiration which leads to the Krebs cycle. However, if oxygen is not present, fermentation of the pyruvate molecule will occur. In the presence of oxygen, when acetyl-CoA is produced, the molecule then enters the citric acid cycle (Krebs cycle) inside the mitochondrial matrix, and is oxidized to CO_2 while at the same time reducing NAD to NADH. NADH can be used by the electron transport chain to create further ATP as part of oxidative phosphorylation. To fully oxidize the equivalent of one glucose molecule, two acetyl-CoA must be metabolized by the Krebs cycle. Two waste products, H_2O and CO_2, are created during this cycle.

The citric acid cycle is an 8-step process involving 18 different enzymes and co-enzymes. During the cycle, acetyl-CoA (2 carbons) + oxaloacetate (4 carbons) yields citrate (6 carbons), which is rearranged to a more reactive form called isocitrate (6 carbons). Isocitrate is modified to become α-ketoglutarate (5 carbons), succinyl-CoA, succinate, fumarate, malate, and, finally, oxaloacetate.

The net gain of high-energy compounds from one cycle is 3 NADH, 1 $FADH_2$, and 1 GTP; the GTP may subsequently be used to produce ATP. Thus, the total yield from 1 glucose molecule (2 pyruvate molecules) is 6 NADH, 2 $FADH_2$, and 2 ATP.

Oxidative Phosphorylation

In eukaryotes, oxidative phosphorylation occurs in the mitochondrial cristae. It comprises the electron transport chain that establishes a proton gradient (chemiosmotic potential) across the boundary of inner membrane by oxidizing the NADH produced from the Krebs cycle. ATP is synthesized by the ATP synthase enzyme when the chemiosmotic gradient is used to drive the phosphorylation of ADP. The electrons are finally transferred to exogenous oxygen and, with the addition of two protons, water is formed.

Efficiency of ATP Production

The table below describes the reactions involved when one glucose molecule is fully oxidized into carbon dioxide. It is assumed that all the reduced coenzymes are oxidized by the electron transport chain and used for oxidative phosphorylation.

Step	coenzyme yield	ATP yield	Source of ATP
Glycolysis preparatory phase		−2	Phosphorylation of glucose and fructose 6-phosphate uses two ATP from the cytoplasm.
Glycolysis pay-off phase		4	Substrate-level phosphorylation
	2 NADH	3 or 5	Oxidative phosphorylation : Each NADH produces net 1.5 ATP (instead of usual 2.5) due to NADH transport over the mitochondrial membrane
Oxidative decarboxylation of pyruvate	2 NADH	5	Oxidative phosphorylation
Krebs cycle		2	Substrate-level phosphorylation
	6 NADH	15	Oxidative phosphorylation
	2 $FADH_2$	3	Oxidative phosphorylation
Total yield		**30 or 32 ATP**	From the complete oxidation of one glucose molecule to carbon dioxide and oxidation of all the reduced coenzymes.

Although there is a theoretical yield of 38 ATP molecules per glucose during cellular respiration, such conditions are generally not realized because of losses such as the cost of moving pyruvate (from glycolysis), phosphate, and ADP (substrates for ATP synthesis) into the mitochondria. All are actively transported using carriers that utilize the stored energy in the proton electrochemical gradient.

- Pyruvate is taken up by a specific, low Km transporter to bring it into the mitochondrial matrix for oxidation by the pyruvate dehydrogenase complex.
- The **phosphate carrier** (PiC) mediates the electroneutral exchange (antiport) of phosphate ($H_2PO_4^-$; P_i) for OH^- or symport of phosphate and protons (H^+) across the inner membrane, and the driving force for moving phosphate ions into the mitochondria is the proton motive force.
- The **ATP-ADP translocase** (also called adenine nucleotide translocase, ANT) is an antiporter and exchanges ADP and ATP across the inner membrane. The driving force is due to the ATP (−4) having a more negative charge than the ADP (−3), and thus it dissipates some of the electrical component of the proton electrochemical gradient.

The outcome of these transport processes using the proton electrochemical gradient is that more than 3 H^+ are needed to make 1 ATP. Obviously this reduces the theoretical efficiency of the whole process and the likely maximum is closer to 28–30 ATP molecules. In practice the efficiency may be even lower because the inner membrane of the mitochondria is slightly leaky to protons. Other factors may also dissipate the proton gradient creating an apparently leaky mitochondria. An uncoupling protein known as thermogenin is expressed in some cell types and is a channel that can transport protons. When this protein is active in the inner membrane it short circuits the coupling between the electron transport chain and ATP synthesis. The potential energy from the proton gradient is not used to make ATP but generates heat. This is particularly important in brown fat thermogenesis of newborn and hibernating mammals.

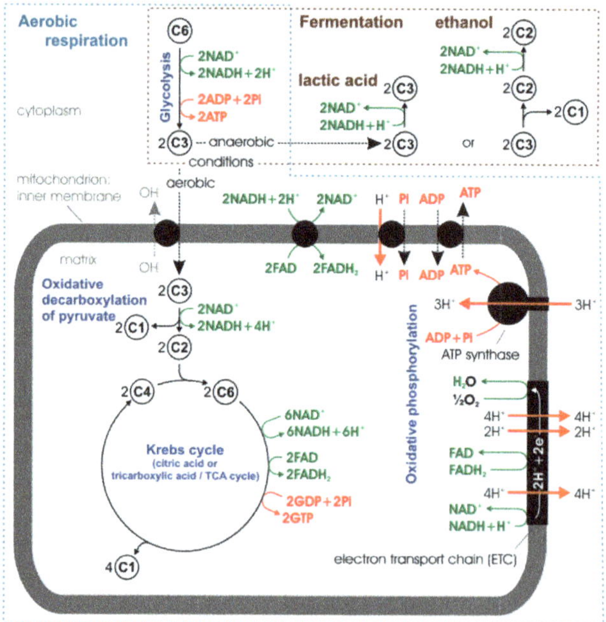

Stoichiometry of aerobic respiration and most known fermentation types in eucaryotic cell. Numbers in circles indicate counts of carbon atoms in molecules, C6 is glucose $C_6H_{12}O_6$, C1 carbon dioxide CO_2. Mitochondrial outer membrane is omitted.

According to some of newer sources the ATP yield during aerobic respiration is not 36–38, but only about 30–32 ATP molecules / 1 molecule of glucose , because:

- ATP : NADH+H^+ and ATP : $FADH_2$ ratios during the oxidative phosphorylation appear to be not 3 and 2, but 2.5 and 1.5 respectively. Unlike in the substrate-level phosphorylation, the stoichiometry here is difficult to establish.
- ATP synthase produces 1 ATP / 3 H^+. However the exchange of matrix ATP for cytosolic ADP and Pi (antiport with OH^- or symport with H^+) mediated by ATP–ADP translocase and phosphate carrier consumes 1 H^+ / 1 ATP as a result of regeneration of the transmembrane potential changed during this transfer, so the net ratio is 1 ATP : 4 H^+.
- The mitochondrial electron transport chain proton pump transfers across the inner membrane 10 H^+ / 1 NADH+H^+ (4 + 2 + 4) or 6 H^+ / 1 $FADH_2$ (2 + 4).

So the final stoichiometry is

1 NADH+H^+ : 10 H^+ : 10/4 ATP = 1 NADH+H^+ : 2.5 ATP

1 $FADH_2$: 6 H^+ : 6/4 ATP = 1 $FADH_2$: 1.5 ATP

- ATP : NADH+H^+ coming from glycolysis ratio during the oxidative phosphorylation is
- 1.5, as for $FADH_2$, if hydrogen atoms ($2H^+$+$2e^-$) are transferred from cytosolic NADH+H^+ to mitochondrial FAD by the glycerol phosphate shuttle located in the inner mitochondrial membrane.

- 2.5 in case of malate-aspartate shuttle transferring hydrogen atoms from cytosolic $NADH+H^+$ to mitochondrial NAD^+

So finally we have, per molecule of glucose

- Substrate-level phosphorylation: 2 ATP from glycolysis + 2 ATP (directly GTP) from Krebs cycle
- Oxidative phosphorylation
- 2 $NADH+H^+$ from glycolysis: 2 × 1.5 ATP (if glycerol phosphate shuttle transfers hydrogen atoms) or 2 × 2.5 ATP (malate-aspartate shuttle)
- 2 $NADH+H^+$ from the oxidative decarboxylation of pyruvate and 6 from Krebs cycle: 8 × 2.5 ATP
- 2 $FADH_2$ from the Krebs cycle: 2 × 1.5 ATP

Altogether this gives 4 + 3 (or 5) + 20 + 3 = 30 (or 32) ATP per molecule of glucose

The total ATP yield in ethanol or lactic acid fermentation is only 2 molecules coming from glycolysis, because pyruvate is not transferred to the mitochondrion and finally oxidized to the carbon dioxide (CO_2), but reduced to ethanol or lactic acid in the cytoplasm.

Fermentation

Without oxygen, pyruvate (pyruvic acid) is not metabolized by cellular respiration but undergoes a process of fermentation. The pyruvate is not transported into the mitochondrion, but remains in the cytoplasm, where it is converted to waste products that may be removed from the cell. This serves the purpose of oxidizing the electron carriers so that they can perform glycolysis again and removing the excess pyruvate. Fermentation oxidizes NADH to NAD+ so it can be re-used in glycolysis. In the absence of oxygen, fermentation prevents the buildup of NADH in the cytoplasm and provides NAD+ for glycolysis. This waste product varies depending on the organism. In skeletal muscles, the waste product is lactic acid. This type of fermentation is called lactic acid fermentation. In strenuous exercise, when energy demands exceed energy supply, the respiratory chain cannot process all of the hydrogen atoms joined by NADH. During anaerobic glycolysis, NAD+ regenerates when pairs of hydrogen combine with pyruvate to form lactate. Lactate formation is catalyzed by lactate dehydrogenase in a reversible reaction. Lactate can also be used as an indirect precursor for liver glycogen. During recovery, when oxygen becomes available, NAD+ attaches to hydrogen from lactate to form ATP. In yeast, the waste products are ethanol and carbon dioxide. This type of fermentation is known as alcoholic or ethanol fermentation. The ATP generated in this process is made by substrate-level phosphorylation, which does not require oxygen.

Fermentation is less efficient at using the energy from glucose: only 2 ATP are produced per glucose, compared to the 38 ATP per glucose nominally produced by aerobic respiration. This is because the waste products of fermentation still contain chemical potential energy that can be released by oxidation. Ethanol, for example, can be burned in an internal combustion engine like gasoline. Glycolytic ATP, however, is created more quickly. For prokaryotes to continue a rapid growth rate when they are shifted from an aerobic environment to an anaerobic environment, they must increase the rate of the glycolytic reactions. For multicellular organisms, during short bursts of strenuous activity, muscle cells use fermentation to supplement the ATP production from the slower aerobic respiration, so fermentation may be used by a cell even before the oxygen levels are depleted, as is the case in sports that do not require athletes to pace themselves, such as sprinting.

Anaerobic Respiration

Cellular respiration is the process by which biological fuels are oxidised in the presence of an inorganic electron acceptor (such as oxygen) to produce large amounts of energy, to drive the bulk production of ATP.

Anaerobic respiration is used by some microorganisms in which neither oxygen (aerobic respiration) nor pyruvate derivatives (fermentation) is the final electron acceptor. Rather, an inorganic acceptor such as sulfate or nitrate is used. Such organisms are typically found in unusual places such as underwater caves or near hydrothermal vents at the bottom of the ocean.

Anabolic Pathway (Anabolism)

In contrast to catabolic pathways, are the **anabolic pathways** that require an input of energy in order to conduct the construction of macromolecules such as polypeptides, nucleic acids, proteins, polysaccharides, and lipids. The isolated reaction of anabolism is unfavorable in a cell due to a positive Gibbs Free Energy ($+\Delta G$); thus, an input of chemical energy through a coupling with an exergonic reaction is necessary. The coupled reaction of the catabolic pathway affects the thermodynamics of the reaction by lowering the overall activation energy of an anabolic pathway and allowing the reaction to take place. Otherwise, an endergonic reaction is non-spontaneous.

An anabolic pathway is a biosynthetic pathway, meaning that it combines smaller molecules to form larger and more complex ones. An example is the reversed pathway of glycolysis, otherwise known as gluconeogenesis, which occurs in the liver and sometimes in the kidney in order to maintain proper glucose concentration in the blood and to be able to supply the brain and muscle tissues with adequate amount of glucose. Although gluconeogenesis is similar to the reverse pathway of glycolysis, it contains three distinct enzymes from glycolysis that allow the pathway to occur spontaneously. An example of the pathway for gluconeogenesis is illustrated in the image titled "Gluconeogenesis Mechanism".

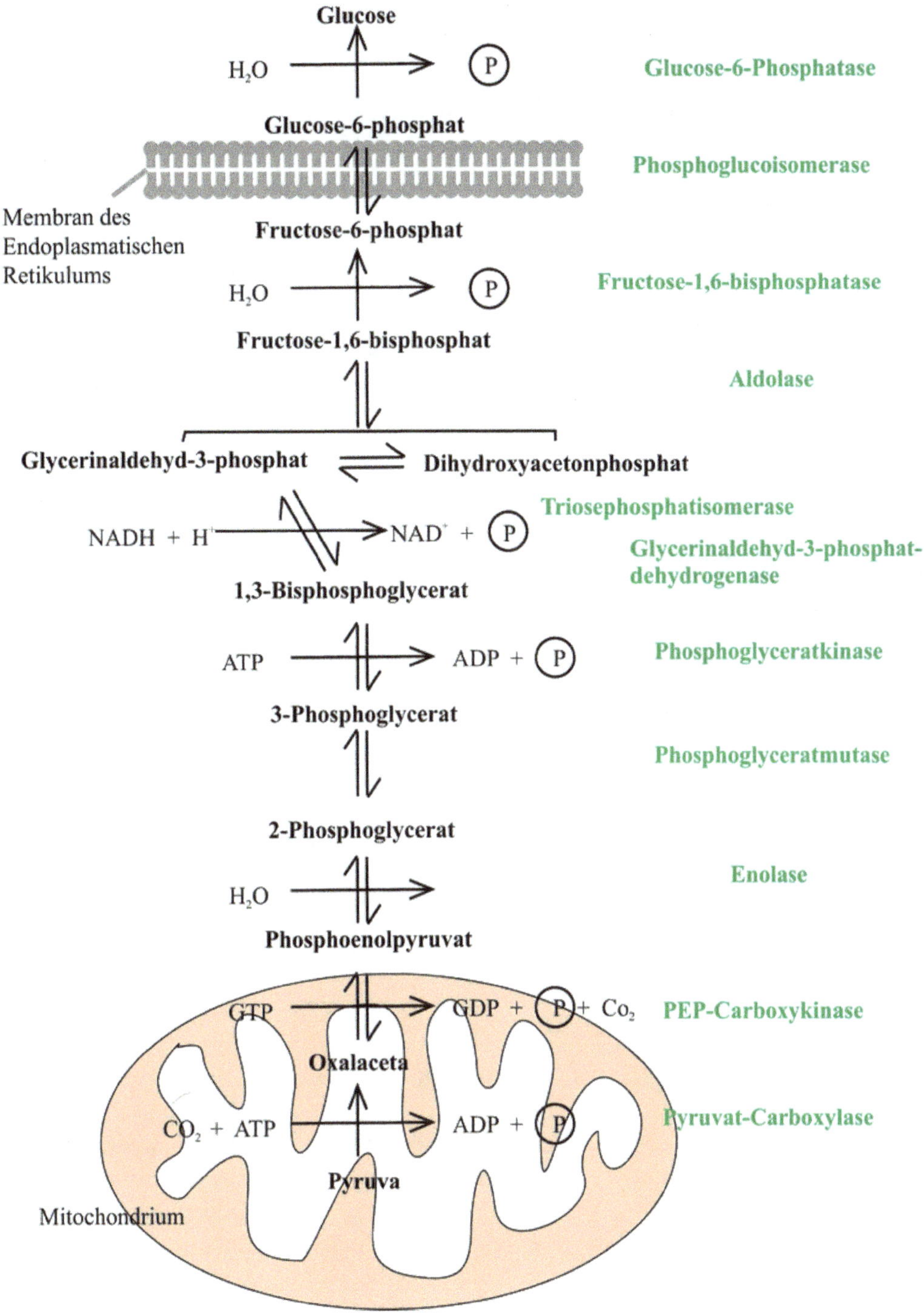

Gluconeogenesis Mechanism

Amphibolic Pathway

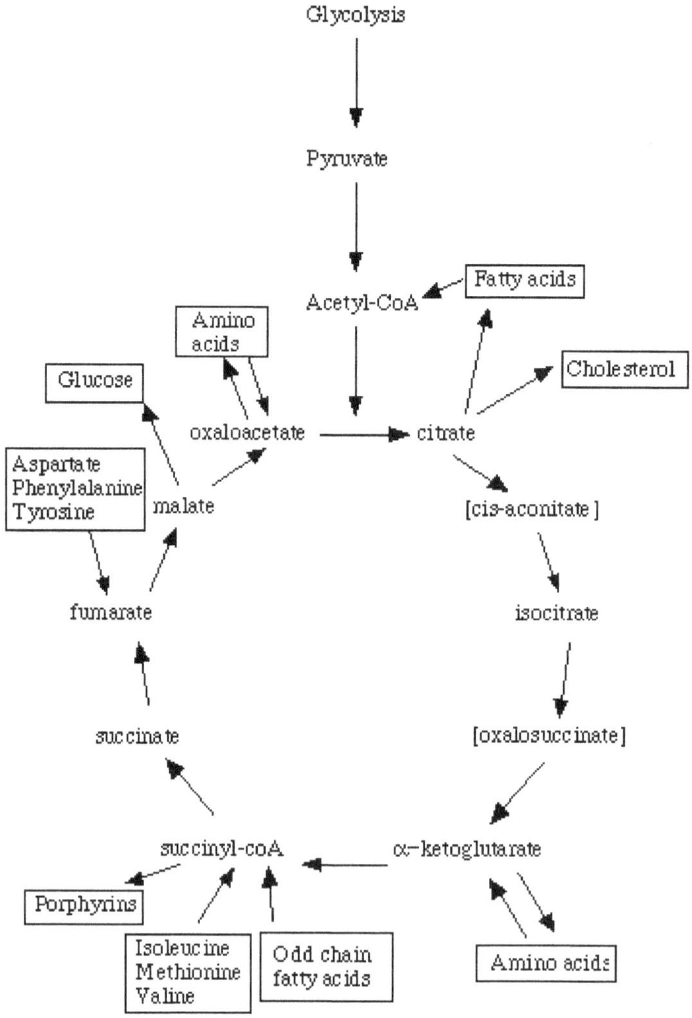

Amphibolic Properties of the Citric Acid Cycle

An **amphibolic pathway** is one that can be either catabolic or anabolic based on the availability of or the need for energy. The currency of energy in a biological cell is adenosine triphosphate (ATP), which stores its energy in the phosphoanhydride bonds. The energy is utilized to conduct biosynthesis, facilitate movement, and regulate active transport inside of the cell. Examples of amphibolic pathways are the citric acid cycle and the glyoxylate cycle. These sets of chemical reactions contain both energy producing and utilizing pathways. To the right is an illustration of the amphibolic properties of the TCA cycle.

The glyoxylate shunt pathway is an alternative to the tricarboxylic acid (TCA) cycle, for it redirects the pathway of TCA to prevent full oxidation of carbon compounds, and to preserve high energy carbon sources as future energy sources. This pathway occurs only in plants and bacteria and transpires in the absence of glucose molecules.

Regulation

The flux of the entire pathway is regulated by the rate-determining steps. These are the slowest steps in a network of reactions. The rate-limiting step occurs near the beginning of the pathway and is regulated by feedback inhibition, which ultimately controls the overall rate of the pathway. The metabolic pathway in the cell is regulated by covalent or non-covalent modifications. A covalent modification involves an addition or removal of a chemical bond, whereas a non-covalent modification (also known as allosteric regulation) is the binding of the regulator to the enzyme via hydrogen bonds, electrostatic interactions, and Van Der Waals forces.

The rate of turnover in a metabolic pathway, otherwise known as the metabolic flux, is regulated based on the stoichiometric reaction model, the utilization rate of metabolites, and the translocation pace of molecules across the lipid bilayer. The regulation methods are based on experiments involving 13C-labeling, which is then analyzed by Nuclear Magnetic Resonance (NMR) or gas chromatography-mass spectrometry (GC-MS)-derived mass compositions. The aforementioned techniques synthesize a statistical interpretation of mass distribution in proteinogenic amino acids to the catalytic activities of enzymes in a cell.

REFERENCES

1. Cox, David L. Nelson, Michael M. (2008). Lehninger principles of biochemistry (5th ed.). New York: W.H. Freeman. p. 26. ISBN 978-0-7167-7108-1.
2. Nicholson, Donald E. (March 1971). An Introduction to Metabolic Pathways by S. DAGLEY (Vol. 59, No. 2 ed.). Sigma Xi, The Scientific Research Society. p. 266.
3. Pratt, Donald Voet, Judith G. Voet, Charlotte W. (2013). Fundamentals of Biochemistry: Life at the Molecular Level (4th ed.). Hoboken, NJ: Wiley. pp. 441–442. ISBN 978-0470-54784-7.
4. ^ Jump up to:a b Reece, Jane B. (2011). Campbell biology / Jane B. Reece ... et al.. (9th ed.). Boston: Benjamin Cummings. p. 143. ISBN 978-0-321-55823-7.
5. Berg, Jeremy M.; Tymoczko, John L.; Stryer, Lubert; Gatto, Gregory J. (2012). Biochemistry (7th ed.). New York: W.H. Freeman. p. 429. ISBN 1429229365.
6. Clarke, Jeremy M. Berg; John L. Tymoczko; Lubert Stryer. Web content by Neil D. (2002). Biochemistry (5. ed., 4. print. ed.). New York, NY u.a.: W. H. Freeman. pp. 578–579. ISBN 0716730510.
7. Eichhorn, Peter H. Raven ; Ray F. Evert ; Susan E. (2011). Biology of plants (8. ed.). New York, NY: Freeman. pp. 100–106. ISBN 978-1-4292-1961-7.
8. Pratt, Donald Voet, Judith G. Voet, Charlotte W. (2013). Fundamentals of biochemistry : life at the molecular level (4th ed.). Hoboken, NJ: Wiley. pp. 474–478. ISBN 978-0470-54784-7.
9. Cox, David L. Nelson, Michael M. (2008). Lehninger principles of biochemistry (5th ed.). New York: W.H. Freeman. pp. 25–27. ISBN 978-0-7167-7108-1.

10. Cox, David L. Nelson, Michael M. (2008). Lehninger principles of biochemistry (5th ed.). New York: W.H. Freeman. p. 25. ISBN 978-0-7167-7108-1.
11. Clarke, Jeremy M. Berg; John L. Tymoczko; Lubert Stryer. Web content by Neil D. (2002). Biochemistry (5. ed., 4. print. ed.). New York, NY u.a.: W. H. Freeman. p. 570. ISBN 0716730510.
12. Berg, Jeremy M.; Tymoczko, John L.; Stryer, Lubert; Gatto, Gregory J. (2012). Biochemistry (7th ed.). New York: W.H. Freeman. pp. 480–482. ISBN 9781429229364.
13. Clarke, Jeremy M. Berg; John L. Tymoczko; Lubert Stryer. Web content by Neil D. (2002). Biochemistry (5. ed., 4. print. ed.). New York, NY u.a. W. H. Freeman. p. 570. ISBN 0-7167-3051-0.
14. Clarke, Jeremy M. Berg; John L. Tymoczko; Lubert Stryer. Web content by Neil D. (2002). Biochemistry (5. ed., 4. print. ed.). New York, NY u.a.: W. H. Freeman. p. 571. ISBN 0-7167-3051-0.
15. Pratt, Donald Voet, Judith G. Voet, Charlotte W. (2013). Fundamentals of biochemistry : life at the molecular level (4th ed.). Hoboken, NJ: Wiley. p. 572. ISBN 978-0470-54784-7.
16. Choffnes, Eileen R.; Relman,, David A.; Academies, Leslie Pray, rapporteurs, Forum on Microbial Threat, Board on Global Health, Institute of Medicine of the National (2011). The science and applications of synthetic and systems biology workshop summary. Washington, D.C.: National Academies Press. p. 135. ISBN 978-0-309-21939-6.
17. Cox, David L. Nelson, Michael M. (2008). Lehninger principles of biochemistry (5th ed.). New York: W.H. Freeman. pp. 577–578. ISBN 978-0-7167-7108-1.
18. Kruger, ed. by Nicholas J.; Hill,, Steve A.; Ratcliffe, R. George (1999). Regulation of primary metabolic pathways in plants : White, David (1995). The physiology and biochemistry of prokaryotes. New York u.a.: Oxford Univ. Press. p. 133. ISBN 0-19-508439-X.
19. Weckwerth, edited by Wolfram (2006). Metabolomics methods and protocols. Totowa, N.J.: Humana Press. p. 177. ISBN 1597452440.
20. Weckwerth, edited by Wolfram (2006). Metabolomics methods and protocols. Totowa, N.J.: Humana Press. p. 178. ISBN 1597452440.
21. Bailey, Regina. "Cellular Respiration".
22. Rich, P. R. (2003). "The molecular machinery of Keilin's respiratory chain". Biochemical Society Transactions. 31 (Pt 6): 1095–1105. doi:10.1042/BST0311095. PMID 14641005.
23. Reece1 Urry2 Cain3 Wasserman4 Minorsky5 Jackson6, Jane1 Lisa2 Michael3 Steven4 Peter5 Robert6 (2010). Campbell Biology Ninth Edition. Pearson Education, Inc. p. 168.
24. "Cellular Respiration" (PDF).
25. Porter, R.; Brand, M. (1 September 1995). "Mitochondrial proton conductance and H+/O ratio are independent of electron transport rate in isolated hepatocytes".

The Biochemical Journal (Free full text). 310 (Pt 2): 379–382. doi:10.1042/bj3100379. ISSN 0264-6021. PMC 1135905 . PMID 7654171.

26. Stryer, Lubert (1995). Biochemistry (fourth ed.). New York – Basingstoke: W. H. Freeman and Company. ISBN 978-0716720096.

CHAPTER 4

Metabolic Networks

Chapter Contents

The new approaches and questions that the genomes make possible are usually referred to as functional genomics. The task is to define the function of a gene (or its protein) in the life processes of the organism, where function refers to the role it plays in a larger context. But what are these life processes? The most obvious example is the metabolism of an organism, the basic chemical system that generates essential components such as amino acids, sugars and lipids, and the energy required to synthesize them and to use them in creating proteins and cellular structures. This system of connected chemical reactions is a metabolic network.

INTRODUCTION

A metabolic network is the complete set of metabolic and physical processes that determine the physiological and biochemical properties of a cell. As such, these networks comprise the chemical reactions of metabolism, the metabolic pathways, as well as the regulatory interactions that guide these reactions.

With the sequencing of complete genomes, it is now possible to reconstruct the network of biochemical reactions in many organisms, from bacteria to human. Several of these networks are available online: Kyoto Encyclopedia of Genes and Genomes (KEGG), EcoCyc , BioCyc and metaTIGER . Metabolic networks are powerful tools for studying and modelling metabolism.

METABOLIC NETWORK MODELLING

Metabolic network **reconstruction and simulation** allows for an in-depth insight into the molecular mechanisms of a particular organism. In particular, these models correlate the genome with molecular physiology. A reconstruction breaks down metabolic pathways (such as glycolysis and the Citric acid cycle) into their respective reactions and enzymes, and analyzes them within the perspective of the entire network. In simplified terms, a reconstruction collects all of the relevant metabolic information of an organism and compiles it in a mathematical model. Validation and analysis of reconstructions can allow identification of key features of metabolism such as growth yield, resource distribution, network robustness, and gene essentiality. This knowledge can then be applied to create novel biotechnology.

In general, the process to build a reconstruction is as follows:

- Draft a reconstruction
- Refine the model
- Convert model into a mathematical/computational representation
- Evaluate and debug model through experimentation

Metabolic network showing interactions between enzymes and metabolites in the *Arabidopsis thaliana* citric acid cycle. Enzymes and metabolites are the red dots and interactions between them are the lines.

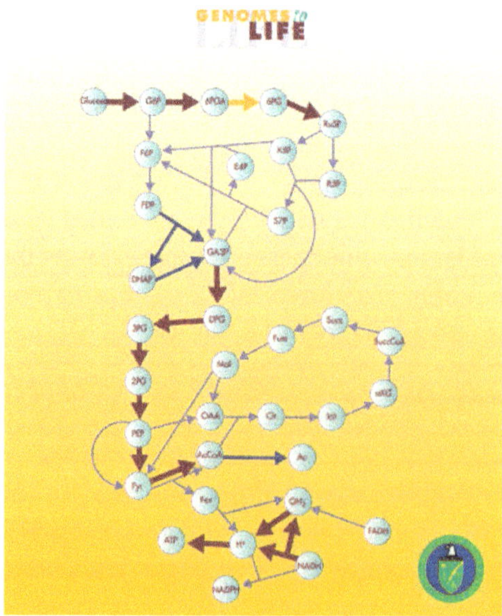

Metabolic Network Model for Escherichia coli.

Genome-Scale Metabolic Reconstruction

A metabolic reconstruction provides a highly mathematical, structured platform on which to understand the systems biology of metabolic pathways within an organism. The integration of biochemical metabolic pathways with rapidly available, unannotated genome sequences has developed what are called genome-scale metabolic models. Simply put, these models correspond metabolic genes with metabolic pathways. In general, the more information about physiology, biochemistry and genetics is available for the target organism, the better the predictive capacity of the reconstructed models. Mechanically speaking, the process of reconstructing prokaryotic and eukaryotic metabolic networks is essentially the same. Having said this, eukaryote reconstructions are typically more challenging because of the size of genomes, coverage of knowledge, and the multitude of cellular compartments. The first genome-scale metabolic model was generated in 1995 for *Haemophilus influenzae*. The first multicellular organism, *C. elegans*, was reconstructed in 1998. Since then, many reconstructions have been formed. For a list of reconstructions that have been converted into a model and experimentally validated, see http://sbrg.ucsd.edu/InSilicoOrganisms/OtherOrganisms.

Organism	Genes in Genome	Genes in Model	Reactions	Metabolites	Date of reconstruction	Reference
Haemophilus influenzae	1,775	296	488	343	June 1999	
Escherichia coli	4,405	660	627	438	May 2000	
Saccharomyces cerevisiae	6,183	708	1,175	584	February 2003	
Mus musculus	28,287	473	1220	872	January 2005	
Homo sapiens	21,090	3,623	3,673	--	January 2007	
Mycobacterium tuberculosis	4,402	661	939	828	June 2007	
Bacillus subtilis	4,114	844	1,020	988	September 2007	
Synechocystis sp. PCC6803	3,221	633	831	704	October 2008	
Salmonella typhimurium	4,489	1,083	1,087	774	April 2009	
Arabidopsis thaliana	27,379	1,419	1,567	1,748	February 2010	

Drafting a Reconstruction

Resources

Because the timescale for the development of reconstructions is so recent, most reconstructions have been built manually. However, now, there are quite a few resources that allow for the semi-automatic assembly of these reconstructions that are utilized due to the time and effort necessary for a reconstruction. An initial fast reconstruction can be developed automatically using resources like PathoLogic or ERGO in combination with encyclopedias like MetaCyc, and then manually updated by using resources like PathwayTools. These semi-automatic methods allow for a fast draft to be created while allowing the fine tune adjustments required once new experimental data is found. It is only in this manner that the field of metabolic reconstructions will keep up with the ever-increasing numbers of annotated genomes.

Databases

- **Kyoto Encyclopedia of Genes and Genomes (KEGG)**: a bioinformatics database containing information on genes, proteins, reactions, and pathways. The 'KEGG Organisms' section, which is divided into eukaryotes and prokaryotes, encompasses many organisms for which gene and DNA information can be searched by typing in the enzyme of choice.
- **BioCyc, EcoCyc, and MetaCyc**: BioCyc Is a collection of 3,000 pathway/genome databases (as of Oct 2013), with each database dedicated to one organism. For example, EcoCyc is a highly detailed bioinformatics database on the genome and metabolic reconstruction of *Escherichia coli*, including thorough descriptions of *E. coli* signaling pathways and regulatory network. The EcoCyc database can serve as a paradigm and model for any reconstruction. Additionally, MetaCyc, an encyclopedia of experimentally defined metabolic pathways and enzymes, contains 2,100 metabolic pathways and 11,400 metabolic reactions (Oct 2013).
- **ENZYME**: An enzyme nomenclature database (part of the ExPASy proteonomics server of the Swiss Institute of Bioinformatics). After searching for a particular enzyme on the database, this resource gives you the reaction that is catalyzed. ENZYME has direct links to other gene/enzyme/literature databases such as KEGG, BRENDA, and PUBMED.
- **BRENDA**: A comprehensive enzyme database that allows for an enzyme to be searched by name, EC number, or organism.
- **BiGG**: A knowledge base of biochemically, genetically, and genomically structured genome-scale metabolic network reconstructions.
- **metaTIGER**: Is a collection of metabolic profiles and phylogenomic information on a taxonomically diverse range of eukaryotes which provides novel facilities for viewing and comparing the metabolic profiles between organisms.

Database	**Scope**				
	Enzymes	Genes	Reactions	Pathways	Metabolites
KEGG	X	X	X	X	X
BioCyc	X	X	X	X	X
MetaCyc	X		X	X	X
ENZYME	X		X		X
BRENDA	X		X		X
BiGG		X		X	X

This table quickly compares the scope of each database.

Tools for Metabolic Modeling

- **Pathway Tools**: A bioinformatics software package that assists in the construction of pathway/genome databases such as EcoCyc. Developed by Peter Karp and associates at the SRI International Bioinformatics Research Group, Pathway Tools has several components. Its PathoLogic module takes an annotated genome for an organism and infers probable metabolic reactions and pathways to produce a new pathway/genome database. Its MetaFlux component can generate a quantitative metabolic model from that pathway/genome database using flux-balance analysis. Its Navigator component provides extensive query and visualization tools, such as visualization of metabolites, pathways, and the complete metabolic network.

- **ERGO**: A subscription-based service developed by Integrated Genomics. It integrates data from every level including genomic, biochemical data, literature, and high-throughput analysis into a comprehensive user friendly network of metabolic and nonmetabolic pathways.
- **KEGGtranslator**: an easy-to-use stand-alone application that can visualize and convert KEGG files (KGML formatted XML-files) into multiple output formats. Unlike other translators, KEGGtranslator supports a plethora of output formats, is able to augment the information in translated documents (e.g., MIRIAM annotations) beyond the scope of the KGML document, and amends missing components to fragmentary reactions within the pathway to allow simulations on those. KEGGtranslator converts these files to SBML, BioPAX, SIF, SBGN, SBML with qualitative modeling extension, GML, GraphML, JPG, GIF, LaTeX, etc.

KEGG pathways can directly be obtained from within the application.

- **Model SEED**: An online resource for the analysis, comparison, reconstruction, and curation of genome-scale metabolic models. Users can submit genome sequences to the RAST annotation system, and the resulting annotation can be automatically piped into the Model SEED to produce a draft metabolic model. The Model SEED automatically constructs a network of metabolic reactions, gene-protein-reaction associations for each reaction, and a biomass composition reaction for each genome to produce a model of microbial metabolism that can be simulated using Flux Balance Analysis.
- **MetaMerge**: algorithm for semi-automatically reconciling a pair of existing metabolic network reconstructions into a single metabolic network model.

Tools for Literature

- **PUBMED**: This is an online library developed by the National Center for Biotechnology Information, which contains a massive collection of medical journals. Using the link provided by ENZYME, the search can be directed towards the organism of interest, thus recovering literature on the enzyme and its use inside of the organism.

Methodology to Draft a Reconstruction

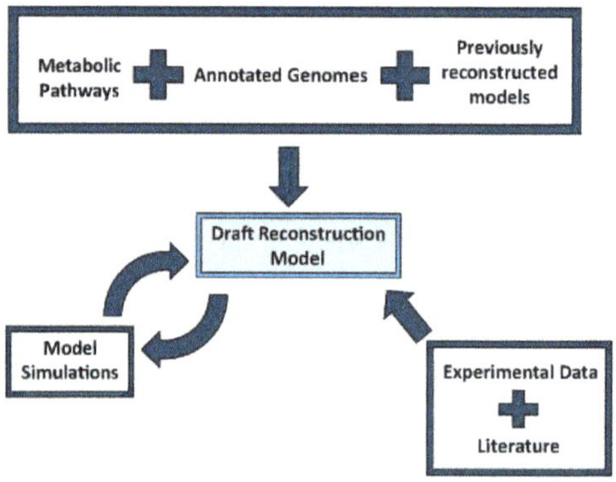

This is a visual representation of the metabolic network reconstruction process.

A reconstruction is built by compiling data from the resources above. Database tools such as KEGG and BioCyc can be used in conjunction with each other to find all the metabolic genes in the organism of interest. These genes will be compared to closely related organisms that have already developed reconstructions to find homologous genes and reactions. These homologous genes and reactions are carried over from the known reconstructions to form the draft reconstruction of the organism of interest. Tools such as ERGO, Pathway Tools and Model SEED can compile data into pathways to form a network of metabolic and non-metabolic pathways. These networks are then verified and refined before being made into a mathematical simulation.

The predictive aspect of a metabolic reconstruction hinges on the ability to predict the biochemical reaction catalyzed by a protein using that protein's amino acid sequence as an input, and to infer the structure of a metabolic network based on the predicted set of reactions. A network of enzymes and metabolites is drafted to relate sequences and function. When an uncharacterized protein is found in the genome, its amino acid sequence is first compared to those of previously characterized proteins to search for homology. When a homologous protein is found, the proteins are considered to have a common ancestor and their functions are inferred as being similar. However, the quality of a reconstruction model is dependent on its ability to accurately infer phenotype directly from sequence, so this rough estimation of protein function will not be sufficient. A number of algorithms and bioinformatics resources have been developed for refinement of sequence homology-based assignments of protein functions:

- **InParanoid**: Identifies eukaryotic orthologs by looking only at in-paralogs.
- **CDD**: Resource for the annotation of functional units in proteins. Its collection of domain models utilizes 3D structure to provide insights into sequence/structure/function relationships.

- **InterPro**: Provides functional analysis of proteins by classifying them into families and predicting domains and important sites.
- **STRING**: Database of known and predicted protein interactions.

Once proteins have been established, more information about the enzyme structure, reactions catalyzed, substrates and products, mechanisms, and more can be acquired from databases such as KEGG, MetaCyc and NC-IUBMB. Accurate metabolic reconstructions require additional information about the reversibility and preferred physiological direction of an enzyme-catalyzed reaction which can come from databases such as BRENDA or MetaCyc database.

Model Refinement

An initial metabolic reconstruction of a genome is typically far from perfect due to the high variability and diversity of microorganisms. Often, metabolic pathway databases such as KEGG and MetaCyc will have "holes", meaning that there is a conversion from a substrate to a product (i.e., an enzymatic activity) for which there is no known protein in the genome that encodes the enzyme that facilitates the catalysis. What can also happen in semi-automatically drafted reconstructions is that some pathways are falsely predicted and don't actually occur in the predicted manner. Because of this, a systematic verification is made in order to make sure no inconsistencies are present and that all the entries listed are correct and accurate.Furthermore, previous literature can be researched in order to support any information obtained from one of the many metabolic reaction and genome databases. This provides an added level of assurance for the reconstruction that the enzyme and the reaction it catalyzes do actually occur in the organism.

Enzyme promiscuity and spontaneous chemical reactions can damage metabolites. This metabolite damage, and its repair or pre-emption, create energy costs that need to be incorporated into models. It is likely that many genes of unknown function encode proteins that repair or pre-empt metabolite damage, but most genome-scale metabolic reconstructions only include a fraction of all genes.

Any new reactions not present in the databases need to be added to the reconstruction. This is an iterative process that cycles between the experimental phase and the coding phase. As new information is found about the target organism, the model will be adjusted to predict the metabolic and phenotypical output of the cell. The presence or absence of certain reactions of the metabolism will affect the amount of reactants/products that are present for other reactions within the particular pathway. This is because products in one reaction go on to become the reactants for another reaction, i.e. products of one reaction can combine with other proteins or compounds to form new proteins/compounds in the presence of different enzymes or catalysts.

Francke *et al.* provide an excellent example as to why the verification step of the project needs to be performed in significant detail. During a metabolic network reconstruction of *Lactobacillus plantarum*, the model showed that succinyl-CoA was one of the reactants for a reaction that was a part of the biosynthesis of methionine. However, an understanding of the physiology of the organism would have revealed that due to an incomplete tricarboxylic acid pathway, *Lactobacillus plantarum* does not actually produce succinyl-CoA, and the correct reactant for that part of the reaction was acetyl-CoA.

Therefore, systematic verification of the initial reconstruction will bring to light several inconsistencies that can adversely affect the final interpretation of the reconstruction, which is to accurately comprehend the molecular mechanisms of the organism. Furthermore, the simulation step also ensures that all the reactions present in the reconstruction are properly balanced. To sum up, a reconstruction that is fully accurate can lead to greater insight about understanding the functioning of the organism of interest.

Metabolic Network Simulation

A metabolic network can be broken down into a stoichiometric matrix where the rows represent the compounds of the reactions, while the columns of the matrix correspond to the reactions themselves. Stoichiometry is a quantitative relationship between substrates of a chemical reaction. In order to deduce what the metabolic network suggests, recent research has centered on a few approaches, such as extreme pathways, elementary mode analysis, flux balance analysis, and a number of other constraint-based modeling methods.

Extreme Pathways

Price, Reed, and Papin, from the Palsson lab, use a method of singular value decomposition (SVD) of extreme pathways in order to understand regulation of a human red blood cell metabolism. Extreme pathways are convex basis vectors that consist of steady state functions of a metabolic network. For any particular metabolic network, there is always a unique set of extreme pathways available. , Price, Reed, and Papin, define a constraint-based approach, where through the help of constraints like mass balance and maximum reaction rates, it is possible to develop a 'solution space' where all the feasible options fall within. Then, using a kinetic model approach, a single solution that falls within the extreme pathway solution space can be determined. Therefore, in their study, Price, Reed, and Papin, use both constraint and kinetic approaches to understand the human red blood cell metabolism.

Elementary Mode Analysis

Elementary mode analysis closely matches the approach used by extreme pathways. Similar to extreme pathways, there is always a unique set of elementary modes available for a particular metabolic network. These are the smallest sub-networks that allow a metabolic reconstruction network to function in steady state. According to Stelling (2002),elementary modes can be used to understand cellular objectives for the overall metabolic network., elementary mode analysis takes into account stoichiometrics and thermodynamics when evaluating whether a particular metabolic route or network is feasible and likely for a set of proteins/enzymes.

Minimal Metabolic Behaviors (MMBs)

In 2009, Larhlimi and Bockmayr presented a new approach called "minimal metabolic behaviors" for the analysis of metabolic networks. Like elementary modes or extreme pathways, these are uniquely determined by the network, and yield a complete description of the flux cone. However, the new description is much more compact. In contrast with elementary modes and extreme pathways, which use an inner description based on generating vectors of the flux cone, MMBs are using an outer description of the flux cone. This approach is based on sets of non-negativity constraints. These can be identified with irreversible reactions, and thus have a direct biochemical interpretation. One can characterize a metabolic network by MMBs and the reversible metabolic space.

Dynamic Simulation and Parameter Estimation

In order to perform a dynamic simulation with such a network it is necessary to construct an ordinary differential equation system that describes the rates of change in each metabolite's concentration or amount. To this end, a rate law, i.e., a kinetic equation that determines the rate of reaction based on the concentrations of all reactants is required for each reaction. Software packages that include numerical integrators, such as COPASI or SBMLsimulator, are then able to simulate the system dynamics given an initial condition. Often these rate laws contain kinetic parameters with uncertain values. In many cases it is desired to estimate these parameter values with respect to given time-series data of metabolite concentrations. The system is then supposed to reproduce the given data. For this purpose the distance between the given data set and the result of the simulation, i.e., the numerically or in few cases analytically obtained solution of the differential equation system is computed. The values of the parameters are then estimated to minimize this distance. One step further, it may be desired to estimate the mathematical structure of the differential equation system because the real rate laws are not known for the reactions within the system under study. To this end, the program SBMLsqueezer allows automatic creation of appropriate rate laws for all reactions with the network.

Synthetic Accessibility

Synthetic accessibility is a simple approach to network simulation whose goal is to predict which metabolic gene knockouts are lethal. The synthetic accessibility approach uses the topology of the metabolic network to calculate the sum of the minimum number of steps needed to traverse the metabolic network graph from the inputs, those metabolites available to the organism from the environment, to the outputs, metabolites needed by the organism to survive. To simulate a gene knockout, the reactions enabled by the gene are removed from the network and the synthetic accessibility metric is recalculated. An increase in the total number of steps is predicted to cause lethality. Wunderlich and Mirny showed this simple, parameter-free approach predicted knockout lethality in *E. coli* and *S. cerevisiae* as well as elementary mode analysis and flux balance analysis in a variety of media.

Applications of a Reconstruction

- Several inconsistencies exist between gene, enzyme, reaction databases, and published literature sources regarding the metabolic information of an organism. A reconstruction is a systematic verification and compilation of data from various sources that takes into account all of the discrepancies.
- The combination of relevant metabolic and genomic information of an organism.
- Metabolic comparisons can be performed between various organisms of the same species as well as between different organisms.
- Analysis of synthetic lethality
- Predict adaptive evolution outcomes
- Use in metabolic engineering for high value outputs

Reconstructions and their corresponding models allow the formulation of hypotheses about the presence of certain enzymatic activities and the production of metabolites that can be experimentally tested, complementing the primarily discovery-based approach of traditional microbial biochemistry with hypothesis-driven research. The results these experiments can uncover novel pathways and metabolic activities and decipher between discrepancies in previous experimental data. Information about the chemical reactions of metabolism and the genetic background of various metabolic properties (sequence to structure to function) can be utilized by genetic engineers to modify organisms to produce high value outputs whether those products be medically relevant like pharmaceuticals; high value chemical intermediates such as terpenoids and isoprenoids; or biotechnological outputs like biofuels.

Metabolic network reconstructions and models are used to understand how an organism or parasite functions inside of the host cell. For example, if the parasite serves to compromise the immune system by lysing macrophages, then the goal of metabolic reconstruction/simulation would be to determine the metabolites that are essential to the organism's proliferation inside of macrophages. If the proliferation cycle is inhibited, then the parasite would not continue to evade the host's immune system. A reconstruction model serves as a first step to deciphering the complicated mechanisms surrounding disease. These models can also look at the minimal genes necessary for a cell to maintain virulence. The next step would be to use the predictions and postulates generated from a reconstruction model and apply it to discover novel biological functions such as drug-engineering and drug delivery techniques.

FLUX BALANCE ANALYSIS

Flux balance analysis (FBA) is a mathematical method for simulating metabolism in genome-scale reconstructions of metabolic networks. In comparison to traditional methods of modeling, FBA is less intensive in terms of the input data required for constructing the model. Simulations performed using FBA are computationally inexpensive and can calculate steady-state metabolic fluxes for large models (over 2000 reactions) in a few seconds on modern personal computers.

FBA finds applications in bioprocess engineering to systematically identify modifications to the metabolic networks of microbes used in fermentation processes that improve product yields of industrially important chemicals such as ethanol and succinic acid. It has also been used for the identification of putative drug targets in cancer and pathogens, rational design of culture media, and more recently host–pathogen interactions. The results of FBA can be visualized using flux maps similar to the image on the right, which illustrates the steady-state fluxes carried by reactions in glycolysis. The thickness of the arrows is proportional to the flux through the reaction.

FBA formalizes the system of equations describing the concentration changes in a metabolic network as the dot product of a matrix of the stoichiometric coefficients (the stoichiometric matrix **S**) and the vector **v** of the unsolved fluxes. The right-hand side of the dot product is a vector of zeros representing the system at steady state. Linear programming is then used to calculate a solution of fluxes corresponding to the steady state.

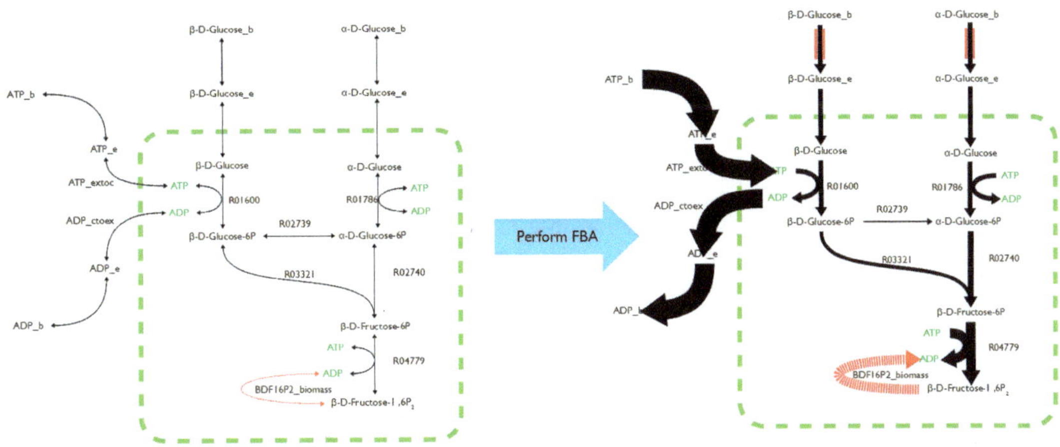

The results of FBA on a prepared metabolic network of the top six reactions of glycolysis. The predicted flux through each reaction is proportional to the width of the line. Objective function in red, constraints on alpha-D-glucose and beta-D-glucose import represented as red bars.

Some of the earliest work in FBA dates back to the early 1980s. Papoutsakis demonstrated that it was possible to construct flux balance equations using a metabolic map. It was Watson, however, who first introduced the idea of using linear programming and an objective function to solve for the fluxes in a pathway. The first significant study was subsequently published by Fell and Small, who used flux balance analysis together with more elaborate objective functions to study the constraints in fat synthesis.

Simulations

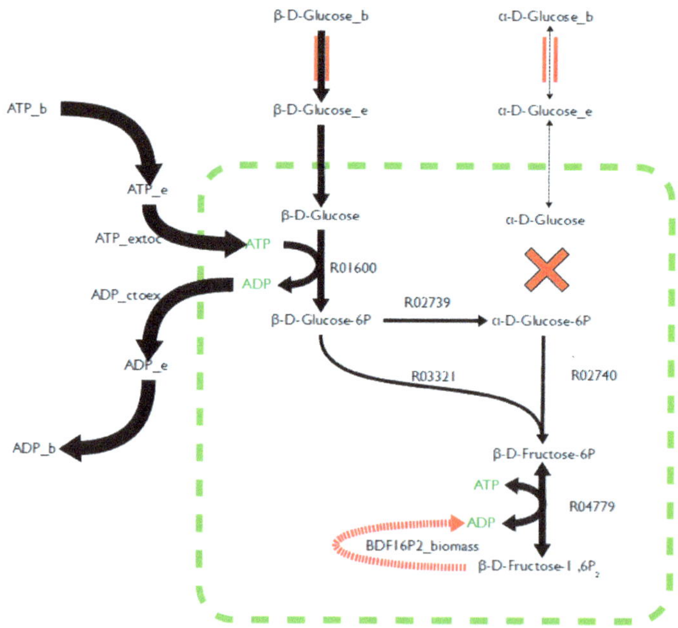

An example of a non lethal gene deletion in a sample metabolic network with fluxes shown by the weight of the reaction lines as calculated by FBA. Here the flux through the objective function is halved but is still present.

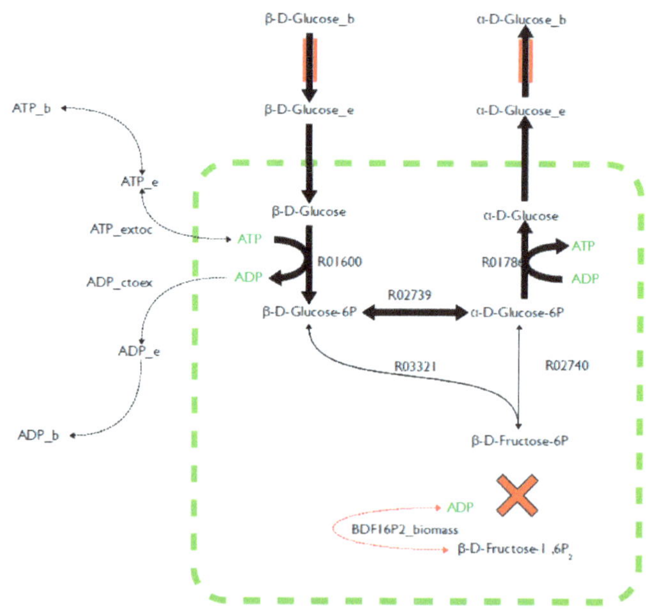

An example of a lethal gene deletion in a sample metabolic network with fluxes shown by the weight of the reaction lines as calculated by FBA. Here there is no flux through the objective function, simulating that the pathway is no longer functional.

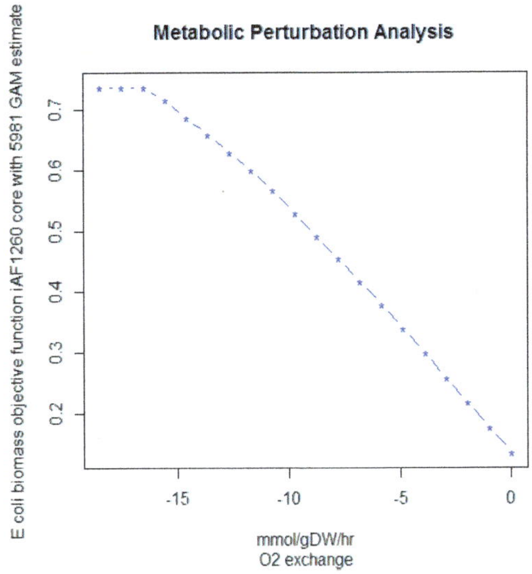

Reaction inhibition: Plot of FBA predicted growth rate (y-axis) to decreasing influx of Oxygen (x-axis) in an E.coli FBA model.

A 3-D Phenotypic Phase Plane showing the effect of varying glucose and glycerol input fluxes on the growth rate of Mycobacterium tuberculosis. The X axis represents glycerol influx and the Y axis represents glucose influx, the height of the surface (red) represents the value of the growth flux for each combination of the input fluxes.

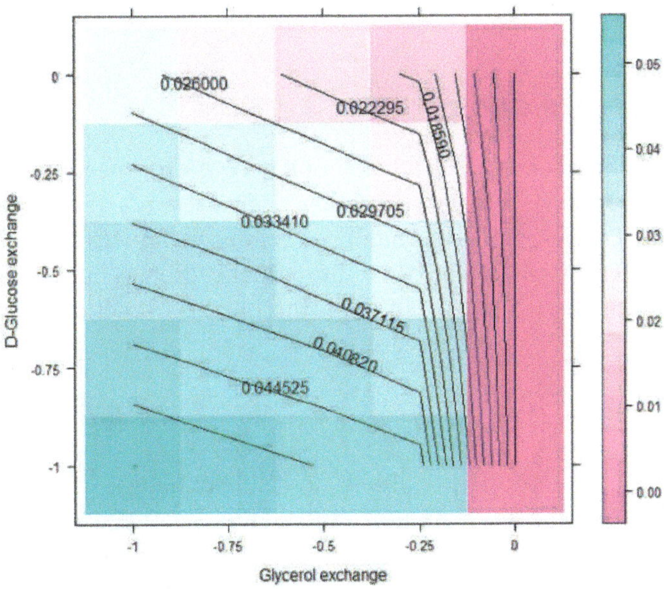

A levelplot version of the Phenotypic Phase Plane showing the effect of varying glucose and glycerol input fluxes on the growth rate of Mycobacterium tuberculosis. The X axis represents glycerol influx and the Y axis represents glucose influx, the color represents the value of the growth flux.

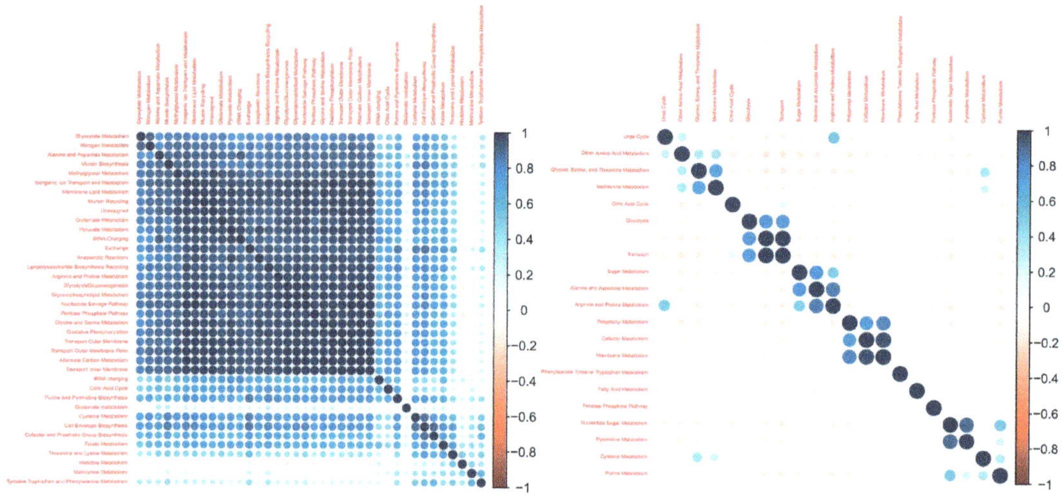

Comparison of correlation plots of lethal Pairwise reaction deletions across different subsystems for E.coli(left) and M.tuberculosis(right).

FBA is not computationally intensive, taking on the order of seconds to calculate optimal fluxes for biomass production for a typical network (around 2000 reactions). This means that the effect of deleting reactions from the network and/or changing flux constraints can be sensibly modelled on a single computer.

Gene/Reaction Deletion and Perturbation Studies

Single Reaction Deletion

A frequently used technique to search a metabolic network for reactions that are particularly critical to the production of biomass. By removing each reaction in a network in turn and measuring the predicted flux through the biomass function, each reaction can be classified as either essential (if the flux through the biomass function is substantially reduced) or non-essential (if the flux through the biomass function is unchanged or only slightly reduced).

Pairwise Reaction Deletion

Pairwise reaction deletion of all possible pairs of reactions is useful when looking for drug targets, as it allows the simulation of multi-target treatments, either by a single drug with multiple targets or by drug combinations. Double deletion studies can also quantify the synthetic lethal interactions between different pathways providing a measure of the contribution of the pathway to overall network robustness.

Single and Multiple Gene Deletions

Genes are connected to enzyme-catalyzed reactions by Boolean expressions known as Gene-Protein-Reaction expressions (GPR). Typically a GPR takes the form (Gene A AND Gene B) to indicate that the products of genes A and B are protein sub-units that assemble to form the complete protein and therefore the absence of either would result in deletion of the reaction. On the other hand, if the GPR is (Gene A OR Gene B) it implies that the products of genes A and B are isozymes.

Therefore, it is possible to evaluate the effect of single or multiple gene deletions by evaluation of the GPR as a Boolean expression. If the GPR evaluates to **false**, the reaction is constrained to zero in the model prior to performing FBA. Thus gene knockouts can be simulated using FBA.

Interpretation of Gene and Reaction Deletion Results

The utility of reaction inhibition and deletion analyses becomes most apparent if a gene-protein-reaction matrix has been assembled for the network being studied with FBA. The gene-protein-reaction matrix is a binary matrix connecting genes with the proteins made from them. Using this matrix, reaction essentiality can be converted into gene essentiality indicating the gene defects which may cause a certain disease phenotype or the proteins/enzymes which are essential (and thus what enzymes are the most promising drug targets in pathogens). However, the gene-protein-reaction matrix does not specify the Boolean relationship between genes with respect to the enzyme, instead it merely indicates an association between them. Therefore, it should be used only if the Boolean GPR expression is unavailable.

Reaction Inhibition

The effect of inhibiting a reaction, rather than removing it entirely, can be simulated in FBA by restricting the allowed flux through it. The effect of an inhibition can be classified as lethal or non-lethal by applying the same criteria as in the case of a deletion where a suitable threshold is used to distinguish "substantially reduced" from "slightly reduced". Generally the choice of threshold is arbitrary but a reasonable estimate can be obtained from growth experiments where the simulated inhibitions/deletions are actually performed and growth rate is measured.

Growth Media Optimization

To design optimal growth media with respect to enhanced growth rates or useful by-product secretion, it is possible to use a method known as Phenotypic Phase Plane analysis. PhPP involves applying FBA repeatedly on the model while co-varying the nutrient uptake constraints and observing the value of the objective function (or by-product fluxes). PhPP makes it possible to find the optimal combination of nutrients that favor a particular phenotype or a mode of metabolism resulting in higher growth rates or secretion of industrially useful by-products. The predicted growth rates of bacteria in varying media have been shown to correlate well with experimental results. as well as to define precise minimal media for the culture of *Salmonella typhimurium*.

Mathematical Description

In contrast to the traditionally followed approach of metabolic modeling using coupled ordinary differential equations, flux balance analysis requires very little information in terms of the enzyme kinetic parameters and concentration of metabolites in the system. It achieves this by making two assumptions, steady state and optimality. The first assumption is that the modeled system has entered a steady state, where the metabolite concentrations no longer change, i.e. in each metabolite node the producing and consuming fluxes cancel each other out. The second assumption is that the organism has been optimized through evolution for some biological goal, such as optimal growth or conservation of resources. The steady-state assumption reduces the system to a set of linear equations, which is then solved to find a flux distribution that satisfies the steady-state condition subject to the stoichiometry constraints while maximizing the value of a pseudo-reaction (the objective function) representing the conversion of biomass precursors into biomass.

The steady-state assumption dates to the ideas of material balance developed to model the growth of microbial cells in fermenters in bioprocess engineering. During microbial growth, a substrate consisting of a complex mixture of carbon, hydrogen, oxygen and nitrogen sources along with trace elements are consumed to generate biomass. The material balance model for this process becomes:

$$\textbf{Input} = \textbf{Output} + \textbf{Accumulation}$$

If we consider the system of microbial cells to be at steady state then we may set the accumulation term to zero and reduce the material balance equations to simple algebraic equations. In such a system, substrate becomes the input to the system which is consumed and biomass is produced becoming the output from the system. The material balance may then be represented as:

$$\textbf{Input} = \textbf{Output}$$
$$\textbf{Input} - \textbf{Output} = 0$$

Mathematically, the algebraic equations can be represented as a dot product of a matrix of coefficients and a vector of the unknowns. Since the steady-state assumption puts the accumulation term to zero. The system can be written as:

$$A \cdot \mathbf{x} = \mathbf{0}$$

Extending this idea to metabolic networks, it is possible to represent a metabolic network as a stoichiometry balanced set of equations. Moving to the matrix formalism, we can represent the equations as the dot product of a matrix of stoichiometry coefficients (stoichiometric matrix S) and the vector of fluxes $\mathbf{v}$ as the unknowns and set the right hand side to 0 implying the steady state.

$$S \cdot \mathbf{v} = \mathbf{0}$$

Metabolic networks typically have more reactions than metabolites and this gives an under-determined system of linear equations containing more variables than equations. The standard approach to solve such under-determined systems is to apply linear programming.

Linear programs are problems that can be expressed in canonical form:

$$\begin{array}{ll} \text{maximize} & \mathbf{c}^{\mathrm{T}}\mathbf{x} \\ \text{subject to} & A\mathbf{x} \leq \mathbf{b} \\ \text{and} & \mathbf{x} \geq \mathbf{0} \end{array}$$

where **x** represents the vector of variables (to be determined), **c** and **b** are vectors of (known) coefficients, A is a (known) matrix of coefficients, and (.) Tis the matrix transpose. The expression to be maximized or minimized is called the objective function (cTx in this case). $A\mathbf{x} \leq \mathbf{b}$ are the constraints which specify a convex polytope over which the objective function is to be optimized. Linear Programming requires the definition of an objective function. The optimal solution to the LP problem is considered to be the solution which maximizes or minimizes the value of the objective function depending on the case in point. In the case of flux balance analysis, the objective function **Z** for the LP is often defined as biomass production. Biomass production is simulated by an equation representing a lumped reaction that converts various biomass precursors into one unit of biomass.

Therefore, the canonical form of a Flux Balance Analysis problem would be:

$$\begin{array}{ll} \text{maximize} & \mathbf{c}^{\mathrm{T}}\mathbf{v} \\ \text{subject to} & S\mathbf{v} = \mathbf{0} \\ \text{and} & \mathbf{lowerbound} \leq \mathbf{v} \leq \mathbf{upperbound} \end{array}$$

where **v** represents the vector of fluxes (to be determined), S is a (known) matrix of coefficients. The expression to be maximized or minimized is called the *objective function* ($\mathbf{c}^{\mathrm{T}}\mathbf{v}$ in this case). The inequalities $\mathbf{lowerbound} \leq \mathbf{v}$ and $\mathbf{v} \leq \mathbf{upperbound}$ define, respectively, the minimal and the maximal rates of flux for every reaction corresponding to the columns of the S matrix. These rates can be experimentally determined to constrain and improve the predictive accuracy of the model even further or they can be specified to an arbitrarily high value indicating no constraint on the flux through the reaction.

The main advantage of the flux balance approach is that it does not require any knowledge of the metabolite concentrations, or more importantly, the enzyme kinetics of the system; the homeostasis assumption precludes the need for knowledge of metabolite concentrations at any time as long as that quantity remains constant, and additionally it removes the need for specific rate laws since it assumes that at steady state, there is no change in the size of the metabolite pool in the system. The stoichiometric coefficients alone are sufficient for the mathematical maximization of a specific objective function.

The objective function is essentially a measure of how each component in the system contributes to the production of the desired product. The product itself depends on the purpose of the model, but one of the most common examples is the study of total biomass. A notable example of the success of FBA is the ability to accurately predict the growth rate of the prokaryote *E. coli* when cultured in different conditions. In this case, the metabolic system was optimized to maximize the biomass objective function. However this model can be used to optimize the production of any product, and is often used to determine the output level of some biotechnologically relevant product. The model itself can be experimentally verified by cultivating organisms using a chemostat or similar tools to ensure that nutrient concentrations are held constant. Measurements of the production of the desired objective can then be used to correct the model. A good description of the basic concepts of FBA can be found in the freely available supplementary material to Edwards et al. 2001 which can be found at the Nature website. Further sources include the book Systems Biology by B. Palsson dedicated to the subject and a useful tutorial and paper by J. Orth. Many other sources of information on the technique exist in published scientific literature including Lee et al. 2006, Feist et al. 2008, and Lewis et al. 2012.

Model Preparation and Refinement

A comprehensive guide to creating, preparing and analysing a metabolic model using FBA, in addition to other techniques, was published by Thiele and Palsson in 2010. The key parts of model preparation are: creating a metabolic network without gaps, adding constraints to the model, and finally adding an objective function (often called the Biomass function), usually to simulate the growth of the organism being modelled.

Metabolic Network and Software Tools

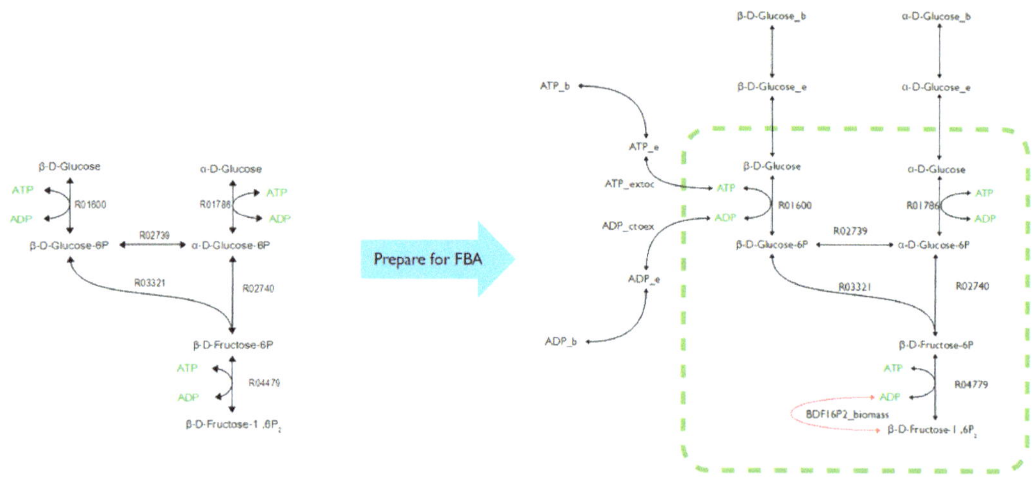

The first six reactions in Glycolysis prepared for FBA through the addition of an objective function (red) and the import and export of nutrients (ATP, ADP, BDG, ADG) across the system boundary (dashed green line).

Metabolic networks can vary in scope from those describing a single pathway, up to the cell, tissue or organism. The main requirement of a metabolic network that forms the basis of an FBA-ready network is that it contains no gaps. This typically means that extensive manual curation is required, making the preparation of a metabolic network for flux-balance analysis a process that can take months or years. However, recent advances such as so-called gap-filling methods can reduce the required time to weeks or months.

Software packages for creation of FBA models include Pathway Tools/MetaFlux, Simpheny, and MetNetMaker.

Generally models are created in BioPAX or SBML format so that further analysis or visualization can take place in other software although this is not a requirement.

Constraints

A key part of FBA is the ability to add constraints to the flux rates of reactions within networks, forcing them to stay within a range of selected values. This lets the model more accurately simulate real metabolism. The constraints belong to two subsets from a biological perspective; boundary constraints that limit nutrient uptake/excretion and internal constraints that limit the flux through reactions within the organism. In mathematical terms, the application of constraints can be considered to reduce the solution space of the FBA model. In addition to constraints applied at the edges of a metabolic network, constraints can be applied to reactions deep within the network. These constraints are usually simple; they may constrain the direction of a reaction due to energy considerations or constrain the maximum speed of a reaction due to the finite speed of all reactions in nature.

Growth Media Constraints

Organisms, and all other metabolic systems, require some input of nutrients. Typically the rate of uptake of nutrients is dictated by their availability (a nutrient that is not present cannot be absorbed), their concentration and diffusion constants (higher concentrations of quickly-diffusing metabolites are absorbed more quickly) and the method of absorption (such as active transport or facilitated diffusion versus simple diffusion).

If the rate of absorption (and/or excretion) of certain nutrients can be experimentally measured then this information can be added as a constraint on the flux rate at the edges of a metabolic model. This ensures that nutrients that are not present or not absorbed by the organism do not enter its metabolism (the flux rate is constrained to zero) and also means that known nutrient uptake rates are adhered to by the simulation. This provides a secondary method of making sure that the simulated metabolism has experimentally verified properties rather than just mathematically acceptable ones.

Thermodynamical Reaction Constraints

In principle, all reactions are reversible however in practice reactions often effectively occur in only one direction. This may be due to significantly higher concentration of reactants compared to the concentration of the products of the reaction. But more often it happens because the products of a reaction have a much lower free energy than the reactants and therefore the forward direction of a reaction is favored more.

For ideal reactions,

$$-\infty < v_i < \infty$$

For certain reactions a thermodynamic constraint can be applied implying direction (in this case forward)

$$0 < v_i < \infty$$

Realistically the flux through a reaction cannot be infinite (given that enzymes in the real system are finite) which implies that,

$$0 < v_i < v_{\max}$$

Experimentally Measured Flux Constraints

Certain flux rates can be measured experimentally (v i,m and the fluxes within a metabolic model can be constrained, within some error ( ) these known flux rates are accurately reproduced in the simulation.

$$v_{i,m} - \varepsilon < v_i < v_{i,m} + \varepsilon$$

Flux rates are most easily measured for nutrient uptake at the edge of the network. Measurements of internal fluxes is possible using radioactively labelled or NMR visible metabolites.

Constrained FBA-ready metabolic models can be analyzed using software such as the COBRA toolbox(requires MATLAB), SurreyFBA, or the web-based FAME. Additional software packages have been listed elsewhere. A comprehensive review of all such software and their functionalities has been recently reviewed.

An open-source alternative is available in the R (programming language) as the packages abcdeFBA or sybil for performing FBA and other constraint based modeling techniques.

Objective Function

FBA can give a large number of mathematically acceptable solutions to the steady-state problem $(S\vec{v}=0)$. However solutions of biological interest are the ones which produce the desired metabolites in the correct proportion. The objective function defines the proportion of these metabolites. For instance when modelling the growth of an organism the objective function is generally defined as biomass. Mathematically, it is a column in the stoichiometry matrix the entries of which place a "demand" or act as a "sink" for biosynthetic precursors such as fatty acids, amino acids and cell wall components which are present on the corresponding rows of the **S** matrix. These entries represent experimentally measured, dry weight proportions of cellular components. Therefore, this column becomes a lumped reaction that simulates growth and reproduction. Therefore, the accuracy of experimental measurements plays an essential role in the correct definition of the biomass function and makes the results of FBA biologically applicable by ensuring that the correct proportion of metabolites are produced by metabolism.

When modeling smaller networks the objective function can be changed accordingly. An example of this would be in the study of the carbohydrate metabolism pathways where the objective function would probably be defined as a certain proportion of ATP and NADH and thus simulate the production of high energy metabolites by this pathway.

Optimization of the Objective/Biomass Function

Linear programming can be used to find a single optimal solution. The most common biological optimization goal for a whole-organism metabolic network would be to choose the flux vector $\vec{v}$ hat maximises the flux through a biomass function composed of the constituent metabolites of the organism placed into the stoichiometric matrix and denoted v_{biomass} or simply v_b

$$\max_{\vec{v}} v_b \qquad \text{s.t.} \qquad \mathbf{S}\vec{v}=0$$

In the more general case any reaction can be defined and added to the biomass function with either the condition that it be maximised or minimised if a single "optimal" solution is desired. Alternatively, and in the most general case, a vector $\vec{c}$ can be introduced, which defines the weighted set of reactions that the linear programming model should aim to maximise or minimise,

$$\max_{\vec{v}} \vec{v}\cdot\vec{c} \qquad \text{s.t.} \qquad \mathbf{S}\vec{v}=0.$$

In the case of there being only a single separate biomass function/reaction within the stoichiometric matrix $\vec{c}$ would simplify to all zeroes with a value of 1 (or any non-zero value) in the position corresponding to that biomass function. Where there were multiple separate objective functions $\vec{c}$ would simplify to all zeroes with weighted values in the positions corresponding to all objective functions.

Reducing the Solution Space – Biological Considerations for the System

The analysis of the null space of matrices is implemented in software packages specialized for matrix operations such as Matlab and Octave. Determination of the null space of s tells us all the possible collections of flux vectors (or linear combinations thereof) that balance fluxes within the biological network. The advantage of this approach becomes evident in biological systems which are described by differential equation systems with many unknowns. The velocities in the differential equations above v_1 *and* v_2 are dependent on the reaction rates of the underlying equations. The velocities are generally taken from the Michaelis–Menten kinetic theory, which involves the kinetic parameters of the enzymes catalyzing the reactions and the concentration of the metabolites themselves. Isolating enzymes from living organisms and measuring their kinetic parameters is a difficult task, as is measuring the internal concentrations and diffusion constants of metabolites within an organism. Therefore, the differential equation approach to metabolic modeling is beyond the current scope of science for all but the most studied organisms. FBA avoids this impediment by applying the homeostatic assumption, which is a reasonably approximate description of biological systems.

Although FBA avoids that biological obstacle, the mathematical issue of a large solution space remains. FBA has a two-fold purpose. Accurately representing the biological limits of the system and returning the flux distribution closest to the natural fluxes within the target system/organism. Certain biological principles can help overcome the mathematical difficulties. While the stoichiometric matrix is almost always under-determined initially (meaning that the solution space to $s\vec{v}=0$ is very large), the size of the solution space can be reduced and be made more reflective of the biology of the problem through the application of certain constraints on the solutions.

Extensions

The success of FBA and the realization of its limitations has led to extensions that attempt to mediate the limitations of the technique.

Flux Variability Analysis

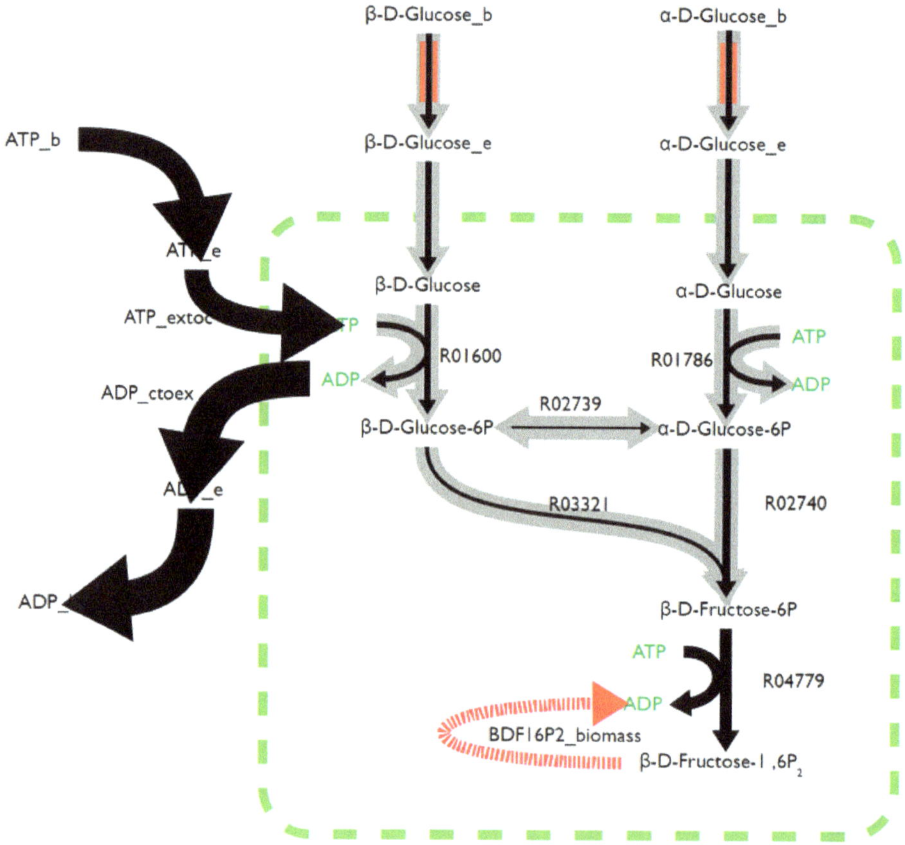

		R2739_c	R03321_c	R02740_c	R01600_c	R01786_c	R04779_c	ATP_extoc_Tr	ADP_ctoex_tr	BDG_extoc_tr	ADG_extoc_tr	BDF16P2_biomass_tr
FBA		9	16	34	25	25	50	50	75	25	25	50
FVA	min	-50	0	0	0	0	50	50	75	0	0	50
	max	50	50	50	50	50	50	50	75	50	50	50

Visual and numerical representation of FVA on a complete network.

The optimal solution to the flux-balance problem is rarely unique with many possible, and equally optimal, solutions existing. Flux variability analysis (FVA), built into virtually all current analysis software, returns the boundaries for the fluxes through each reaction that can, paired with the right combination of other fluxes, produce the optimal solution.

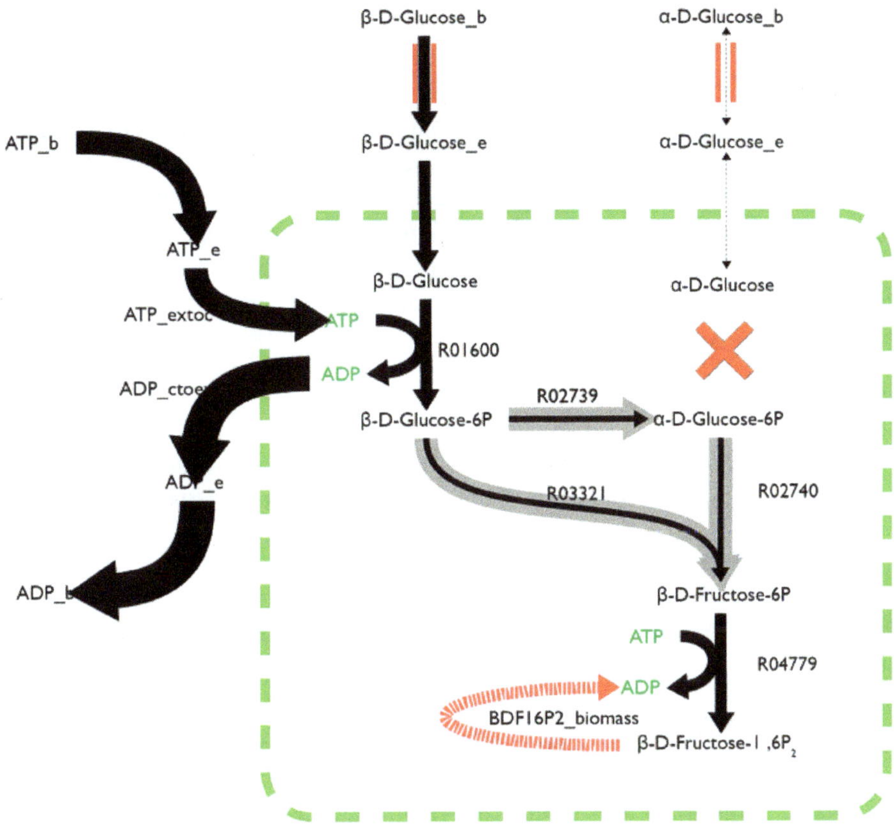

		R2739_c	R03321_c	R02740_c	R01600_c	R01786_c	R04779_c	ATP_extoc_Tr	ADP_ctoex_tr	BDG_extoc_tr	ADG_extoc_tr	BDF16P2_biomass_tr
FBA		25	25	25	50	0	50	50	75	50	0	50
FVA	min	0	0	0	50	0	50	50	75	50	0	50
	max	50	50	50	50	0	50	50	75	50	0	50

Visual and numerical representation of FVA on a network with non-lethal deletion.

Reactions which can support a low variability of fluxes through them are likely to be of a higher importance to an organism and FVA is a promising technique for the identification of reactions that are highly important.

Minimization of Metabolic Adjustment (MOMA)

When simulating knockouts or growth on media, FBA gives the final steady-state flux distribution. This final steady state is reached in varying time-scales. For example, the predicted growth rate of *E. coli* on glycerol as the primary carbon source did not match the FBA predictions, however on sub-culturing for 40 days or 700 generations the growth rate adaptively evolved to match the FBA prediction.

Sometimes it is of interest to find out what is the immediate effect of a perturbation or knockout, since it takes time for regulatory changes to occur and for the organism to re-organize fluxes to optimally utilize a different carbon source or circumvent the effect of the knockout. MOMA predicts the immediate sub-optimal flux distribution following the perturbation by minimizing the distance (Euclidean) between the wild-type FBA flux distribution and the mutant flux distribution using quadratic programming. This yields an optimization problem of the form.

$$\min \|\mathbf{v_w} - \mathbf{v_d}\|^2 \qquad s.t. \quad \mathbf{S} \cdot \mathbf{v_d} = 0$$

where v_w represents the wild-type (or unperturbed state) flux distribution and v_d represents the flux distribution on gene deletion that is to be solved for. This simplifies to:

$$\min \frac{1}{2} \mathbf{v_d}^T \mathbf{I} \mathbf{v_d} + (-\mathbf{v_w}) \cdot \mathbf{v_d} \qquad s.t. \quad \mathbf{S} \cdot \mathbf{v_d} = 0$$

This is the MOMA solution which represents the flux distribution immediately post-perturbation.

Regulatory On-Off Minimization (ROOM)

ROOM attempts to improve the prediction of the metabolic state of an organism after a gene knockout. It follows the same premise as MOMA that an organism would try to restore a flux distribution as close as possible to the wild-type after a knockout. However it further hypothesizes that this steady state would be reached through a series of transient metabolic changes by the regulatory network and that the organism would try to minimize the number of regulatory changes required to reach the wild-type state. Instead of using a distance metric minimization however it uses a Mixed Integer Linear Programming method.

Dynamic FBA

Dynamic FBA attempts to add the ability for models to change over time, thus in some ways avoiding the strict steady state condition of pure FBA. Typically the technique involves running an FBA simulation, changing the model based on the outputs of that simulation, and rerunning the simulation. By repeating this process an element of feedback is achieved over time.

Comparison with other Techniques

FBA provides a less simplistic analysis than Choke Point Analysis while requiring far less information on reaction rates and a much less complete network reconstruction than a full dynamic simulation would require. In filling this niche, FBA has been shown to be a very useful technique for analysis of the metabolic capabilities of cellular systems.

Choke Point Analysis

Unlike choke point analysis which only considers points in the network where metabolites are produced but not consumed or vice versa, FBA is a true form of metabolic network modelling because it considers the metabolic network as a single complete entity (the stoichiometric matrix) at all stages of analysis. This means that network effects, such as chemical reactions in distant pathways affecting each other, can be reproduced in the model. The upside to the inability of choke point analysis to simulate network effects is that it considers each reaction within a network in isolation and thus can suggest important reactions in a network even if a network is highly fragmented and contains many gaps.

Dynamic Metabolic Simulation

Unlike dynamic metabolic simulation, FBA assumes that the internal concentration of metabolites within a system stays constant over time and thus is unable to provide anything other than steady-state solutions. It is unlikely that FBA could, for example, simulate the functioning of a nerve cell. Since the internal concentration of metabolites is not considered within a model, it is possible that an FBA solution could contain metabolites at a concentration too high to be biologically acceptable. This is a problem that dynamic metabolic simulations would probably avoid. One advantage of the simplicity of FBA over dynamic simulations is that they are far less computationally expensive, allowing the simulation of large numbers of perturbations to the network. A second advantage is that the reconstructed model can be substantially simpler by avoiding the need to consider enzyme rates and the effect of complex interactions on enzyme kinetics.

REFERENCES

1. Franke; Siezen, Teusink (2005). "Reconstructing the metabolic network of a bacterium from its genome.". Trends in Microbiology. 13 (11): 550–558. doi:10.1016/j.tim.2005.09.001. PMID 16169729.
2. Thiele, Ines; Bernhard Ø Palsson (January 2010). "A protocol for generating a high-quality genome-scale metabolic reconstruction". Nature Protocols. 5 (1): 93–121. doi:10.1038/nprot.2009.203. PMC 3125167 . PMID 20057383.
3. Fleischmann, R. D.; Adams, M. D.; White, O; Clayton, R. A.; Kirkness, E. F.; Kerlavage, A. R.; Bult, C. J.; Tomb, J. F.; Dougherty, B. A.; Merrick, J. M. (1995). "Whole-genome random sequencing and assembly of Haemophilus influenzae Rd". Science. 269 (1995): 496–512. doi:10.1126/science.7542800. PMID 7542800.
4. The C. elegans Sequencing Consortium (1998). "Genome Sequence of the Nematode C. elegans: A Platform for Investigating Biology". Science. 282 (5396): 2012–2018. doi:10.1126/science.282.5396.2012. PMID 9851916.
5. Edwards, J. S.; et al. (May 2000). "The Escherichia coli MG1655 in silico

metabolic genotype: Its definition, characteristics, and capabilities". PNAS. 97 (10): 5528–5533. doi:10.1073/pnas.97.10.5528. PMC 25862 . PMID 10805808.

6. Forster, J.; et al. (February 2003). "Genome-Scale Reconstruction of the Saccharomyces cerevisiae Metabolic Network". Genome Research. 13 (2): 244–253. doi:10.1101/gr.234503. PMC 420374 . PMID 12566402. Missing |last4= in Authors list (help)
7. Sheikh, Kashif; et al. (January 2005). "Modeling Hybridoma Cell Metabolism Using a Generic Genome-Scale Metabolic Model of Mus musculus". Biotechnology Resources. 21 (1): 112–121. doi:10.1021/bp0498138.
8. Romero, Pedro; Jonathan Wagg; Michelle L Green; Dale Kaiser; Markus Krummenacker; Peter D Karp (June 2004). "Computational prediction of human metabolic pathways from the complete human genome". Genome Biology. 6 (1): R2. doi:10.1186/gb-2004-6-1-r2. PMC 549063 . PMID 15642094.
9. Duarte, N. C.; et al. (January 2007). "Global reconstruction of the human metabolic network based on genomic and bibliomic data". PNAS. 104 (6): 1777–1782. doi:10.1073/pnas.0610772104. PMC 1794290 . PMID 17267599.
10. Jamshidi, Neema; B. O. Palsson (June 2007). "Investigating the metabolic capabilities of Mycobacterium tuberculosis H". BMC Systems Biology. 1: 26. doi:10.1186/1752-0509-1-26. PMC 1925256 . PMID 17555602.
11. Oh, Y.-K.; et al. (September 2007). "Genome-scale Reconstruction of Metabolic Network in Bacillus subtilis Based on High-throughput Phenotyping and Gene Essentiality Data". Journal of Biological Chemistry. 282 (39): 28791–28799. doi:10.1074/jbc.M703759200. PMID 17573341.
12. Fu, Pengcheng (October 2008). "Genome-scale modeling of Synechocystis sp. PCC 6803 and prediction of pathway insertion". Journal of Chemical Technology and Biotechnology. 84 (4): 473–483. doi:10.1002/jctb.2065.
13. Raghunathan, Anu; et al. (April 2009). "Constraint-based analysis of metabolic capacity of Salmonella typhimurium during host-pathogen interaction". BMC Systems Biology. 3: 38. doi:10.1186/1752-0509-3-38. PMC 2678070 . PMID 19356237.
14. de Oliveira Dal'Molin, C. G.; Quek, L.-E.; Palfreyman, R. W.; Brumbley, S. M.; Nielsen, L. K. (February 2010). "AraGEM, a Genome-Scale Reconstruction of the Primary Metabolic Network in Arabidopsis". Plant Physiology. 152 (2): 579–589. doi:10.1104/pp.109.148817. PMC 2815881 . PMID 20044452.
15. Karp; et al. (January 2010). "Pathway Tools version 13.0: Integrated Software for Pathway/Genome Informatics and Systems Biology". Briefings in Bioinformatics. 11 (1): 40–79. doi:10.1093/bib/bbp043. PMC 2810111 . PMID 19955237.
16. Wrzodek, Clemens; Büchel, Finja; Ruff, Manuel; Dräger, Andreas; Zell, Andreas (2013). "Precise generation of systems biology models from KEGG pathways". BMC Systems Biology. 7 (1): 15. doi:10.1186/1752-0509-7-15.
17. Wrzodek, Clemens; Dräger, Andreas; Zell, Andreas (23 June 2011). "KEGGtranslator: visualizing and converting the KEGG PATHWAY database to various formats". Bioinformatics. 27 (16): 2314–2315. doi:10.1093/bioinformatics/

btr377. PMID 21700675.

18. Chaouiya, Claudine; Bérenguier, Duncan; Keating, Sarah M; Naldi, Aurélien; van Iersel, Martijn P; Rodriguez, Nicolas; Dräger, Andreas; Büchel, Finja; Cokelaer, Thomas; Kowal, Bryan; Wicks, Benjamin; Gonçalves, Emanuel; Dorier, Julien; Page, Michel; Monteiro, Pedro T; von Kamp, Axel; Xenarios, Ioannis; de Jong, Hidde; Hucka, Michael; Klamt, Steffen; Thieffry, Denis; Le Novère, Nicolas; Saez-Rodriguez, Julio; Helikar, Tomáš (2013). "SBML qualitative models: a model representation format and infrastructure to foster interactions between qualitative modelling formalisms and tools". BMC Systems Biology. 7 (1): 135. doi:10.1186/1752-0509-7-135.
19. Henry, CS; DeJongh M; Best AA; Frybarger PM; Linsay B; Stevens RL (September 2010). "High-throughput Generation and Optimization of Genome-scale Metabolic Models". Nature Biotechnology. 28 (9): 977–982. doi:10.1038/nbt.1672. PMID 20802497.
20. Chindelevitch, Leonid; Sarah Stanley; Deborah Hung; Aviv Regev; Bonnie Berger (January 2012). "MetaMerge: scaling up genome-scale metabolic reconstructions with application to Mycobacterium tuberculosis". Genome Biology. 13 (r6): R6. doi:10.1186/gb-2012-13-1-r6. Archived from
21. Ivanova, N.; A. Lykidis (2009). "Metabolic Reconstruction". Encyclopedia of Microbiology, 3rd Ed.: 607–621. doi:10.1016/B978-012373944-5.00010-9. ISBN 9780123739445.
22. Linster, Carole L.; Van Schaftingen, Emile; Hanson, Andrew D. (2013-02-01). "Metabolite damage and its repair or pre-emption". Nature Chemical Biology. 9 (2): 72–80. doi:10.1038/nchembio.1141. ISSN 1552-4469. PMID 23334546.
23. Hanson, Andrew D.; Henry, Christopher S.; Fiehn, Oliver; de Crécy-Lagard, Valérie (2015-11-19). "Metabolite Damage and Metabolite Damage Control in Plants". Annual Review of Plant Biology. 67: 131–52. doi:10.1146/annurev-arplant-043015-111648. ISSN 1545-2123. PMID 26667673.
24. Papin, JA; Stelling, J; Price, ND; Klamt, S; Schuster, S; Palsson, BO (Aug 2004). "Comparison of network-based pathway analysis methods". Trends Biotechnol. 22 (8): 400–5. doi:10.1016/j.tibtech.2004.06.010. PMID 15283984.
25. Lewis, N.E.; Nagarajan, H.; Palsson (2012). "Constraining the metabolic genotype–phenotype relationship using a phylogeny of in silico methods". Nature Reviews Microbiology. 10: 291–305. doi:10.1038/nrmicro2737.
26. CoBRA Methods - Constraint-based analysis
27. Price, Nathan; Jennifer Reed; Jason Papin; Sharon Wiback; Bernhard O Palsson (November 2003). "Network-based analysis of metabolic regulation in the human red blood cell". Journal of Theoretical Biology. 225 (2): 185–194. doi:10.1016/s0022-5193(03)00237-6. PMID 14575652.
28. Papin, Jason; Nathan Price; Bernhard O Palsson (December 2002). "Extreme Pathway Lengths and Reaction Participation in Genome-Scale Metabolic Networks". Genome Research. 12 (12): 1889–1900. doi:10.1101/gr.327702. PMC 187577 . PMID 12466293.

29. Papin, Jason; Nathan Price; Bernhard O Palsson (August 2004). "Comparison of network-based pathway analysis methods". Trends in Biotechnology. 22 (8): 400–405. doi:10.1016/j.tibtech.2004.06.010. PMID 15283984.
30. Schuster, S; Fell DA; Dandekar T (March 2000). "A general definition of metabolic pathways useful for systematic organization and analysis of complex metabolic networks". Nature Biotechnology. 18 (3): 326–332. doi:10.1038/73786. PMID 10700151.
31. Stelling, J; Klamt S; Bettenbrock K; Schuster S; Gilles ED (November 2002). "Metabolic network structure determines key aspects of functionality and regulation.". Nature. 420 (6912): 190–193. doi:10.1038/nature01166. PMID 12432396.
32. Ullah, E; Aeron S; Hassoun S (2015). "gEFM: An Algorithm for Computing Elementary Flux Modes Using Graph Traversal.". IEEE/ACM Transactions on Computational Biology and Bioinformatics: 1. doi:10.1109/TCBB.2015.2430344.
33. Larhlimi, A; Bockmayr, A. (2009). "A new constraint-based description of the steady-state flux cone of metabolic networks". Discrete Applied Mathematics. 157 (10): 2257–2266. doi:10.1016/j.dam.2008.06.039.
34. Dräger, A; Kronfeld M; Ziller MJ; Supper J; Planatscher H; Magnus JB; Oldiges M; Kohlbacher O; Zell A (January 2009). "Modeling metabolic networks in C. glutamicum: a comparison of rate laws in combination with various parameter optimization strategies". BMC Systems Biology. 3 (5): 5. doi:10.1186/1752-0509-3-5. PMC 2661887 . PMID 19144170.
35. Dräger, Andreas; Hassis, Nadine; Supper, Jochen; Schröder, Adrian; Zell, Andreas (2008). "SBMLsqueezer: A CellDesigner plug-in to generate kinetic rate equations for biochemical networks". BMC Systems Biology. 2 (1): 39. doi:10.1186/1752-0509-2-39.
36. Wunderlich, Z; Leonid Mirny (September 2006). "Using the topology of metabolic networks to predict viability of mutant strains". Biophysical Journal. 91 (6): 2304–11. doi:10.1529/biophysj.105.080572. PMID 16782788.
37. Costanzo, M; et al. (2010). "The Genetic Landscape of a Cell". Science. 327 (5964): 425–431. doi:10.1126/science.1180823. PMID 20093466.
38. Fong, SS; Marciniak JY; Palsson BØ (November 2003). "Description and interpretation of adaptive evolution of Escherichia coli K-12 MG1655 by using a genome-scale in silico metabolic model". Journal of Bacteriology. 185 (21): 6400–6408. doi:10.1128/JB.185.21.6400-6408.2003. PMC 219384 . PMID 14563875.
39. Ivanova, A; A. Lykidis (2009). Metabolic Reconstruction. Encyclopedia of Microbiology, 3rd Edition: 607–621. doi:10.1016/B978-012373944-5.00010-9. ISBN 9780123739445.
40. Ranganathan, Sridhar; Suthers, Patrick F.; Maranas, Costas D. (2010). OptForce: An Optimization Procedure for Identifying All Genetic Manipulations Leading to Targeted Overproductions. PLoS Comput Biol. 6 (4): e1000744. doi:10.1371/journal.pcbi.1000744.

41. Lewis, NE; Abdel-Haleem, AM (2013). The evolution of genome-scale models of cancer metabolism. Front. Physiol. 4: 237. doi:10.3389/fphys.2013.00237.
42. Raman, Karthik; Yeturu, Kalidas; Chandra, Nagasuma (2008). targetTB: A Target Identification Pipeline for Mycobacterium tuberculosis Through an Interactome, Reactome and Genome-scale Structural Analysis. BMC Systems Biology. 2 (1): 109. doi:10.1186/1752-0509-2-109.
43. Yang, Hong; Roth, Charles M.; Ierapetritou, Marianthi G. (2009). A rational design approach for amino acid supplementation in hepatocyte culture. Biotechnology and Bioengineering. 103: 1176–1191. doi:10.1002/bit.22342.
44. Raghunathan, Anu; Shin, Sookil; Daefler, Simon (2010). Systems Approach to Investigating Host-pathogen Interactions in Infections with the Biothreat Agent Francisella. Constraints-based Model of Francisella tularensis. BMC Systems Biology. 4 (1): 118. doi:10.1186/1752-0509-4-118.
45. Papoutsakis, ET (1984). Equations and calculations for fermentations of butyric acid bacteria. Biotech and Bioeng. 26 (2): 174–187. doi:10.1002/bit.260260210.
46. Watson MR (1984) Metabolic maps for the Apple II. 12, 1093-1094
47. Fell, DA; Small, JR (1986). Fat synthesis in adipose tissue. An examination of stoichiometric constraints. Biochem J. 238 (3): 781–786. doi:10.1042/bj2380781.
48. Edwards, J.; Ibarra, R.; Palsson, B. (2001). In silico predictions of Escherichia coli metabolic capabilities are consistent with experimental data. Nature Biotechnology. 19: 125–130. doi:10.1038/84379. PMID 11175725.
49. Raghunathan, A.; et al. (2009). Constraint-based analysis of metabolic capacity of Salmonella typhimurium during host-pathogen interaction. BMC systems biology. 3: 38. doi:10.1186/1752-0509-3-38. PMC 2678070 . PMID 19356237.
50. (http://www.nature.com/nbt/web_extras/supp_info/nbt0201_125/info_frame.html)
51. Palsson, B.O. Systems Biology: Properties of Reconstructed Networks. 334(Cambridge University Press: 2006).
52. Orth, J.D.; Thiele, I.; Palsson, B.Ø. (2010). What is flux balance analysis?. Nature Biotechnology. 28: 245–248. doi:10.1038/nbt.1614. PMC 3108565 . PMID 20212490.
53. Lee, J.M.; Gianchandani, E.P.; Papin, J.A. (2006). Flux balance analysis in the era of metabolomics. Briefings in bioinformatics. 7: 140–50. doi:10.1093/bib/bbl007.
54. Feist, A.M.; Palsson, B.Ø. (2008). The growing scope of applications of genome-scale metabolic reconstructions using Escherichia coli. Nature Biotechnology. 26: 659–67. doi:10.1038/nbt1401.
55. Lewis, N.E.; Nagarajan, H.; Palsson, B.Ø. (2012). Constraining the metabolic genotype–phenotype relationship using a phylogeny of in silico methods. Nature Reviews Microbiology. 10: 291–305. doi:10.1038/nrmicro2737.
56. Thiele, I.; Palsson, B.Ø. (2010). A protocol for generating a high-quality genome-scale metabolic reconstruction. Nature protocols. 5: 93–121. doi:10.1038/nprot.2009.203. PMC 3125167 . PMID 20057383.

57. Karp, P.D.; Paley, S.M.; Krummenacker, M.; et al. (2010). Pathway Tools version 13.0: Integrated Software for Pathway/Genome Informatics and Systems Biology. Briefings in Bioinformatics. 11: 40–79. doi:10.1093/bib/bbp043. PMC 2810111 . PMID 19955237.
58. Latendresse, M.; Krummenacker, M.; Trupp, M.; Karp, P.D. Construction and completion of flux balance models from pathway databases. Bioinformatics. 28 (388-96): 2012. doi:10.1093/bioinformatics/btr681.
59. Schilling, C.H. et al. SimPheny: A Computational Infrastructure for Systems Biology. (2008).
60. http://www.genomatica.com/technology/technologySuite.html
61. http://www.metnetmaker.com
62. Becker, S.A.; et al. (2007). Quantitative prediction of cellular metabolism with constraint-based models: the COBRA Toolbox. Nature protocols. 2: 727–38. doi:10.1038/nprot.2007.99.
63. Gevorgyan, A; Bushell, ME; Avignone-Rossa, C; Kierzek, AM (2011). SurreyFBA: a command line tool and graphics user interface for constraint-based modeling of genome-scale metabolic reaction networks. Bioinformatics. 27 (3): 433–4. doi:10.1093/bioinformatics/btq679. PMID 21148545.
64. Boele, J; Olivier, BG; Teusink, B (2012). FAME: the Flux Analysis and Modeling Environment. BMC Syst Biol. 6 (1): 8. doi:10.1186/1752-0509-6-8. PMC 3317868 . PMID 22289213.
65. http://cobramethods.wikidot.com/
66. Lakshmanan, M; Koh, G; Chung, BK; Lee, DY (Jan 2014). Software applications for flux balance analysis.. Briefings in bioinformatics. 15 (1): 108–22. doi:10.1093/bib/bbs069. PMID 23131418.
67. Gelius-Dietrich, G.; Amer Desouki, A.; Fritzemeier, C.J.; Lercher, M.J. (2013). sybil – Efficient constraint-based modelling in R.. BMC Systems Biology. 7 (1): 125. doi:10.1186/1752-0509-7-125. Software available at https://cran.r-project.org/package=sybil
68. Gangadharan A. Rohatgi N. abcdeFBA: Functions for Constraint Based Simulation using Flux Balance Analysis and informative analysis of the data generated during simulation. Available at: https://cran.r-project.org/web/packages/abcdeFBA/
69. Kotte, O.; Zaugg, J. B.; Heinemann, M. (2010). Bacterial adaptation through distributed sensing of metabolic fluxes. Molecular Systems Biology. 6 (355): 355. doi:10.1038/msb.2010.10.
70. Ibarra, Rafael U.; Edwards, Jeremy S.; Palsson, Bernhard O. (2002). Escherichia Coli K-12 Undergoes Adaptive Evolution to Achieve in Silico Predicted Optimal Growth. Nature. 420 (6912): 186–189. doi:10.1038/nature01149.
71. Segrè, Daniel; Vitkup, Dennis; Church, George M. (2002). Analysis of Optimality in Natural and Perturbed Metabolic Networks. Proceedings of the National Academy of Sciences. 99 (23): 15112–15117. doi:10.1073/pnas.232349399.

PMC 137552 . PMID 12415116.

72. Shlomi, Tomer, Omer Berkman, and Eytan Ruppin. Regulatory On/off Minimization of Metabolic Flux Changes After Genetic Perturbations. Proceedings of the National Academy of Sciences of the United States of America 102, no. 21 (May 24, 2005): 7695–7700. doi:10.1073/pnas.0406346102.

CHAPTER 5

Carbohydrate Metabolism

Chapter Contents

- **Introduction**
- **Diabetes Mellitus**
- **Lactose Intolerance**
- **Galactosemia**
- **Glycogen Storage Disease**

Carbohydrate metabolism begins with digestion in the small intestine where monosaccharides are absorbed into the blood stream. Blood sugar concentrations are controlled by three hormones: insulin, glucagon, and epinephrine. If the concentration of glucose in the blood is too high, insulin is secreted by the pancreas.

INTRODUCTION

Carbohydrate metabolism denotes the various biochemical processes responsible for the formation, breakdown and interconversion of carbohydrates in living organisms.

The most important carbohydrate is glucose, a simple sugar (monosaccharide) that is metabolized by nearly all known organisms. Glucose and other carbohydrates are part of a wide variety of metabolic pathways across species: plants synthesize carbohydrates from carbon dioxide and water by photosynthesis, storing the absorbed energy internally, often in the form of starch or lipids. Plant components are consumed by animals and fungi, and used as fuel for cellular respiration. Oxidation of one gram of carbohydrate yields approximately 4 kcal of energy, while the oxidation of one gram of lipids yields about 9 kcal. Energy obtained from metabolism (e.g., oxidation of glucose) is usually stored temporarily within cells in the form of ATP. Organisms capable of aerobic respiration metabolize glucose and oxygen to release energy with carbon dioxide and water as byproducts.

Carbohydrates can be chemically divided into two types: complex and simple. Simple carbohydrates consist of single or double sugar units (monosaccharides and disaccharides, respectively). Sucrose or table sugar (a disaccharide) is a common example of a simple carbohydrate. Complex carbohydrates contain three or more sugar units linked in a chain, with most containing hundreds to thousands of sugar units. They are digested by enzymes to release the simple sugars. Starch, for example, is a polymer of glucose units and is typically broken down to glucose. Cellulose is also a polymer of glucose but it cannot be digested by most organisms. Bacteria that produce enzymes to digest cellulose live inside the gut of some mammals, such as cows, and when these mammals eat plants, the cellulose is broken down by the bacteria and some of it is released into the gut.

Doctors and scientists once believed that eating complex carbohydrates instead of sugars would help maintain lower blood glucose. Numerous studies suggest, however, that both sugars and starch produce an unpredictable range of glycemic and insulinemic responses. While some studies support a more rapid absorption of sugars relative to starches other studies reveal that many carbohydrates such as those found in white bread, some types of white rice, and potatoes have glycemic indices similar to simple carbohydrates such as sucrose.Sucrose, for example, has a glycemic index (83) lower than expected because the sucrose molecule is half fructose, which has little effect on blood glucose. The value of classifying carbohydrates as simple or complex is questionable. The glycemic index is a better predictor of a carbohydrate›s effect on blood glucose.

Carbohydrates are a superior short-term fuel for organisms because they are simpler to metabolize than fats or those amino acids (components of proteins) that can be used for fuel. In animals, the most important carbohydrate is glucose. The concentration of glucose in the blood is used as the main control for the central metabolic hormone, insulin. Starch, and cellulose in a few organisms (e.g., some animals (such as termites) and some microorganisms (such as protists and bacteria)), both being glucose polymers, are disassembled during digestion and absorbed as glucose. Some simple carbohydrates have their own enzymatic oxidation pathways, as do only a few of the more complex carbohydrates. The disaccharide lactose, for instance, requires the enzyme lactase to be broken into its monosaccharide components; many animals lack this enzyme in adulthood.

Carbohydrates are typically stored as long polymers of glucose molecules with glycosidic bonds for structural support (e.g. chitin, cellulose) or for energy storage (e.g. glycogen, starch). However, the strong affinity of most carbohydrates for water makes storage of large quantities of carbohydrates inefficient due to the large molecular weight of the solvated water-carbohydrate complex. In most organisms, excess carbohydrates are regularly catabolised to form acetyl-CoA, which is a feed stock for the fatty acid synthesis pathway; fatty acids, triglycerides, and other lipids are commonly used for long-term energy storage. The hydrophobic character of lipids makes them a much more compact form of energy storage than hydrophilic carbohydrates. However, animals, including humans, lack the necessary enzymatic machinery and so do not synthesize glucose from lipids (with a few exceptions, e.g. glycerol).

All carbohydrates share a general formula of approximately $C_nH_{2n}O_n$; glucose is $C_6H_{12}O_6$. Monosaccharides may be chemically bonded together to form disaccharides such as sucrose and longer polysaccharides such as starch and cellulose.

Catabolism

Oligosaccharides and/or polysaccharides are typically cleaved into smaller monosaccharides by enzymes called glycoside hydrolases. The monosaccharide units then enter monosaccharide catabolism. Organisms vary in the range of monosaccharides they can absorb and use and they can also vary in the range of more complex carbohydrates they are capable of disassembling.

Metabolic Pathways

- Carbon fixation, or photosynthesis, in which CO_2 is reduced to carbohydrate.
- Glycolysis - the oxidation metabolism of glucose molecules to obtain ATP and pyruvate
- Pyruvate from glycolysis enters the Krebs cycle, also known as the citric acid cycle, in aerobic organisms after moving through pyruvate dehydrogenase complex.
- The pentose phosphate pathway, which acts in the conversion of hexoses into pentoses and in NADPH regeneration. NADPH is an essential antioxidant in cells which prevents oxidative damage and acts as precursor for production of many biomolecules.
- Glycogenesis - the conversion of excess glucose into glycogen as a cellular storage mechanism; this prevents excessive osmotic pressure buildup inside the cell
- Glycogenolysis - the breakdown of glycogen into glucose, which provides a glucose supply for glucose-dependent tissues.
- Gluconeogenesis - de novo synthesis of glucose molecules from simple organic compounds. An example in humans is the conversion of a few amino acids in cellular protein to glucose.

Metabolic use of glucose is highly important as an energy source for muscle cells and in the brain, and red blood cells.

Energy Production

Typically, a breakdown of one molecule of glucose by aerobic respiration (i.e. involving both glycolysis and Krebs cycle) is about 33-35 ATP. This is categorized as:

- Anaerobic breakdown by glycolysis - yielding 8-10 ATP
- Aerobic respiration by Krebs cycle - yielding 25 ATP

Glucoregulation

Glucoregulation is the maintenance of steady levels of glucose in the body; it is part of homeostasis, and so keeps a constant internal environment around cells in the body.

The hormone insulin is the primary regulatory signal in animals, suggesting that the basic mechanism is very old and very central to animal life. When present, it causes many tissue cells to take up glucose from the circulation, causes some cells to store glucose internally in the form of glycogen, causes some cells to take in and hold lipids, and in many cases controls cellular electrolyte balances and amino acid uptake as well. Its absence turns off glucose uptake into cells, reverses electrolyte adjustments, begins glycogen breakdown and glucose release into the circulation by some cells, begins lipid release from lipid storage cells, etc. The level of circulatory glucose (known informally as "blood sugar") is the most important signal to the insulin-producing cells. Because the level of circulatory glucose is largely determined by the intake of dietary carbohydrates, diet controls major aspects of metabolism via insulin. In humans, insulin is made by beta cells in the pancreas, fat is stored in adipose tissue cells, and glycogen is both stored and released as needed by liver cells. Regardless of insulin levels, no glucose is released to the blood from internal glycogen stores from muscle cells.

The hormone glucagon, on the other hand, has an effect opposite to that of insulin, forcing the conversion of glycogen in liver cells to glucose, which is then released into the blood. Muscle cells, however, lack the ability to export glucose into the blood. The release of glucagon is precipitated by low levels of blood glucose. Other hormones, notably growth hormone, cortisol, and certain catecholamines (such as epinepherine) have glucoregulatory actions similar to glucagon.

DIABETES MELLITUS

Diabetes mellitus (DM), commonly referred to as **diabetes**, is a group of metabolic diseases in which there are high blood sugar levels over a prolonged period. Symptoms of high blood sugar include frequent urination, increased thirst, and increased hunger. If left untreated, diabetes can cause many complications. Acute complications can include diabetic ketoacidosis, nonketotic hyperosmolar coma, or death. Serious long-term complications include heart disease, stroke, chronic kidney failure, foot ulcers, and damage to the eyes.

Diabetes is due to either the pancreas not producing enough insulin or the cells of the body not responding properly to the insulin produced. There are three main types of diabetes mellitus:

- Type 1 DM results from the pancreas's failure to produce enough insulin. This form was previously referred to as "insulin-dependent diabetes mellitus" (IDDM) or "juvenile diabetes". The cause is unknown.
- Type 2 DM begins with insulin resistance, a condition in which cells fail to respond to insulin properly. As the disease progresses a lack of insulin may also develop. This form was previously referred to as "non insulin-dependent diabetes mellitus" (NIDDM) or "adult-onset diabetes". The most common cause is excessive body weight and not enough exercise.

- Gestational diabetes is the third main form and occurs when pregnant women without a previous history of diabetes develop high blood-sugar levels.

Prevention and treatment involve maintaining a healthy diet, regular physical exercise, a normal body weight, and avoiding use of tobacco. Control of blood pressure and maintaining proper foot care are important for people with the disease. Type 1 DM must be managed with insulin injections. Type 2 DM may be treated with medications with or without insulin. Insulin and some oral medications can cause low blood sugar. Weight loss surgery in those with obesity is sometimes an effective measure in those with type 2 DM. Gestational diabetes usually resolves after the birth of the baby.

As of 2015, an estimated 415 million people had diabetes worldwide, with type 2 DM making up about 90% of the cases. This represents 8.3% of the adult population, with equal rates in both women and men. As of 2014, trends suggested the rate would continue to rise. Diabetes at least doubles a person's risk of early death. From 2012 to 2015, approximately 1.5 to 5.0 million deaths each year resulted from diabetes. The global economic cost of diabetes in 2014 was estimated to be US$612 billion. In the United States, diabetes cost $245 billion in 2012.

Signs and Symptoms

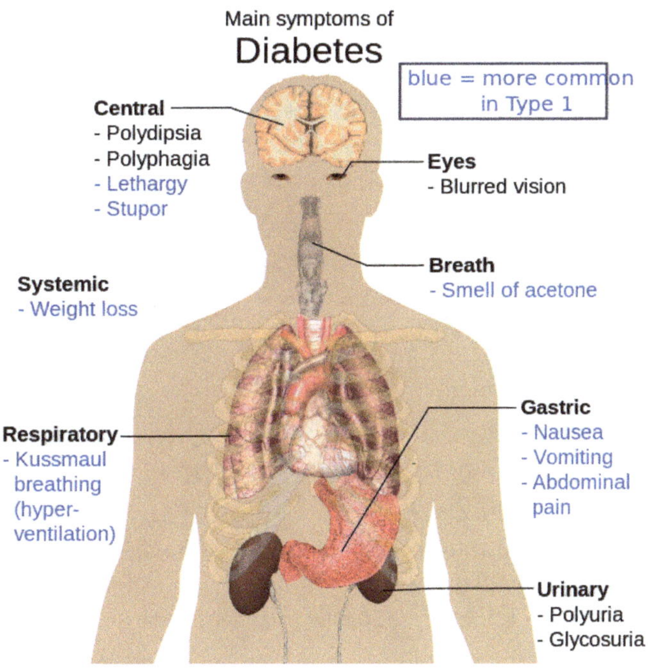

Overview of the most significant symptoms of diabetes

The classic symptoms of untreated diabetes are weight loss, polyuria (increased urination), polydipsia (increased thirst), and polyphagia (increased hunger). Symptoms may develop rapidly (weeks or months) in type 1 DM, while they usually develop much more slowly and may be subtle or absent in type 2 DM.

Several other signs and symptoms can mark the onset of diabetes although they are not specific to the disease. In addition to the known ones above, they include blurry vision, headache, fatigue, slow healing of cuts, and itchy skin. Prolonged high blood glucose can cause glucose absorption in the lens of the eye, which leads to changes in its shape, resulting in vision changes. A number of skin rashes that can occur in diabetes are collectively known as diabetic dermadromes.

Diabetic Emergencies

Low blood sugar is common in persons with type 1 and type 2 DM. Most cases are mild and are not considered medical emergencies. Effects can range from feelings of unease, sweating, trembling, and increased appetite in mild cases to more serious issues such as confusion, changes in behavior such as aggressiveness, seizures, unconsciousness, and (rarely) permanent brain damage or death in severe cases. Moderate hypoglycemia may easily be mistaken for drunkenness;rapid breathing and sweating, cold, pale skin are characteristic of hypoglycemia but not definitive. Mild to moderate cases are self-treated by eating or drinking something high in sugar. Severe cases can lead to unconsciousness and must be treated with intravenous glucose or injections with glucagon.

People (usually with type 1 DM) may also experience episodes of diabetic ketoacidosis, a metabolic disturbance characterized by nausea, vomiting and abdominal pain, the smell of acetone on the breath, deep breathing known as Kussmaul breathing, and in severe cases a decreased level of consciousness.

A rare but equally severe possibility is hyperosmolar nonketotic state, which is more common in type 2 DM and is mainly the result of dehydration.

Complications

All forms of diabetes increase the risk of long-term complications. These typically develop after many years (10–20) but may be the first symptom in those who have otherwise not received a diagnosis before that time.

The major long-term complications relate to damage to blood vessels. Diabetes doubles the risk of cardiovascular disease and about 75% of deaths in diabetics are due to coronary artery disease. Other "macrovascular" diseases are stroke, and peripheral vascular disease.

The primary complications of diabetes due to damage in small blood vessels include damage to the eyes, kidneys, and nerves. Damage to the eyes, known as diabetic retinopathy, is caused by damage to the blood vessels in the retina of the eye, and can result in gradual vision loss and blindness. Damage to the kidneys, known as diabetic nephropathy, can lead to tissue scarring, urine protein loss, and eventually chronic kidney disease, sometimes requiring dialysis or kidney transplant. Damage to the nerves of the body, known as diabetic neuropathy, is the most common complication of diabetes. The symptoms can include numbness, tingling, pain, and altered pain sensation, which can lead to damage to the skin. Diabetes-related foot problems (such as diabetic foot ulcers) may occur, and can be difficult to treat, occasionally requiring amputation. Additionally, proximal diabetic neuropathy causes painful muscle wasting and weakness.

There is a link between cognitive deficit and diabetes. Compared to those without diabetes, those with the disease have a 1.2 to 1.5-fold greater rate of decline in cognitive function.

Causes

Diabetes mellitus is classified into four broad categories: type 1, type 2, gestational diabetes, and "other specific types". The "other specific types" are a collection of a few dozen individual causes. Diabetes is a more variable disease than once thought and people may have combinations of forms. The term "diabetes", without qualification, usually refers to diabetes mellitus.

Type 1

Type 1 diabetes mellitus is characterized by loss of the insulin-producing beta cells of the islets of Langerhans in the pancreas, leading to insulin deficiency. This type can be further classified as immune-mediated or idiopathic. The majority of type 1 diabetes is of the immune-mediated nature, in which a T-cell-mediated autoimmune attack leads to the loss of beta cells and thus insulin. It causes approximately 10% of diabetes mellitus cases in North America and Europe. Most affected people are otherwise healthy and of a healthy weight when onset occurs. Sensitivity and responsiveness to insulin are usually normal, especially in the early stages. Type 1 diabetes can affect children or adults, but was traditionally termed "juvenile diabetes" because a majority of these diabetes cases were in children.

"Brittle" diabetes, also known as unstable diabetes or labile diabetes, is a term that was traditionally used to describe the dramatic and recurrent swings in glucose levels, often occurring for no apparent reason in insulin-dependent diabetes. This term, however, has no biologic basis and should not be used. Still, type 1 diabetes can be accompanied by irregular and unpredictable high blood sugar levels, frequently with ketosis, and sometimes with serious low blood sugar levels. Other complications include an impaired counterregulatory response to low blood sugar, infection, gastroparesis (which leads to erratic absorption of dietary carbohydrates), and endocrinopathies (e.g., Addison's disease). These phenomena are believed to occur no more frequently than in 1% to 2% of persons with type 1 diabetes.

Type 1 diabetes is partly inherited, with multiple genes, including certain HLA genotypes, known to influence the risk of diabetes. The increase of incidence of type 1 diabetes reflects the modern lifestyle. In genetically susceptible people, the onset of diabetes can be triggered by one or more environmental factors, such as a viral infection or diet. Several viruses have been implicated, but to date there is no stringent evidence to support this hypothesis in humans. Among dietary factors, data suggest that gliadin (a protein present in gluten) may play a role in the development of type 1 diabetes, but the mechanism is not fully understood.

Type 2

Type 2 DM is characterized by insulin resistance, which may be combined with relatively reduced insulin secretion. The defective responsiveness of body tissues to insulin is believed to involve the insulin receptor. However, the specific defects are not known. Diabetes mellitus cases due to a known defect are classified separately. Type 2 DM is the most common type of diabetes mellitus.

In the early stage of type 2, the predominant abnormality is reduced insulin sensitivity. At this stage, high blood sugar can be reversed by a variety of measures and medications that improve insulin sensitivity or reduce the liver's glucose production.

Type 2 DM is due primarily to lifestyle factors and genetics. A number of lifestyle factors are known to be important to the development of type 2 DM, including obesity (defined by a body mass index of greater than 30), lack of physical activity, poor diet, stress, and urbanization. Excess body fat is associated with 30% of cases in those of Chinese and Japanese descent, 60–80% of cases in those of European and African descent, and 100% of Pima Indians and Pacific Islanders. Even those who are not obese often have a high waist–hip ratio.

Dietary factors also influence the risk of developing type 2 DM. Consumption of sugar-sweetened drinks in excess is associated with an increased risk. The type of fats in the diet is also important, with saturated fats and trans fatty acids increasing the risk and polyunsaturated and monounsaturated fat decreasing the risk. Eating lots of white rice also may increase the risk of diabetes. A lack of exercise is believed to cause 7% of cases.

Gestational Diabetes

Gestational diabetes mellitus (GDM) resembles type 2 DM in several respects, involving a combination of relatively inadequate insulin secretion and responsiveness. It occurs in about 2–10% of all pregnancies and may improve or disappear after delivery. However, after pregnancy approximately 5–10% of women with gestational diabetes are found to have diabetes mellitus, most commonly type 2. Gestational diabetes is fully treatable, but requires careful medical supervision throughout the pregnancy. Management may include dietary changes, blood glucose monitoring, and in some cases, insulin may be required.

Though it may be transient, untreated gestational diabetes can damage the health of the fetus or mother. Risks to the baby include macrosomia (high birth weight), congenital heart and central nervous system abnormalities, and skeletal muscle malformations. Increased levels of insulin in a fetus's blood may inhibit fetal surfactant production and cause respiratory distress syndrome. A high blood bilirubin level may result from red blood cell destruction. In severe cases, perinatal death may occur, most commonly as a result of poor placental perfusion due to vascular impairment. Labor induction may be indicated with decreased placental function. A Caesarean section may be performed if there is marked fetal distress or an increased risk of injury associated with macrosomia, such as shoulder dystocia.

Other Types

Prediabetes indicates a condition that occurs when a person's blood glucose levels are higher than normal but not high enough for a diagnosis of type 2 DM. Many people destined to develop type 2 DM spend many years in a state of prediabetes.

Latent autoimmune diabetes of adults (LADA) is a condition in which type 1 DM develops in adults. Adults with LADA are frequently initially misdiagnosed as having type 2 DM, based on age rather than etiology.

Some cases of diabetes are caused by the body's tissue receptors not responding to insulin (even when insulin levels are normal, which is what separates it from type 2 diabetes); this form is very uncommon. Genetic mutations (autosomal or mitochondrial) can lead to defects in beta cell function. Abnormal insulin action may also have been genetically determined in some cases. Any disease that causes extensive damage to the pancreas may lead to diabetes (for example, chronic pancreatitis and cystic fibrosis). Diseases associated with excessive secretion of insulin-antagonistic hormones can cause diabetes (which is typically resolved once the hormone excess is removed). Many drugs impair insulin secretion and some toxins damage pancreatic beta cells. The ICD-10 (1992) diagnostic entity, malnutrition-related diabetes mellitus (MRDM or MMDM, ICD-10 code E12), was deprecated by the World Health Organization when the current taxonomy was introduced in 1999.

Other forms of diabetes mellitus include congenital diabetes, which is due to genetic defects of insulin secretion, cystic fibrosis-related diabetes, steroid diabetes induced by high doses of glucocorticoids, and several forms of monogenic diabetes.

"Type 3 diabetes" has been suggested as a term for Alzheimer›s disease as the underlying processes may involve insulin resistance by the brain.

The following is a comprehensive list of other causes of diabetes:

<table>
<tr>
<td>

- Genetic defects of β-cell function
  - Maturity onset diabetes of the young
  - Mitochondrial DNA mutations
- Genetic defects in insulin processing or insulin action
  - Defects in proinsulin conversion
  - Insulin gene mutations
  - Insulin receptor mutations
- Exocrine pancreatic defects
  - Chronic pancreatitis
  - Pancreatectomy
  - Pancreatic neoplasia
  - Cystic fibrosis
  - Hemochromatosis
  - Fibrocalculous pancreatopathy

</td>
<td>

- Endocrinopathies
  - Growth hormone excess (acromegaly)
  - Cushing syndrome
  - Hyperthyroidism
  - Pheochromocytoma
  - Glucagonoma
- Infections
  - Cytomegalovirus infection
  - Coxsackievirus B
- Drugs
  - Glucocorticoids
  - Thyroid hormone
  - β-adrenergic agonists
  - Statins

</td>
</tr>
</table>

Pathophysiology

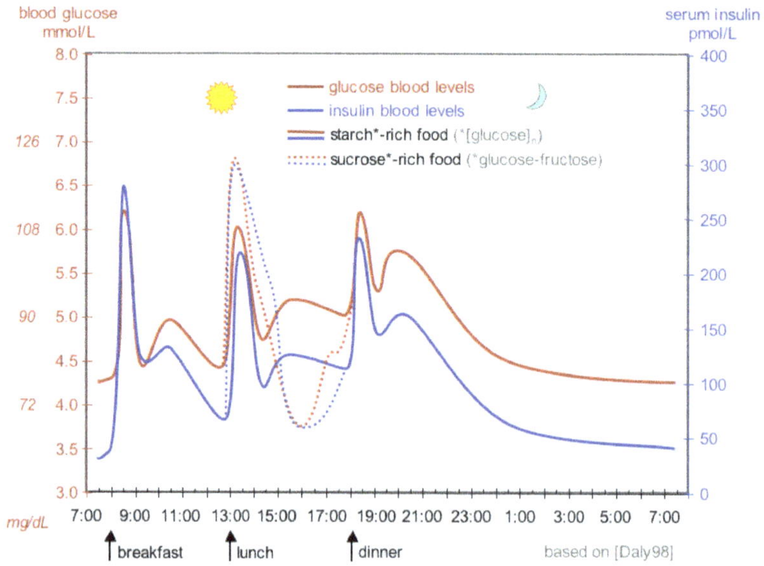

The fluctuation of blood sugar (red) and the sugar-lowering hormone insulin (blue) in humans during the course of a day with three meals — one of the effects of a sugar-rich vs a starch-rich meal is highlighted.

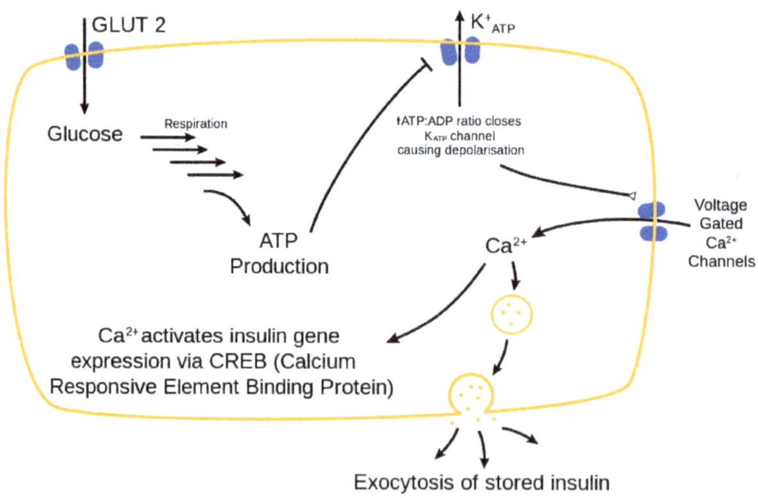

Mechanism of insulin release in normal pancreatic beta cells — insulin production is more or less constant within the beta cells. Its release is triggered by food, chiefly food containing absorbable glucose.

Insulin is the principal hormone that regulates the uptake of glucose from the blood into most cells of the body, especially liver, adipose tissue and muscle, except smooth muscle, in which insulin acts via the IGF-1. Therefore, deficiency of insulin or the insensitivity of its receptors plays a central role in all forms of diabetes mellitus.

The body obtains glucose from three main places: the intestinal absorption of food, the breakdown of glycogen, the storage form of glucose found in the liver, and gluconeogenesis, the generation of glucose from non-carbohydrate substrates in the body. Insulin plays a critical role in balancing glucose levels in the body. Insulin can inhibit the breakdown of glycogen or the process of gluconeogenesis, it can stimulate the transport of glucose into fat and muscle cells, and it can stimulate the storage of glucose in the form of glycogen.

Insulin is released into the blood by beta cells (β-cells), found in the islets of Langerhans in the pancreas, in response to rising levels of blood glucose, typically after eating. Insulin is used by about two-thirds of the body's cells to absorb glucose from the blood for use as fuel, for conversion to other needed molecules, or for storage. Lower glucose levels result in decreased insulin release from the beta cells and in the breakdown of glycogen to glucose. This process is mainly controlled by the hormone glucagon, which acts in the opposite manner to insulin.

If the amount of insulin available is insufficient, if cells respond poorly to the effects of insulin (insulin insensitivity or insulin resistance), or if the insulin itself is defective, then glucose will not be absorbed properly by the body cells that require it, and it will not be stored appropriately in the liver and muscles. The net effect is persistently high levels of blood glucose, poor protein synthesis, and other metabolic derangements, such as acidosis.

When the glucose concentration in the blood remains high over time, the kidneys will reach a threshold of reabsorption, and glucose will be excreted in the urine (glycosuria). This increases the osmotic pressure of the urine and inhibits reabsorption of water by the kidney, resulting in increased urine production (polyuria) and increased fluid loss. Lost blood volume will be replaced osmotically from water held in body cells and other body compartments, causing dehydration and increased thirst (polydipsia).

Diagnosis

WHO diabetes diagnostic criteria edit

Condition	**2 hour glucose**	**Fasting glucose**	**HbA_{1c}**	
Unit	mmol/l(mg/dl)	mmol/l(mg/dl)	mmol/mol	DCCT %
Normal	<7.8 (<140)	<6.1 (<110)	<42	<6.0
Impaired fasting glycaemia	<7.8 (<140)	≥6.1(≥110) & <7.0(<126)	42-46	6.0–6.4
Impaired glucose tolerance	≥7.8 (≥140)	<7.0 (<126)	42-46	6.0–6.4
Diabetes mellitus	≥11.1 (≥200)	≥7.0 (≥126)	≥48	≥6.5

Diabetes mellitus is characterized by recurrent or persistent high blood sugar, and is diagnosed by demonstrating any one of the following:

- Fasting plasma glucose level ≥ 7.0 mmol/l (126 mg/dl)

- Plasma glucose ≥ 11.1 mmol/l (200 mg/dl) two hours after a 75 g oral glucose load as in a glucose tolerance test
- Symptoms of high blood sugar and casual plasma glucose ≥ 11.1 mmol/l (200 mg/dl)
- Glycated hemoglobin (HbA_{1C}) ≥ 48 mmol/mol (≥ 6.5 DCCT %).

A positive result, in the absence of unequivocal high blood sugar, should be confirmed by a repeat of any of the above methods on a different day. It is preferable to measure a fasting glucose level because of the ease of measurement and the considerable time commitment of formal glucose tolerance testing, which takes two hours to complete and offers no prognostic advantage over the fasting test. According to the current definition, two fasting glucose measurements above 126 mg/dl (7.0 mmol/l) is considered diagnostic for diabetes mellitus.

Per the World Health Organization people with fasting glucose levels from 6.1 to 6.9 mmol/l (110 to 125 mg/dl) are considered to have impaired fasting glucose. people with plasma glucose at or above 7.8 mmol/l (140 mg/dl), but not over 11.1 mmol/l (200 mg/dl), two hours after a 75 g oral glucose load are considered to have impaired glucose tolerance. Of these two prediabetic states, the latter in particular is a major risk factor for progression to full-blown diabetes mellitus, as well as cardiovascular disease. The American Diabetes Association since 2003 uses a slightly different range for impaired fasting glucose of 5.6 to 6.9 mmol/l (100 to 125 mg/dl).

Glycated hemoglobin is better than fasting glucose for determining risks of cardiovascular disease and death from any cause.

The rare disease diabetes insipidus has similar symptoms to diabetes mellitus, but without disturbances in the sugar metabolism (insipidus means "without taste" in Latin) and does not involve the same disease mechanisms. Diabetes is a part of the wider condition known as metabolic syndrome.

Prevention

There is no known preventive measure for type 1 diabetes. Type 2 diabetes — which accounts for 85-90% of all cases — can often be prevented or delayed by maintaining a normal body weight, engaging in physical exercise, and consuming a healthful diet. Higher levels of physical activity (more than 90 minutes per day) reduce the risk of diabetes by 28%.Dietary changes known to be effective in helping to prevent diabetes include maintaining a diet rich in whole grains and fiber, and choosing good fats, such as the polyunsaturated fats found in nuts, vegetable oils, and fish. Limiting sugary beverages and eating less red meat and other sources of saturated fat can also help prevent diabetes. Tobacco smoking is also associated with an increased risk of diabetes and its complications, so smoking cessation can be an important preventive measure as well.

The relationship between type 2 diabetes and the main modifiable risk factors (excess weight, unhealthy diet, physical inactivity and tobacco use) is similar in all regions of the world. There is growing evidence that the underlying determinants of diabetes are a reflection of the major forces driving social, economic and cultural change: globalization, urbanization, population aging, and the general health policy environment.

Management

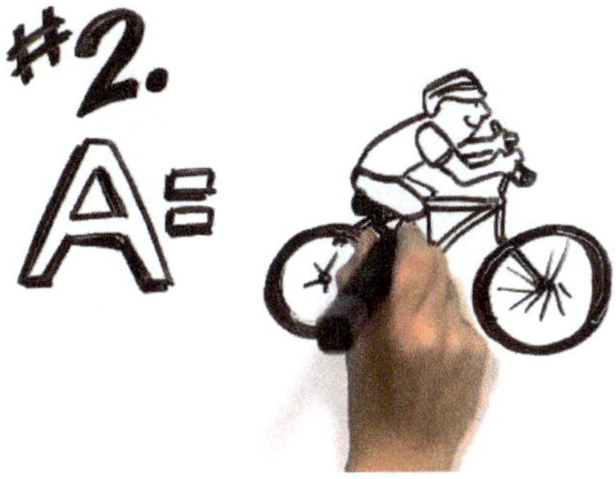

Overview of management

Diabetes mellitus is a chronic disease, for which there is no known cure except in very specific situations. Management concentrates on keeping blood sugar levels as close to normal, without causing low blood sugar. This can usually be accomplished with a healthy diet, exercise, weight loss, and use of appropriate medications (insulin in the case of type 1 diabetes; oral medications, as well as possibly insulin, in type 2 diabetes).

Learning about the disease and actively participating in the treatment is important, since complications are far less common and less severe in people who have well-managed blood sugar levels. The goal of treatment is an HbA_{1C} level of 6.5%, but should not be lower than that, and may be set higher. Attention is also paid to other health problems that may accelerate the negative effects of diabetes. These include smoking, elevated cholesterol levels, obesity, high blood pressure, and lack of regular exercise. Specialized footwear is widely used to reduce the risk of ulceration, or re-ulceration, in at-risk diabetic feet. Evidence for the efficacy of this remains equivocal, however.

Lifestyle

People with diabetes can benefit from education about the disease and treatment, good nutrition to achieve a normal body weight, and exercise, with the goal of keeping both short-term and long-term blood glucose levels within acceptable bounds. In addition, given the associated higher risks of cardiovascular disease, lifestyle modifications are recommended to control blood pressure.

Medications

Medications used to treat diabetes do so by lowering blood sugar levels. There are a number of different classes of anti-diabetic medications. Some are available by mouth, such as metformin, while others are only available by injection such as GLP-1 agonists. Type 1 diabetes can only be treated with insulin, typically with a combination of regular and NPH insulin, or synthetic insulin analogs.

Metformin is generally recommended as a first line treatment for type 2 diabetes, as there is good evidence that it decreases mortality. It works by decreasing the liver's production of glucose. Several other groups of drugs, mostly given by mouth, may also decrease blood sugar in type II DM. These include agents that increase insulin release, agents that decrease absorption of sugar from the intestines, and agents that make the body more sensitive to insulin. When insulin is used in type 2 diabetes, a long-acting formulation is usually added initially, while continuing oral medications. Doses of insulin are then increased to effect.

Since cardiovascular disease is a serious complication associated with diabetes, some have recommended blood pressure levels below 130/80 mmHg. However, evidence supports less than or equal to somewhere between 140/90 mmHg to 160/100 mmHg; the only additional benefit found for blood pressure targets beneath this range was an isolated decrease in stroke risk, and this was accompanied by an increased risk of other serious adverse events. A 2016 review found potential harm to treating lower than 140 mmHg. Among medications that lower blood pressure, angiotensin converting enzyme inhibitors (ACEIs) improve outcomes in those with DM while the similar medications angiotensin receptor blockers (ARBs) do not. Aspirin is also recommended for people with cardiovascular problems, however routine use of aspirin has not been found to improve outcomes in uncomplicated diabetes.

Surgery

A pancreas transplant is occasionally considered for people with type 1 diabetes who have severe complications of their disease, including end stage kidney disease requiring kidney transplantation.

Weight loss surgery in those with obesity and type two diabetes is often an effective measure. Many are able to maintain normal blood sugar levels with little or no medications following surgery and long-term mortality is decreased. There however is some short-term mortality risk of less than 1% from the surgery. The body mass index cutoffs for when surgery is appropriate are not yet clear. It is recommended that this option be considered in those who are unable to get both their weight and blood sugar under control.

Support

In countries using a general practitioner system, such as the United Kingdom, care may take place mainly outside hospitals, with hospital-based specialist care used only in case of complications, difficult blood sugar control, or research projects. In other circumstances, general practitioners and specialists share care in a team approach. Home telehealth support can be an effective management technique.

Epidemiology

As of 2016, 422 million people have diabetes worldwide, up from an estimated 382 million people in 2013 and from 108 million in 1980. Accounting for the shifting age structure of the global population, the prevalence of diabetes is 8.5% among adults, nearly double the rate of 4.7% in 1980. Type 2 makes up about 90% of the cases. Some data indicate rates are roughly equal in women and men, but male excess in diabetes has been found in many populations with higher type 2 incidence, possibly due to sex-related differences in insulin sensitivity, consequences of obesity and regional body fat deposition, and other contributing factors such as high blood pressure, tobacco smoking, and alcohol intake.

The World Health Organization (WHO) estimates that diabetes mellitus resulted in 1.5 million deaths in 2012, making it the 8th leading cause of death. However another 2.2 million deaths worldwide were attributable to high blood glucose and the increased risks of cardiovascular disease and other associated complications (e.g. kidney failure), which often lead to premature death and are often listed as the underlying cause on death certificates rather than diabetes. For example, in 2014, the International Diabetes Federation (IDF) estimated that diabetes resulted in 4.9 million deaths worldwide, using modeling to estimate the total amount of deaths that could be directly or indirectly attributed to diabetes.

Diabetes mellitus occurs throughout the world but is more common (especially type 2) in more developed countries. The greatest increase in rates has however been seen in low- and middle-income countries, where more than 80% of diabetic deaths occur.The fastest prevalence increase is expected to occur in Asia and Africa, where most people with diabetes will probably live in 2030. The increase in rates in developing countries follows the trend of urbanization and lifestyle changes, including increasingly sedentary lifestyles, less physically demanding work and the global nutrition transition, marked by increased intake of foods that are high energy-dense but nutrient-poor (often high in sugar and saturated fats, sometimes referred to as the "Western-style" diet).

Etymology

The word diabetes comes from Latin diabētēs, which in turn comes from Ancient Greek διαβήτης (diabētēs) which literally means "a passer through; a siphon." Ancient Greek physician Aretaeus of Cappadocia (fl. 1st century CE) used that word, with the intended meaning "excessive discharge of urine", as the name for the disease. Ultimately, the word comes from Greek διαβαίνειν (diabainein), meaning "to pass through," which is composed of δια- (dia-), meaning "through" and βαίνειν (bainein), meaning "to go". The word "diabetes" is first recorded in English, in the form diabete, in a medical text written around 1425.

The word mellitus comes from the classical Latin word mellītus, meaning "mellite" (i.e. sweetened with honey; honey-sweet). The Latin word comes from mell-, which comes from mel, meaning "honey"; sweetness; pleasant thing, and the suffix -ītus, whose meaning is the same as that of the English suffix "-ite". It was Thomas Willis who in 1675 added "mellitus" to the word "diabetes" as a designation for the disease, when he noticed the urine of a diabetic had a sweet taste (glycosuria). This sweet taste had been noticed in urine by the ancient Greeks, Chinese, Egyptians, Indians, and Persians.

Society and Culture

The 1989 "St. Vincent Declaration" was the result of international efforts to improve the care accorded to those with diabetes. Doing so is important not only in terms of quality of life and life expectancy but also economically—expenses due to diabetes have been shown to be a major drain on health—and productivity-related resources for healthcare systems and governments.

Several countries established more and less successful national diabetes programmes to improve treatment of the disease.

People with diabetes who have neuropathic symptoms such as numbness or tingling in feet or hands are twice as likely to be unemployed as those without the symptoms.

In 2010, diabetes-related emergency room (ER) visit rates in the United States were higher among people from the lowest income communities (526 per 10,000 population) than from the highest income communities (236 per 10,000 population). Approximately 9.4% of diabetes-related ER visits were for the uninsured.

Naming

The term "type 1 diabetes" has replaced several former terms, including childhood-onset diabetes, juvenile diabetes, and insulin-dependent diabetes mellitus (IDDM). Likewise, the term "type 2 diabetes" has replaced several former terms, including adult-onset diabetes, obesity-related diabetes, and noninsulin-dependent diabetes mellitus (NIDDM). Beyond these two types, there is no agreed-upon standard nomenclature.

Diabetes mellitus is also occasionally known as "sugar diabetes" to differentiate it from diabetes insipidus.

Other Animals

In animals, diabetes is most commonly encountered in dogs and cats. Middle-aged animals are most commonly affected. Female dogs are twice as likely to be affected as males, while according to some sources, male cats are also more prone than females. In both species, all breeds may be affected, but some small dog breeds are particularly likely to develop diabetes, such as Miniature Poodles. The symptoms may relate to fluid loss and polyuria, but the course may also be insidious. Diabetic animals are more prone to infections. The long-term complications recognized in humans are much rarer in animals. The principles of treatment (weight loss, oral antidiabetics, subcutaneous insulin) and management of emergencies (e.g. ketoacidosis) are similar to those in humans.

Research

Inhalable insulin has been developed. The original products were withdrawn due to side effects. Afrezza, under development by pharmaceuticals company MannKind Corporation, was approved by the FDA for general sale in June 2014. An advantage to inhaled insulin is that it may be more convenient and easy to use.

Transdermal insulin in the form of a cream has been developed and trials are being conducted on people with type 2 diabetes.

LACTOSE INTOLERANCE

Lactose intolerance is a condition in which people have symptoms due to the decreased ability to digest lactose, a sugar found in milk products. Those affected vary in the amount of lactose they can tolerate before symptoms develop. Symptoms may include abdominal pain, bloating, diarrhea, gas, and nausea. These typically start between half and two hours after drinking milk. Severity depends on the amount a person eats or drinks. It does not cause damage to the gastrointestinal tract.

Lactose intolerance is due to not enough of the enzyme lactase in the small intestines to break lactose down into glucose and galactose. There are four types: primary, secondary, developmental, and congenital. Primary lactose intolerance is when the amount of lactase decline as people age. Secondary lactose intolerance is due to injury to the small intestine such as from infection, celiac disease, inflammatory bowel disease, or other diseases. Developmental lactose intolerance may occur in premature babies and usually improves over a short period of time. Congenital lactose intolerance is an extremely rare genetic disorder in which little or no lactase is made from birth.

Diagnosis may be confirmed if symptoms resolve following eliminating lactose from the diet. Other supporting tests include a hydrogen breath test and a stool acidity test. Other conditions that may produce similar symptoms include irritable bowel syndrome, celiac disease, and inflammatory bowel disease. Lactose intolerance is different from a milk allergy. Management is typically by decreasing the amount of lactose in the diet or taking lactase supplements. Those affected are usually able to drink at least one cup of milk without developing significant symptoms, with greater amounts tolerated if drunk with a meal or throughout the day.

The number of people with lactose intolerance is unknown. The percentage of the population that has a decrease in lactase as they age is less than 10% in Northern Europe and as high as 95% in parts of Asia and Africa. Onset is typically in late childhood or adulthood. The ability to digest lactose into adulthood is believed to have developed among some human populations in the last 10,000 years.

Terminology

Lactose intolerance primarily refers to a syndrome having one or more symptoms upon the consumption of food substances containing lactose. Individuals may be lactose intolerant to varying degrees, depending on the severity of these symptoms. "Lactose malabsorption" refers to the physiological concomitant of lactase deficiency (i.e., the body does not have sufficient lactase capacity to digest the amount of lactose ingested). Hypolactasia (lactase deficiency) is distinguished from alactasia (total lack of lactase), a rare congenital defect.

Lactose intolerance is not an allergy, because it is not an immune response, but rather a sensitivity to dairy caused by lactase deficiency. Milk allergy, occurring in only 4% of the population, is a separate condition, with distinct symptoms that occur when the presence of milk proteins trigger an immune reaction.

Signs and Symptoms

The principal symptom of lactose intolerance is an adverse reaction to products containing lactose (primarily milk), including abdominal bloating and cramps, flatulence, diarrhea, nausea, borborygmi, and vomiting (particularly in adolescents). These appear one-half to two hours after consumption. The severity of symptoms typically increases with the amount of lactose consumed; most lactose-intolerant people can tolerate a certain level of lactose in their diets without ill effects.

Primary Congenital Alactasia

Primary congenital alactasia, or congenital lactase deficiency (CLD), where the production of lactase is inhibited from birth, can be dangerous in any society because of infants' initial reliance on human breast milk for nutrition until they are weaned onto other foods. Before the 20th century, babies born with CLD often did not survive, but death rates decreased with soybean-derived infant formulas and manufactured lactose-free dairy products.

Causes

Lactose intolerance is a consequence of lactase deficiency, which may be genetic (primary hypolactasia and primary congenital alactasia) or environmentally induced (secondary or acquired hypoalactasia). In either case, symptoms are caused by insufficient levels of lactase in the lining of the duodenum. Lactose, a disaccharide molecule found in milk and dairy products, cannot be directly absorbed through the wall of the small intestine into the bloodstream, so, in the absence of lactase, passes intact into the colon. Bacteria in the colon can metabolise lactose, and the resulting fermentation produces copious amounts of gas (a mixture of hydrogen, carbon dioxide, and methane) that causes the various abdominal symptoms. The unabsorbed sugars and fermentation products also raise the osmotic pressure of the colon, causing an increased flow of water into the bowels (diarrhea). The LCT gene provides the instructions for making lactase. The specific DNA sequence in the MCM6 gene helps control whether the LCT gene is turned on or off. At least several thousand years ago, some humans developed a mutation in the MCM6 gene that keeps the LCT gene turned on even after breast feeding is stopped. People who are lactose intolerant do not have this mutation. The LCT and MCM6 genes are both located on the long arm (q) of chromosome 2 in region 21. The locus can be expressed as 2q21. The lactase deficiency also could be linked to certain heritages. Seventy-five percent of all African American, Jewish, Mexican American, and Native American adults are lactose intolerant. Analysis of the DNA of 94 ancient skeletons in Europe and Russia concluded that the lactose tolerant mutation appeared about 4,300 years ago and spread throughout the European population.

Some human populations have developed lactase persistence, in which lactase production continues into adulthood probably as a response to the benefits of being able to digest milk from farm animals. Some have argued that this links intolerance to natural selection favoring lactase-persistent individuals, but it is also consistent with a physiological response to decrease lactase production when it is not needed in cultures in which dairy products are not an available food source. Although populations in Europe,

India, Arabia, and Africa were first thought to have high rates of lactase persistence because of a single mutation, lactase persistence has been traced to a number of mutations that occurred independently.

Different alleles for lactase persistence have developed at least three times in East African populations, with persistence extending from 26% in Tanzania to 88% in the Beja pastoralist population in Sudan.

Lactose intolerance is classified according to its causes as:

Primary Hypolactasia

Primary hypolactasia, or primary lactase deficiency, is genetic, only affects adults, and is caused by the absence of a lactase persistence allele. In individuals without the lactase persistence allele, less lactase is produced by the body over time, leading to hypolactasia in adulthood. The frequency of lactase persistence, which allows lactose tolerance, varies enormously worldwide, with the highest prevalence in Northwestern Europe, declines across southern Europe and the Middle East and is low in Asia and most of Africa, although it is common in pastoralist populations from Africa.

Secondary Hypolactasia

Secondary hypolactasia or secondary lactase deficiency, also called acquired hypolactasia or acquired lactase deficiency, is caused by an injury to the small intestine. This form of lactose intolerance can occur in both infants and lactase persistent adults and is generally reversible. It may be caused by acute gastroenteritis, coeliac disease, Crohn's disease, ulcerative colitis, chemotherapy, intestinal parasites (such as giardia), or other environmental causes.

Primary Congenital Alactasia

Primary congenital alactasia, also called congenital lactase deficiency, is an extremely rare, autosomal recessive enzyme defect that prevents lactase expression from birth. People with congenital lactase deficiency cannot digest lactose from birth, so cannot digest breast milk. This genetic defect is characterized by a complete lack of lactase (alactasia). About 40 cases have been reported worldwide, mainly limited to Finland.

Diagnosis

To assess lactose intolerance, intestinal function is challenged by ingesting more dairy products than can be readily digested. Clinical symptoms typically appear within 30 minutes, but may take up to two hours, depending on other foods and activities. Substantial variability in response (symptoms of nausea, cramping, bloating, diarrhea, and flatulence) is to be expected, as the extent and severity of lactose intolerance varies among individuals.

The next step is to determine whether it is due to primary lactase deficiency or an underlying disease that causes secondary lactase deficiency. Physicians should investigate the presence of undiagnosed coeliac disease, Crohn disease, or other enteropathies when secondary lactase deficiency is suspected and an infectious gastroenteritis has been ruled out.

Lactose intolerance is distinct from milk allergy, an immune response to cow's milk proteins. They may be distinguished in diagnosis by giving lactose-free milk, producing no symptoms in the case of lactose intolerance, but the same reaction as to normal milk in the presence of a milk allergy. A person can have both conditions. If positive confirmation is necessary, four tests are available.

Hydrogen Breath Test

In a hydrogen breath test, the most accurate lactose intolerance test, after an overnight fast, 25 grams of lactose (in a solution with water) are swallowed. If the lactose cannot be digested, enteric bacteria metabolize it and produce hydrogen, which, along with methane, if produced, can be detected on the patient's breath by a clinical gas chromatograph or compact solid-state detector. The test takes about 2.5 hours to complete. If the hydrogen levels in the patient's breath are high, they may have lactose intolerance. This test is not usually done on babies and very young children, because it can cause severe diarrhea.

Blood Test

In conjunction, measuring blood glucose level every 10 to 15 minutes after ingestion will show a "flat curve" in individuals with lactose malabsorption, while the lactase persistent will have a significant "top", with a typical elevation of 50% to 100%, within one to two hours. However, due to the need for frequent blood sampling, this approach has been largely replaced by breath testing.

After an overnight fast, blood is drawn and then 50 grams of lactose (in aqueous solution) are swallowed. Blood is then drawn again at the 30-minute, 1-hour, 2-hour, and 3-hour marks. If the lactose cannot be digested, blood glucose levels will rise by less than 20 mg/dl.

Stool Acidity Test

This test can be used to diagnose lactose intolerance in infants, for whom other forms of testing are risky or impractical. The infant is given lactose to drink. If the individual is tolerant, the lactose is digested and absorbed in the small intestine; otherwise, it is not digested and absorbed, and it reaches the colon. The bacteria in the colon, mixed with the lactose, cause acidity in stools. Stools passed after the ingestion of the lactose are tested for level of acidity. If the stools are acidic, the infant is intolerant to lactose. Stool pH in lactose intolerance is less than 5.5.

Intestinal Biopsy

An intestinal biopsy can confirm lactase deficiency following discovery of elevated hydrogen in the hydrogen breath test. Modern techniques have enabled a bedside test, identifying presence of lactase enzyme on upper gastrointestinal endoscopy instruments.

However, for research applications such as mRNA measurements, a specialist laboratory is required.

Stool Sugar Chromatography

Chromatography can be used to separate and identify undigested sugars present in faeces. Although lactose may be detected in the faeces of people with lactose intolerance, this test is not considered reliable enough to conclusively diagnose or exclude lactose intolerance.

Genetic Diagnostic

Genetic tests may be useful in assessing whether a person has primary lactose intolerance. Lactase activity persistence in adults is associated with two polymorphisms: C/T 13910 and G/A 22018 located in the MCM6 gene. These polymorphisms may be detected by molecular biology techniques at the DNA extracted from blood or saliva samples; genetic kits specific for this diagnosis are available. The procedure consists of extracting and amplifying DNA from the sample, following with a hybridation protocol in a strip. Colored bands are obtained as final result, and depending on the different combination, it would be possible to determine whether the patient is lactose intolerant. This test allows a noninvasive definitive diagnostic.

Management

When lactose intolerance is due to secondary lactase deficiency, treatment of the underlying disease allows lactase activity to return to normal levels. In people with coeliac disease, lactose intolerance normally revert or improve several months after starting a gluten-free diet, but temporary dietary restriction of lactose may be needed.

Lactose intolerance due to primary lactase deficiency is not considered a condition that requires treatment in societies where the diet contains relatively little dairy. However, those living among societies that are largely lactose-tolerant may find lactose intolerance troublesome. Although no way to reinstate lactase production had been found, some individuals have reported their intolerance varies over time, depending on health status and pregnancy. Some lactose-intolerant women may improve the ability to digest lactose during pregnancy. This might be caused by colonic flora changes during pregnancy. Lactose intolerance can also be managed by ingesting live yogurt cultures containing lactobacilli that are able to digest the lactose in other dairy products. This may explain why many South Asians, though genetically lactose intolerant, are able to consume large quantities of milk without many symptoms of lactose intolerance, since consuming live yogurt cultures is very common among the South Asian population. Lactose intolerance is not usually an absolute condition: the reduction in lactase production, and the amount of lactose that can therefore be tolerated, varies from person to person. Since lactose intolerance poses no further threat to a person's health, the condition is managed by minimizing the occurrence and severity of symptoms. Berdanier and Hargrove recognize four general principles in dealing with lactose intolerance — avoidance of dietary lactose, substitution to maintain nutrient intake, regulation of calcium intake and use of enzyme substitute.

Diet

Individuals vary in the amount of lactose they can tolerate. Label reading is essential, as commercial terminology varies according to language and region.

Lactose is present in two large food categories: conventional dairy products, and as a food additive (casein, caseinate, whey), which may contain traces of lactose.

Dairy Products

Lactose is a water-soluble substance. Fat content and the curdling process affect tolerance of foods. After the curdling process, lactose is found in the water-based portion (along with whey and casein), but not in the fat-based portion. Dairy products that are "reduced-fat" or "fat-free" generally have slightly higher lactose content. Low-fat dairy foods also often have various dairy derivatives added, such as milk solids, increasing the lactose content.

Milk

Human milk has a high lactose content, around 9%. Unprocessed cow milk is about 4.7% lactose. Unprocessed milk from other bovids contains a similar fraction of lactose (goat milk 4.7%, buffalo 4.86%, yak 4.93%, sheep 4.6%)

Butter

The butter-making process separates the majority of milk's water components from the fat components. Lactose, being a water-soluble molecule, will largely be removed, but will still be present in small quantities in the butter unless it is also fermented to produce cultured butter. Clarified butter, however, contains very little lactose and is safe for most lactose-intolerant people.

Yogurt

People can be more tolerant of traditionally made yogurt than milk, because it contains lactase produced by the bacterial cultures used to make the yogurt. Frozen yogurt will contain similarly reduced lactose levels. Greek yogurt is better for lactose intolerant people as more lactose is removed during processing.

Cheeses

Traditionally made hard cheeses, and soft-ripened cheeses may create less reaction than the equivalent amount of milk because of the processes involved. Fermentation and higher fat content contribute to lesser amounts of lactose. Traditionally made Emmental or Cheddar might contain 10% of the lactose found in whole milk. In addition, the ageing methods of traditional cheeses (sometimes over two years) reduce their lactose content to practically nothing. Commercial cheeses, however, are often manufactured by processes that do not have the same lactose-reducing properties. Ageing of some cheeses is governed by regulations; in other cases, no quantitative indication of degree of ageing and concomitant lactose reduction is given, and lactose content is not usually indicated on labels.

Sour Cream

If made in the traditional way, this may be tolerable, but most modern brands add milk solids.

Examples of Lactose Levels in Foods

As industry standardization has not been established concerning lactose content analysis methods (nonhydrated form or the monohydrated form), and considering that dairy content varies greatly according to labeling practices, geography, and manufacturing processes, lactose numbers may not be very reliable. The following table contains a guide to the typical lactose levels found in various foods.

Dairy product	Serving size	Lactose content	Percentage
Milk, regular	250 ml/g	12 g	4.80%
Milk, reduced fat	250 ml/g	13 g	5.20%
Yogurt, plain, regular	200 g	9 g	4.50%
Yogurt, plain, low-fat	200 g	12 g	6.00%
Cheddar cheese	30 g	0.02 g	0.07%
Cottage cheese	30 g	0.1 g	0.33%
Butter	5 g	0.03 g	0.6%
Ice cream	50 g	3 g	6.00%

Lactose in Nondairy Products

Lactose (also present when labels state lactoserum, whey, milk solids, modified milk ingredients, etc.) is a commercial food additive used for its texture, flavor, and adhesive qualities, and is found in foods such as processed meats (sausages/hot dogs, sliced meats, pâtés), gravy stock powder, margarines, sliced breads, breakfast cereals, potato chips,processed foods, medications, prepared meals, meal replacements (powders and bars), protein supplements (powders and bars), and even beers in the milk stout style. Some barbecue sauces and liquid cheeses used in fast-food restaurants may also contain lactose. Lactose is often used as the primary filler (main ingredient) in most Prescription and non-prescription solid pill form medications, though product labeling seldom mentions the presence of 'lactose' or 'milk', and neither do product monograms provided to Pharmacists, and most Pharmacists are unaware of the very wide scale yet common use of lactose in such medications until they contact the supplier or manufacturer for verification.

Kosher products labeled pareve or fleishig are free of milk. However, if a "D" (for "dairy") is present next to the circled "K", "U", or other hechsher, the food product likely contains milk solids, although it may also simply indicate the product was produced on equipment shared with other products containing milk derivatives.

Alternative Products

Plant-based "milks" and derivatives such as soy milk, rice milk, almond milk, coconut milk, hazelnut milk, oat milk, hemp milk, and peanut milk are inherently lactose-free. Low-lactose and lactose-free versions of foods are often available to replace dairy-based foods for those with lactose intolerance.

Lactase Supplementation

When lactose avoidance is not possible, or on occasions when a person chooses to consume such items, then enzymatic lactase supplements may be used.

Lactase enzymes similar to those produced in the small intestines of humans are produced industrially by fungi of the genus Aspergillus. The enzyme, β-galactosidase, is available in tablet form in a variety of doses, in many countries without a prescription. It functions well only in high-acid environments, such as that found in the human gut due to the addition of gastric juices from the stomach. Unfortunately, too much acid can denature it, so it should not be taken on an empty stomach. Also, the enzyme is ineffective if it does not reach the small intestine by the time the problematic food does. Lactose-sensitive individuals can experiment with both timing and dosage to fit their particular needs.

While essentially the same process as normal intestinal lactose digestion, direct treatment of milk employs a different variety of industrially produced lactase. This enzyme, produced by yeast from the genus Kluyveromyces, takes much longer to act, must be thoroughly mixed throughout the product, and is destroyed by even mildly acidic environments. Its main use is in producing the lactose-free or lactose-reduced dairy products sold in supermarkets.

Rehabituation to Dairy Products

For healthy individuals with primary lactose intolerance, it may be possible in some cases for the bacteria in the large intestine to adapt to an altered diet and break down small quantities of lactose more effectively by habitually consuming small amounts of dairy products several times a day over a period of time. This is not suitable for people who have an underlying or chronic illness which may have damaged the intestinal tract in a way which prevents the lactase enzyme from being expressed.

Environmental factors—more specifically, the consumption of lactose—may "play a more important role than genetic factors in the etio-pathogenesis of milk intolerance".

Epidemiology

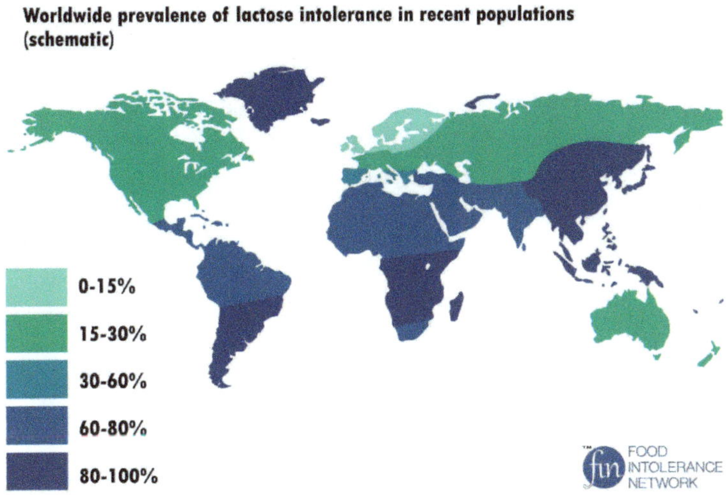

Worldwide rates of lactose intolerance

Overall, about 65% of people experience some form of lactase intolerance as they age past infancy, but there are significant differences between populations and regions, with rates as low as 5% among Northern Europeans and as high as more than 90% of adults in some communities of East Asia.

Lactase persistence is the phenotype associated with various autosomal dominant alleles prolonging the activity of lactase beyond infancy; conversely, lactase nonpersistence is the phenotype associated with primary lactase deficiency. Among mammals, lactase persistence is unique to humans — it evolved relatively recently (in the last 10,000 years) among some populations, and the majority of people worldwide remain lactase nonpersistent. For this reason, lactase persistence is of some interest to the fields of anthropology, human genetics, and archeology, which typically use the genetically derived persistence/non-persistence terminology.

Genetic analysis shows lactase persistence has developed several times in different places independently in an example of convergent evolution.

Recognition of the extent and genetic basis of lactose intolerance is relatively recent. Though its symptoms were described as early as Hippocrates (460-370 BC), until the 1960s, the prevailing assumption in the medical community was that tolerance was the norm and intolerance was either the result of milk allergy, an intestinal pathogen, or else was psychosomatic (it being recognised that some cultures did not practice dairying, and people from those cultures often reacted badly to consuming milk). Two reasons were given for this perception. Firstly, many Western countries have a predominantly European heritage, so have low frequencies of lactose intolerance, and have an extensive cultural history of dairying. Therefore, tolerance actually was the norm in most of the societies investigated by medical researchers at that point. Secondly, within even these societies, lactose intolerance tends to be under-reported: genetically lactase nonpersistent individuals can tolerate varying quantities of lactose before showing symptoms, and their symptoms differ in severity. Most are able to digest a small quantity of milk, for example in tea or coffee, without suffering any adverse effects. Fermented dairy products, such as cheese, also contain dramatically less lactose than plain milk. Therefore, in societies where tolerance is the norm, many people who consume only small amounts of dairy or have only mild symptoms, may be unaware that they cannot digest lactose. Eventually, however, lactose intolerance was recognised in the United States to be correlated with race. Subsequent research revealed intolerance was more common globally than lactase persistence, and that the variation was genetic.

Other Animals

Most mammals normally cease to produce lactase and become lactose intolerant, after weaning.

GALACTOSEMIA

Galactosemia (British galactosaemia) is a rare genetic metabolic disorder that affects an individual's ability to metabolize the sugar galactose properly. Galactosemia follows an autosomal recessive mode of inheritance that confers a deficiency in an enzyme responsible for adequate galactose degradation.

Friedrich Goppert (1870–1927), a German physician, first described the disease in 1917, with its cause as a defect in galactose metabolism being identified by a group led by Herman Kalckar in 1956.

Its incidence is about 1 per 60,000 births for people of European ancestry. In other populations the incidence rate differs. Galactosaemia is about one hundred times more common (1:480 births) within the Irish Traveller population.

Cause

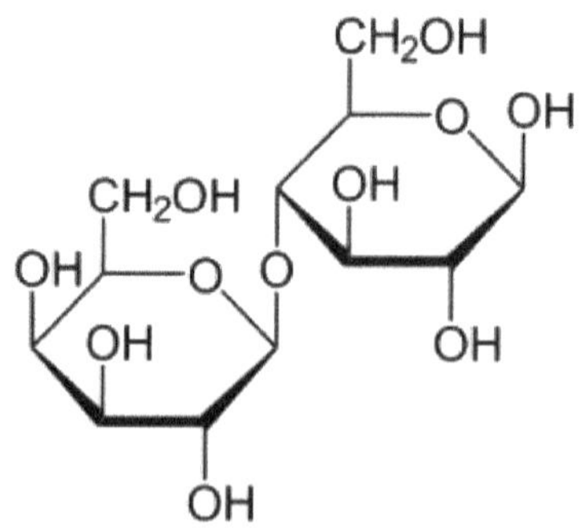

Lactose

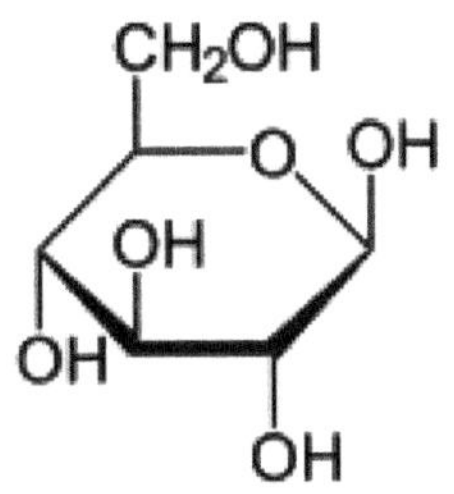

Glucose

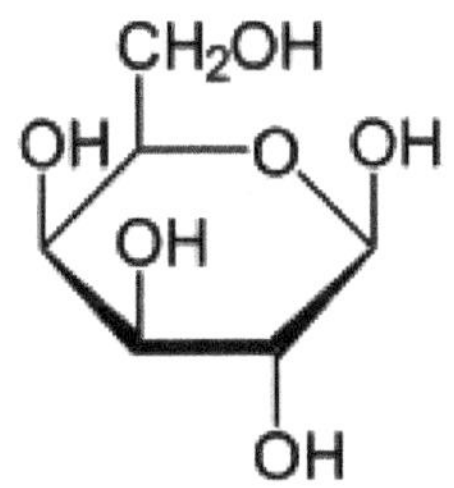

Galactose

Lactose in food (such as dairy products) is broken down by the enzyme lactase into glucose & galactose. In individuals with galactosemia, the enzymes needed for further metabolism of galactose are severely diminished or missing entirely, leading to toxic levels of galactose 1-phosphate in various tissues as in the case of classic galactosemia, resulting in hepatomegaly (an enlarged liver), cirrhosis, renal failure, cataracts, vomiting, seizure, hypoglycemia, lethargy, brain damage, and ovarian failure. Without treatment, mortality in infants with galactosemia is about 75%.

Galactosemia is inherited in an autosomal recessive manner, meaning a child must inherit one defective gene from each parent to show the disease. Heterozygotes are carriers, because they inherit one normal gene & one defective gene. Carriers show no symptoms of galactosemia.

Types

Galactose is converted into glucose by the action of three enzymes, known as the Leloir pathway. There are diseases associated with deficiencies of each of these three enzymes:

Type	Diseases Database	OMIM	Gene	Locus	Enzyme	Name
Type 1	5056	230400	GALT	9p13	galactose-1-phosphate uridyl transferase	classic galactosemia
Type 2	29829	230200	GALK1	17q24	galactokinase	galactokinase deficiency

Type 3	29842	230350	GALE	1p36-p35	UDP galactose epimerase	galactose epimerase deficiency, UDP-Galactose-4-epimerase deficiency

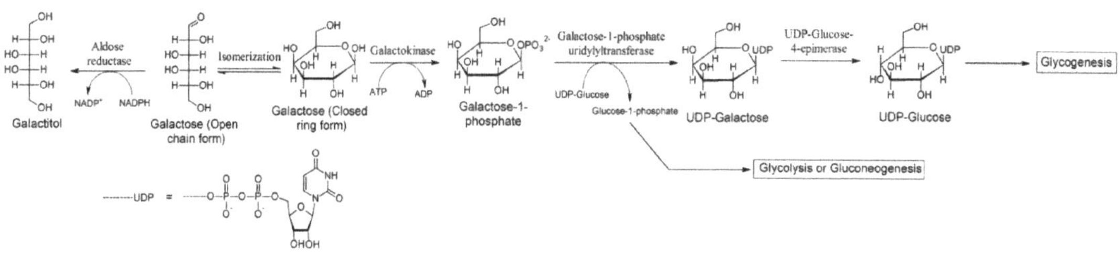

Normal metabolic pathway for galactose in humans.

Accumulation of Galactose

Reduction to Galactitol

In galactosemic patients, the accumulation of galactose becomes the substrate for enzymes that catalyze the polyol pathway of carbohydrate metabolism. The first reaction of this pathway is the reduction of aldoses, types of sugars including galactose, to sugar alcohols. Recent data suggests that aldose reductase is the enzyme responsible for the primary stage of this pathway. Therefore, aldose reductase reduces galactose to its sugar alcohol form, galactitol. Galactitol, however, is not a suitable substrate for the next enzyme in the polyol pathway, polyol dehydrogenase. Thus, galactitol accumulates in body tissues and is excreted in the urine of galactosemic patients. Accumulation of galactitol has been attributed to many of the negative effects of galactosemia, and high concentrations of galactitol have been found in people with classic galactosemia (GALT deficiency or Galactose-1-phosphate uridylyltransferase deficiency), galactokinase deficiency, and epimerase deficiency.

Oxidation to Galactonate

Accumulated galactose can also undergo an alternative reaction: oxidation to galactonate. The mechanism of galactonate formation is still unclear. However, recent studies suggest that galactose dehydrogenase is responsible for converting galactose to galactonolactone, which then spontaneously or enzymatically converts to galactonate. Once formed, galactonate may enter the pentose phosphate pathway. Thus, oxidation to galactonate serves as an alternate pathway for metabolizing galactose. This oxidative pathway renders accumulated galactonate less harmful than accumulated galactitol.

Diagnosis

Infants are routinely screened for galactosemia in the United States, and the diagnosis is made while the person is still an infant. Infants affected by galactosemia typically present with symptoms of lethargy, vomiting, diarrhea, failure to thrive, and jaundice. None of these symptoms are specific to galactosemia, often leading to diagnostic delays. Luckily, most infants are diagnosed on newborn screening. If the family of the baby has a history of galactosemia, doctors can test prior to birth by taking a sample of fluid from around the fetus (amniocentesis) or from the placenta (chorionic villus sampling or CVS).

A galactosemia test is a blood test (from the heel of the infant) or urine test that checks for three enzymes that are needed to change galactose sugar that is found in milk and milk products into glucose, a sugar that the human body uses for energy. A person with galactosemia doesn't have one of these enzymes. This causes high levels of galactose in the blood or urine.

Galactosemia is normally first detected through newborn screening, or NBS. Affected children can have serious, irreversible effects or even die within days from birth. It is important that newborns be screened for metabolic disorders without delay. Galactosemia can even be detected through NBS before any ingestion of galactose-containing formula or breast milk.

Detection of the disorder through newborn screening (NBS) does not depend on protein or lactose ingestion, and, therefore, it should be identified on the first specimen unless the infant has been transfused. A specimen should be taken prior to transfusion. The enzyme is prone to damage if analysis of the sample is delayed or exposed to high temperatures. The routine NBS is accurate for detection of galactosemia. Two screening tests are used to screen infants affected with galactosemia—the Beutler's test and the Hill test. The Beutler's test screens for galactosemia by detecting the level of enzyme of the infant. Therefore, the ingestion of formula or breast milk does not affect the outcome of this part of the NBS, and the NBS is accurate for detecting galactosemia prior to any ingestion of galactose.

Duarte galactosemia is a milder form of classical galactosemia and usually has no long term side effects.

Treatment

The only treatment for classic galactosemia is eliminating lactose and galactose from the diet. Even with an early diagnosis and a restricted diet, however, some individuals with galactosemia experience long-term complications such as speech difficulties, learning disabilities, neurological impairment (e.g. tremors, etc.), and ovarian failure. Symptoms have not been associated with Duarte galactosemia, and many individuals with Duarte galactosemia do not need to restrict their diet at all. However, research corroborates a previously overlooked theory that Duarte galactosemia may lead to language developmental issues in children with no clinical symptoms. Infants with classic galactosemia cannot be breast-fed due to lactose in human breast milk and are usually fed a soy-based formula.

Galactosemia is sometimes confused with lactose intolerance, but galactosemia is a more serious condition. Lactose intolerant individuals have an acquired or inherited shortage of the enzyme lactase, and experience abdominal pains after ingesting dairy products, but no long-term effects. In contrast, a galactosemic individual who consumes galactose can cause permanent damage to their bodies.

Long term complication of galactosemia includes:

- Speech deficits
- Ataxia
- Dysmetria
- Diminished bone density
- Premature ovarian failure
- Cataract

GLYCOGEN STORAGE DISEASE

Glycogen storage disease (GSD, also glycogenosis and dextrinosis) is the result of defects in the processing of glycogen synthesis or breakdown within muscles, liver, and other cell types.

GSD has two classes of cause: genetic and acquired. Genetic GSD is caused by any inborn error of metabolism (genetically defective enzymes) involved in these processes. In livestock, acquired GSD is caused by intoxication with the alkaloid castanospermine.

Types

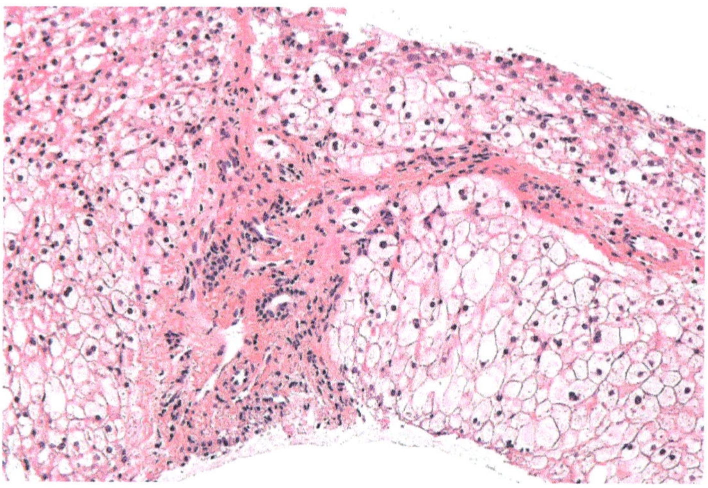

Micrograph of glycogen storage disease with histologic features consistent with Cori disease. Liver biopsy. H&E stain.

There are eleven (11) distinct diseases that are commonly considered to be glycogen storage diseases (some previously thought to be distinct have been reclassified). (Although glycogen synthase deficiency does not result in storage of extra glycogen in the liver, it is often classified with the GSDs as type 0 because it is another defect of glycogen storage and can cause similar problems.)..

- GSD type VIII: In the past, considered a distinct condition. Now classified with VI. Has been described as X-linked recessive.
- GSD type X: In the past, considered a distinct condition. Now classified with VI.

Number	Enzyme deficiency	Eponym	Incidence	Hypo-glycemia?	Hepato-megaly?	Hyperlip-idemia?	Muscle symptoms	Development/ prognosis	Other symptoms
GSD type 0	glycogen synthase	-		Yes	No	No	Occasional muscle cramping	Growth failure in some cases	
GSD type I	glucose-6-phosphatase	von Gierke's disease	1 in 50,000-100,000 births	Yes	Yes	Yes	None	Growth failure	Lactic acidosis, hyperuricemia
GSD type II	acid alpha-glucosidase	Pompe's disease	1 in 40,000 births-50,000	No	Yes	No	Muscle weakness	*Death by age ~2 years (infantile variant)	heart failure
GSD type III	glycogen debranching enzyme	Cori's disease or Forbes' disease	1 in 100,000 births	Yes	Yes	Yes	Myopathy		
GSD type IV	glycogen branching enzyme	Andersen disease	1 to 500,000	No	Yes, also cirrhosis	No	None	Failure to thrive, death at age ~5 years	
GSD type V	muscle glycogen phosphorylase	McArdle disease	1 in 100,000-500,000	No	No	No	Exercise-induced cramps, Rhabdomyolysis		Renal failure by myoglobinuria, second wind phenomenon
GSD type VI	liver glycogen phosphorylase	Hers' disease	1 in 65,000-85,000 births	Yes	Yes	Yes	None	initially benign, growth retardation follows.	
GSD type VII	muscle phosphofructo kinase	Tarui's disease	1 in 1,000,000	No	No	No	Exercise-induced muscle cramps and weakness	growth retardation	Haemolytic anaemia
GSD type IX	Phosphorylase kinase			Yes	Yes	Yes	None	Delayed motor development, Growth retardation	
GSD type XI	glucose transporter, GLUT2	Fanconi-Bickel syndrome		Yes	Yes	No	None		
GSD type XII	Aldolase A	Red cell aldolase deficiency		?	?	?	Exercise intolerance, cramps		
GSD type XIII	β-enolase	-		?	?	?	Exercise intolerance, cramps	Increasing intensity of myalgias over decades	Serum CK: Episodic elevations; Reduced with rest

Prevalence

Overall, according to a study in British Columbia, approximately 2.3 children per 100 000 births (1 in 43,000) have some form of glycogen storage disease. In the United States, they are estimated to occur in 1 per 20,000-25,000 births. A Dutch study estimated it to be 1 in 40,000.

REFERENCES

1. "Diabetes Blue Circle Symbol". International Diabetes Federation. 17 March 2006.
2. "About diabetes". World Health Organization. Archived from the original on 31 March 2014. Retrieved 4 April 2014.
3. "Diabetes Fact sheet N°312". WHO. October 2013. Archived from the original on 26 Aug 2013. Retrieved 25 March 2014.
4. Kitabchi, AE; Umpierrez, GE; Miles, JM; Fisher, JN (Jul 2009). "Hyperglycemic crises in adult patients with diabetes.". Diabetes Care. 32 (7): 1335–43. doi:10.2337/dc09-9032. PMC 2699725 . PMID 19564476.
5. Shoback, edited by David G. Gardner, Dolores (2011). "Chapter 17". Greenspan's basic & clinical endocrinology (9th ed.). New York: McGraw-Hill Medical. ISBN 0-07-162243-8.
6. RSSDI textbook of diabetes mellitus. (Rev. 2nd ed.). New Delhi: Jaypee Brothers Medical Publishers. 2012. p. 235. ISBN 9789350254899.
7. "The top 10 causes of death Fact sheet N°310". World Health Organization. Oct 2013.
8. Rippe, edited by Richard S. Irwin, James M. (2010). Manual of intensive care medicine (5th ed.). Philadelphia: Wolters Kluwer Health/Lippincott Williams & Wilkins. p. 549. ISBN 9780781799928.
9. Picot, J; Jones, J; Colquitt, JL; Gospodarevskaya, E; Loveman, E; Baxter, L; Clegg, AJ (September 2009). "The clinical effectiveness and cost-effectiveness of bariatric (weight loss) surgery for obesity: a systematic review and economic evaluation". Health Technology Assessment (Winchester, England). 13 (41): 1–190, 215–357, iii–iv. doi:10.3310/hta13410. PMID 19726018.
10. Cash, Jill (2014). Family Practice Guidelines (3rd ed.). Springer. p. 396. ISBN 9780826168757.
11. "Update 2015". IDF. International Diabetes Federation. p. 13. Retrieved 21 Mar 2016.
12. Williams textbook of endocrinology (12th ed.). Philadelphia: Elsevier/Saunders. pp. 1371–1435. ISBN 978-1-4377-0324-5.
13. Shi, Yuankai; Hu, Frank B (7 June 2014). "The global implications of diabetes and cancer". The Lancet. 383 (9933): 1947–8. doi:10.1016/S0140-6736(14)60886-2. PMID 24910221.
14. Vos T, Flaxman AD, Naghavi M, Lozano R, Michaud C, Ezzati M, Shibuya K, Salomon JA, Abdalla S, Aboyans V, et al. (Dec 15, 2012). "Years lived with disability (YLDs) for 1160 sequelae of 289 diseases and injuries 1990–2010: a systematic analysis for the Global Burden of Disease Study 2010.". Lancet. 380 (9859): 2163–96. doi:10.1016/S0140-6736(12)61729-2. PMID 23245607.

15. "Annual Report 2014" (PDF). IDF. International Diabetes Federation. Retrieved 13 July 2016.
16. IDF DIABETES ATLAS (PDF) (6th ed.). International Diabetes Federation. 2013. p. 7. ISBN 2930229853.
17. American Diabetes, Association (Apr 2013). "Economic costs of diabetes in the U.S. in 2012.". Diabetes Care. 36 (4): 1033–46. doi:10.2337/dc12-2625. PMC 3609540 . PMID 23468086.
18. Cooke DW, Plotnick L (November 2008). "Type 1 diabetes mellitus in pediatrics". Pediatr Rev. 29 (11): 374–84; quiz 385. doi:10.1542/pir.29-11-374. PMID 18977856.
19. Kenny C (April 2014). "When hypoglycemia is not obvious: diagnosing and treating under-recognized and undisclosed hypoglycemia". Primary care diabetes. 8 (1): 3–11. doi:10.1016/j.pcd.2013.09.002. PMID 24100231.
20. Verrotti A, Scaparrotta A, Olivieri C, Chiarelli F (December 2012). "Seizures and type 1 diabetes mellitus: current state of knowledge". European Journal of Endocrinology. 167 (6): 749–58. doi:10.1530/EJE-12-0699. PMID 22956556. Archived from the original on 2014-11-07.
21. Hsieh, Arthur. "Drunk versus diabetes: How can you tell?". Retrieved 29 June 2016.
22. "Symptoms of Low Blood Sugar". WebMD. Retrieved 29 June 2016.
23. Kitabchi AE, Umpierrez GE, Miles JM, Fisher JN (July 2009). "Hyperglycemic crises in adult patients with diabetes". Diabetes Care. 32 (7): 1335–43. doi:10.2337/dc09-9032. PMC 2699725 . PMID 19564476.
24. Sarwar N, Gao P, Seshasai SR, Gobin R, Kaptoge S, Di Angelantonio E, Ingelsson E, Lawlor DA, Selvin E, Stampfer M, Stehouwer CD, Lewington S, Pennells L, Thompson A, Sattar N, White IR, Ray KK, Danesh J (2010). "Diabetes mellitus, fasting blood glucose concentration, and risk of vascular disease: A collaborative meta-analysis of 102 prospective studies". The Lancet. 375 (9733): 2215–22. doi:10.1016/S0140-6736(10)60484-9. PMC 2904878 . PMID 20609967.
25. O'Gara PT, Kushner FG, Ascheim DD, Casey DE, Chung MK, de Lemos JA, Ettinger SM, Fang JC, Fesmire FM, Franklin BA, Granger CB, Krumholz HM, Linderbaum JA, Morrow DA, Newby LK, Ornato JP, Ou N, Radford MJ, Tamis-Holland JE, Tommaso CL, Tracy CM, Woo YJ, Zhao DX, Anderson JL, Jacobs AK, Halperin JL, Albert NM, Brindis RG, Creager MA, DeMets D, Guyton RA, Hochman JS, Kovacs RJ, Kushner FG, Ohman EM, Stevenson WG, Yancy CW (29 January 2013). "2013 ACCF/AHA guideline for the management of ST-elevation myocardial infarction: a report of the American College of Cardiology Foundation/American Heart Association Task Force on Practice Guidelines.". Circulation. 127 (4): e362–425. doi:10.1161/CIR.0b013e3182742cf6. PMID 23247304.
26. "Diabetes Programme". World Health Organization. Retrieved 22 April 2014.
27. Cukierman, T (8 Nov 2005). "Cognitive decline and dementia in diabetes—

systematic overview of prospective observational studies". Springer-Verlag. Retrieved 28 Apr 2013.

28. Lambert P, Bingley PJ (2002). "What is Type 1 Diabetes?". Medicine. 30: 1–5. doi:10.1383/medc.30.1.1.28264.
29. Tuomi T, Santoro N, Caprio S, Cai M, Weng J, Groop L (2014). "The many faces of diabetes: a disease with increasing heterogeneity". Lancet. 383 (9922): 1084–94. doi:10.1016/S0140-6736(13)62219-9. PMID 24315621.
30. Rother KI (April 2007). "Diabetes treatment—bridging the divide". The New England Journal of Medicine. 356 (15): 1499–501. doi:10.1056/NEJMp078030. PMC 4152979 . PMID 17429082.
31. "Diabetes Mellitus (DM): Diabetes Mellitus and Disorders of Carbohydrate Metabolism: Merck Manual Professional". Merck Publishing. April 2010. Retrieved 2010-07-30.
32. Dorner M, Pinget M, Brogard JM (May 1977). "Essential labile diabetes". MMW Munch Med Wochenschr (in German). 119 (19): 671–4. PMID 406527.
33. Phillips JE, Couper JJ, Penno MA, Harrison LC, ENDIA Study Group (2016). "Type 1 diabetes: a disease of developmental origins.". Pediatr Diabetes (Review). doi:10.1111/pedi.12425. PMID 27526948.
34. Petzold A, Solimena M, Knoch KP (2015). "Mechanisms of Beta Cell Dysfunction Associated With Viral Infection.". Curr Diab Rep (Review). 15 (10): 73. doi:10.1007/s11892-015-0654-x. PMC 4539350 . PMID 26280364. So far, none of the hypotheses accounting for virus-induced beta cell autoimmunity has been supported by stringent evidence in humans, and the involvement of several mechanisms rather than just one is also plausible.
35. Butalia S, Kaplan GG, Khokhar B, Rabi DM (Aug 18, 2016). "Environmental Risk Factors and Type 1 Diabetes: Past, Present, and Future". Can J Diabetes (Review). 40: 586–593. doi:10.1016/j.jcjd.2016.05.002. PMID 27545597.
36. Serena G, Camhi S, Sturgeon C, Yan S, Fasano A (2015). "The Role of Gluten in Celiac Disease and Type 1 Diabetes.". Nutrients. 7 (9): 7143–62. doi:10.3390/nu7095329. PMC 4586524 . PMID 26343710.
37. Visser J, Rozing J, Sapone A, Lammers K, Fasano A (2009). "Tight junctions, intestinal permeability, and autoimmunity: celiac disease and type 1 diabetes paradigms.". Ann N Y Acad Sci. 1165: 195–205. doi:10.1111/j.1749-6632.2009.04037.x. PMC 2886850 . PMID 19538307.
38. Risérus U, Willett WC, Hu FB (January 2009). "Dietary fats and prevention of type 2 diabetes". Progress in Lipid Research. 48 (1): 44–51. doi:10.1016/j.plipres.2008.10.002. PMC 2654180 . PMID 19032965.
39. Malik VS, Popkin BM, Bray GA, Després JP, Hu FB (2010-03-23). "Sugar Sweetened Beverages, Obesity, Type 2 Diabetes and Cardiovascular Disease risk". Circulation. 121 (11): 1356–64. doi:10.1161/CIRCULATIONAHA.109.876185. PMC 2862465 . PMID 20308626.
40. Malik VS, Popkin BM, Bray GA, Després JP, Willett WC, Hu FB (November

2010). "Sugar-Sweetened Beverages and Risk of Metabolic Syndrome and Type 2 Diabetes: A meta-analysis". Diabetes Care. 33 (11): 2477–83. doi:10.2337/dc10-1079. PMC 2963518 . PMID 20693348.

41. Hu EA, Pan A, Malik V, Sun Q (2012-03-15). "White rice consumption and risk of type 2 diabetes: meta-analysis and systematic review". BMJ (Clinical research ed.). 344: e1454. doi:10.1136/bmj.e1454. PMC 3307808 . PMID 22422870.
42. Lee IM, Shiroma EJ, Lobelo F, Puska P, Blair SN, Katzmarzyk PT (1 July 2012). "Effect of physical inactivity on major non-communicable diseases worldwide: an analysis of burden of disease and life expectancy". The Lancet. 380 (9838): 219–29. doi:10.1016/S0140-6736(12)61031-9. PMC 3645500 . PMID 22818936.
43. "National Diabetes Clearinghouse (NDIC): National Diabetes Statistics 2011". U.S. Department of Health and Human Services. Retrieved 22 April 2014.
44. "Definition, Diagnosis and Classification of Diabetes Mellitus and its Complications" (PDF). World Health Organisation. 1999.
45. de la Monte, SM (December 2014). "Type 3 diabetes is sporadic Alzheimer's disease: mini-review.". European neuropsychopharmacology : the journal of the European College of Neuropsychopharmacology. 24 (12): 1954–60. doi:10.1016/j.euroneuro.2014.06.008. PMC 4444430 . PMID 25088942.
46. Unless otherwise specified, reference is: Table 20-5 in Mitchell, Richard Sheppard; Kumar, Vinay; Abbas, Abul K.; Fausto, Nelson. Robbins Basic Pathology (8th ed.). Philadelphia: Saunders. ISBN 1-4160-2973-7.
47. Sattar N, Preiss D, Murray HM, Welsh P, Buckley BM, de Craen AJ, Seshasai SR, McMurray JJ, Freeman DJ, Jukema JW, Macfarlane PW, Packard CJ, Stott DJ, Westendorp RG, Shepherd J, Davis BR, Pressel SL, Marchioli R, Marfisi RM, Maggioni AP, Tavazzi L, Tognoni G, Kjekshus J, Pedersen TR, Cook TJ, Gotto AM, Clearfield MB, Downs JR, Nakamura H, Ohashi Y, Mizuno K, Ray KK, Ford I (February 2010). "Statins and risk of incident diabetes: a collaborative meta-analysis of randomised statin trials". The Lancet. 375 (9716): 735–42. doi:10.1016/S0140-6736(09)61965-6. PMID 20167359.
48. "Insulin Basics". American Diabetes Association. Retrieved 24 April 2014.
49. Shoback, edited by David G. Gardner, Dolores (2011). Greenspan's basic & clinical endocrinology (9th ed.). New York: McGraw-Hill Medical. ISBN 9780071622431.
50. al.], Kim E. Barrett, ... et (2012). Ganong's review of medical physiology. (24th ed.). New York: McGraw-Hill Medical. ISBN 0071780033.
51. al.], Robert K. Murray ... et (2012). Harper's illustrated biochemistry (29th ed.). New York: McGraw-Hill Medical. ISBN 007176576X.
52. Definition and diagnosis of diabetes mellitus and intermediate hyperglycemia: report of a WHO/IDF consultation (PDF). Geneva: World Health Organization. 2006. p. 21. ISBN 978-92-4-159493-6.
53. Vijan, S (March 2010). "Type 2 diabetes". Annals of Internal Medicine. 152 (5): ITC31-15. doi:10.7326/0003-4819-152-5-201003020-01003. PMID 20194231.

54. “”Diabetes Care” January 2010”. American Diabetes Association. Retrieved 2010-01-29.

55. Saydah SH, Miret M, Sung J, Varas C, Gause D, Brancati FL (August 2001). “Postchallenge hyperglycemia and mortality in a national sample of U.S. adults”. Diabetes Care. 24 (8): 1397–402. doi:10.2337/diacare.24.8.1397. PMID 11473076.

56. Definition and diagnosis of diabetes mellitus and intermediate hyperglycemia : report of a WHO/IDF consultation (PDF). World Health Organization. 2006. p. 21. ISBN 978-92-4-159493-6.

57. Santaguida PL, Balion C, Hunt D, Morrison K, Gerstein H, Raina P, Booker L, Yazdi H. “Diagnosis, Prognosis, and Treatment of Impaired Glucose Tolerance and Impaired Fasting Glucose”. Summary of Evidence Report/Technology Assessment, No. 128. Agency for Healthcare Research and Quality. Retrieved 2008-07-20.

58. Bartoli E, Fra GP, Carnevale Schianca GP (Feb 2011). “The oral glucose tolerance test (OGTT) revisited.”. European journal of internal medicine. 22 (1): 8–12. doi:10.1016/j.ejim.2010.07.008. PMID 21238885.

59. Selvin E, Steffes MW, Zhu H, Matsushita K, Wagenknecht L, Pankow J, Coresh J, Brancati FL (2010). “Glycated hemoglobin, diabetes, and cardiovascular risk in nondiabetic adults”. N. Engl. J. Med. 362 (9): 800–11. doi:10.1056/NEJMoa0908359. PMC 2872990 . PMID 20200384.

60. Kyu, Hmwe H; Bachman, Victoria F; Alexander, Lily T; Mumford, John Everett; Afshin, Ashkan; Estep, Kara; Veerman, J Lennert; Delwiche, Kristen; Iannarone, Marissa L; Moyer, Madeline L; Cercy, Kelly; Vos, Theo; Murray, Christopher J L; Forouzanfar, Mohammad H (9 August 2016). “Physical activity and risk of breast cancer, colon cancer, diabetes, ischemic heart disease, and ischemic stroke events: systematic review and dose-response meta-analysis for the Global Burden of Disease Study 2013”. BMJ: i3857. doi:10.1136/bmj.i3857.

61. “The Nutrition Source”. Harvard School of Public Health. Retrieved 24 April 2014.

62. Willi C, Bodenmann P, Ghali WA, Faris PD, Cornuz J (Dec 12, 2007). “Active smoking and the risk of type 2 diabetes: a systematic review and meta-analysis.”. JAMA: The Journal of the American Medical Association. 298 (22): 2654–64. doi:10.1001/jama.298.22.2654. PMID 18073361.

63. World Health Organization, Chronic diseases and their common risk factors. Geneva, 2005. Accessed 30 August 2016.

64. No cure for diabetes (Retrieved May 2015, WebMD website)

65. Nathan DM, Cleary PA, Backlund JY, Genuth SM, Lachin JM, Orchard TJ, Raskin P, Zinman B (December 2005). “Intensive diabetes treatment and cardiovascular disease in patients with type 1 diabetes”. The New England Journal of Medicine. 353 (25): 2643–53. doi:10.1056/NEJMoa052187. PMC 2637991 . PMID 16371630.

66. The Diabetes Control; Complications Trial Research Group (April 1995). “The effect of intensive diabetes therapy on the development and progression of

neuropathy.". Annals of Internal Medicine. 122 (8): 561–8. doi:10.1059/0003-4819-122-8-199504150-00001. PMID 7887548.

67. National Institute for Health and Clinical Excellence. Clinical guideline 66: Type 2 diabetes. London, 2008.

68. Cavanagh PR (2004). "Therapeutic footwear for people with diabetes". Diabetes Metab. Res. Rev. 20 (Suppl 1): S51–5. doi:10.1002/dmrr.435. PMID 15150815.

69. Adler AI, Stratton IM, Neil HA, Yudkin JS, Matthews DR, Cull CA, Wright AD, Turner RC, Holman RR (August 2000). "Association of systolic blood pressure with macrovascular and microvascular complications of type 2 diabetes (UKPDS 36): prospective observational study". BMJ. 321 (7258): 412–9. doi:10.1136/bmj.321.7258.412. PMC 27455 . PMID 10938049.

70. Ripsin CM, Kang H, Urban RJ (2009). "Management of blood glucose in type 2 diabetes mellitus" (PDF). American family physician. 79 (1): 29–36. PMID 19145963.

71. Krentz, AJ; Bailey, CJ (2005). "Oral antidiabetic agents: current role in type 2 diabetes mellitus.". Drugs. 65 (3): 385–411. doi:10.2165/00003495-200565030-00005. PMID 15669880.

72. Consumer Reports; American College of Physicians (April 2012), "Choosing a type 2 diabetes drug - Why the best first choice is often the oldest drug" (PDF), High Value Care, Consumer Reports, retrieved August 14, 2012

73. Nelson, Mark. "Drug treatment of elevated blood pressure". Australian Prescriber (33): 108–112. Retrieved 11 August 2010.

74. Arguedas, JA; Perez, MI; Wright, JM (Jul 8, 2009). Arguedas, Jose Agustin, ed. "Treatment blood pressure targets for hypertension". Cochrane Database of Systematic Reviews (3): CD004349. doi:10.1002/14651858.CD004349.pub2. PMID 19588353.

75. Arguedas, JA; Leiva, V; Wright, JM (Oct 30, 2013). "Blood pressure targets for hypertension in people with diabetes mellitus.". The Cochrane database of systematic reviews. 10: CD008277. doi:10.1002/14651858.cd008277.pub2. PMID 24170669.

76. Brunström, Mattias; Carlberg, Bo (24 February 2016). "Effect of antihypertensive treatment at different blood pressure levels in patients with diabetes mellitus: systematic review and meta-analyses". BMJ: i717. doi:10.1136/bmj.i717.

77. Cheng J, Zhang W, Zhang X, Han F, Li X, He X, Li Q, Chen J (Mar 31, 2014). "Effect of Angiotensin-Converting Enzyme Inhibitors and Angiotensin II Receptor Blockers on All-Cause Mortality, Cardiovascular Deaths, and Cardiovascular Events in Patients With Diabetes Mellitus: A Meta-analysis.". JAMA internal medicine. 174 (5): 773–85. doi:10.1001/jamainternmed.2014.348. PMID 24687000.

78. Pignone M, Alberts MJ, Colwell JA, Cushman M, Inzucchi SE, Mukherjee D, Rosenson RS, Williams CD, Wilson PW, Kirkman MS (June 2010). "Aspirin for primary prevention of cardiovascular events in people with diabetes: a position statement of the American Diabetes Association, a scientific statement

of the American Heart Association, and an expert consensus document of the American College of Cardiology Foundation". Diabetes Care. 33 (6): 1395–402. doi:10.2337/dc10-0555. PMC 2875463 . PMID 20508233.

79. "Pancreas Transplantation". American Diabetes Association. Retrieved 9 April 2014.
80. Picot, J; Jones, J; Colquitt, JL; Gospodarevskaya, E; Loveman, E; Baxter, L; Clegg, AJ (September 2009). "The clinical effectiveness and cost-effectiveness of bariatric (weight loss) surgery for obesity: a systematic review and economic evaluation". Health technology assessment (Winchester, England). 13 (41): 1–190, 215–357, iii–iv. doi:10.3310/hta13410. PMID 19726018.
81. Frachetti, KJ; Goldfine, AB (April 2009). "Bariatric surgery for diabetes management". Current Opinion in Endocrinology, Diabetes and Obesity. 16 (2): 119–24. doi:10.1097/MED.0b013e32832912e7. PMID 19276974.
82. ^ Jump up to:a b Schulman, AP; del Genio, F; Sinha, N; Rubino, F (September–October 2009). ""Metabolic" surgery for treatment of type 2 diabetes mellitus". Endocrine Practice. 15 (6): 624–31. doi:10.4158/EP09170.RAR. PMID 19625245.
83. Colucci, RA (January 2011). "Bariatric surgery in patients with type 2 diabetes: a viable option". Postgraduate Medicine. 123 (1): 24–33. doi:10.3810/pgm.2011.01.2242. PMID 21293081.
84. Dixon, JB; le Roux, CW; Rubino, F; Zimmet, P (16 June 2012). "Bariatric surgery for type 2 diabetes". Lancet. 379 (9833): 2300–11. doi:10.1016/S0140-6736(12)60401-2. PMID 22683132.
85. Polisena J, Tran K, Cimon K, Hutton B, McGill S, Palmer K (2009). "Home telehealth for diabetes management: a systematic review and meta-analysis". Diabetes Obes Metab. 11 (10): 913–30. doi:10.1111/j.1463-1326.2009.01057.x. PMID 19531058.
86. World Health Organization, Global Report on Diabetes. Geneva, 2016.
87. Gale EA, Gillespie KM (2001). "Diabetes and gender". Diabetologia. 44 (1): 3–15. doi:10.1007/s001250051573.
88. Meisinger C, Thorand B, Schneider A; et al. (2002). "Sex differences in risk factors for incident type 2 Diabetes Mellitus: The MONICA Augsburg Cohort Study". JAMA Internal Medicine. 162 (1): 82–89. doi:10.1001/archinte.162.1.82.
89. Public Health Agency of Canada, Diabetes in Canada: Facts and figures from a public health perspective. Ottawa, 2011.
90. Mathers CD, Loncar D (November 2006). "Projections of global mortality and burden of disease from 2002 to 2030". PLoS Med. 3 (11): e442. doi:10.1371/journal.pmed.0030442. PMC 1664601 . PMID 17132052.
91. Wild S, Roglic G, Green A, Sicree R, King H (2004). "Global prevalence of diabetes: Estimates for the year 2000 and projections for 2030". Diabetes Care. 27 (5): 1047–53. doi:10.2337/diacare.27.5.1047. PMID 15111519.
92. Ripoll, Brian C. Leutholtz, Ignacio (2011-04-25). Exercise and disease management (2nd ed.). Boca Raton: CRC Press. p. 25. ISBN 978-1-4398-2759-8.

93. editor, Leonid Poretsky, (2009). Principles of diabetes mellitus (2nd ed.). New York: Springer. p. 3. ISBN 978-0-387-09840-1.
94. Roberts, Jacob (2015). "Sickening sweet". Distillations. 1 (4): 12–15. Retrieved 3 January 2017.
95. Laios K, Karamanou M, Saridaki Z, Androutsos G (2012). "Aretaeus of Cappadocia and the first description of diabetes" (PDF). Hormones. 11 (1): 109–113. PMID 22450352.
96. Oxford English Dictionary. diabetes. Retrieved 2011-06-10.
97. Harper, Douglas (2001–2010). "Online Etymology Dictionary. diabetes.". Retrieved 2011-06-10.
98. Aretaeus, De causis et signis acutorum morborum (lib. 2), Κεφ. β. περ Διαβήτεω (Chapter 2, On Diabetes, Greek original, on Perseus
99. Oxford English Dictionary. mellite. Retrieved 2011-06-10.
100. "MyEtimology. mellitus.". Retrieved 2011-06-10.
101. Oxford English Dictionary. -ite. Retrieved 2011-06-10.
102. Theodore H. Tulchinsky, Elena A. Varavikova (2008). The New Public Health, Second Edition. New York: Academic Press. p. 200. ISBN 0-12-370890-7.
103. Piwernetz K, Home PD, Snorgaard O, Antsiferov M, Staehr-Johansen K, Krans M (May 1993). "Monitoring the targets of the St Vincent Declaration and the implementation of quality management in diabetes care: the DIABCARE initiative. The DIABCARE Monitoring Group of the St Vincent Declaration Steering Committee". Diabetic Medicine. 10 (4): 371–7. doi:10.1111/j.1464-5491.1993.tb00083.x. PMID 8508624.
104. Dubois, HFW; Bankauskaite, V (2005). "Type 2 diabetes programmes in Europe" (PDF). Euro Observer. 7 (2): 5–6.
105. Stewart WF, Ricci JA, Chee E, Hirsch AG, Brandenburg NA (June 2007). "Lost productive time and costs due to diabetes and diabetic neuropathic pain in the US workforce". J. Occup. Environ. Med. 49 (6): 672–9. doi:10.1097/JOM.0b013e318065b83a. PMID 17563611.
106. Washington R.E.; Andrews R.M.; Mutter R.L. (November 2013). "Emergency Department Visits for Adults with Diabetes, 2010". HCUP Statistical Brief #167. Rockville MD: Agency for Healthcare Research and Quality.
107. Parker, Katrina (2008). Living with diabetes. New York: Facts On File. p. 143. ISBN 9781438121086.
108. "Diabetes mellitus". Merck Veterinary Manual, 9th edition (online version). 2005. Retrieved 2011-10-23.
109. Maria Rotella C, Pala L, Mannucci E (Summer 2013). "Role of Insulin in the Type 2 Diabetes Therapy: Past, Present and Future.". International journal of endocrinology and metabolism. 11 (3): 137–144. doi:10.5812/ijem.7551. PMC 3860110 . PMID 24348585.
110. "Press Announcement". FDA. Retrieved 11 February 2016.

111. "Inhaled Insulin Clears Hurdle Toward F.D.A. Approval". New York Times. Retrieved 12 April 2014.
112. in-PharmaTechnologist.com. "World›s first transdermal insulin shows promise". Retrieved 2016-07-03.
113. "PHOSPHAGENICS INITIATES TRIAL OF TRANSDERMAL INSULIN GEL". www.fdanews.com. Retrieved 2016-07-03.
114. "Lactose Intolerance". NIDDK. June 2014. Retrieved 25 October 2016.
115. Heyman MB (2006). "Lactose Intolerance in Infants, Children, and Adolescents". Pediatrics (Review). 118 (3): 1279–1286. doi:10.1542/peds.2006-1721. PMID 16951027.
116. Deng Y, Misselwitz B, Dai N, Fox M (2015). "Lactose Intolerance in Adults: Biological Mechanism and Dietary Management". Nutrients (Review). 7 (9): 8020–35. doi:10.3390/nu7095380. PMC 4586575 . PMID 26393648.
117. Berni Canani R, Pezzella V, Amoroso A, Cozzolino T, Di Scala C, Passariello A (Mar 10, 2016). "Diagnosing and Treating Intolerance to Carbohydrates in Children". Nutrients (Review). 8 (3): pii: E157. doi:10.3390/nu8030157. PMC 4808885 . PMID 26978392.
118. Suchy FJ, Brannon PM, Carpenter TO, Fernandez JR, Gilsanz V, Gould JB, et al. (2010). "NIH consensus development conference statement: Lactose intolerance and health.". NIH Consens State Sci Statements (Consensus Development Conference, NIH. Review). 27 (2): 1–27. PMID 20186234.
119. "How many people are affected or at risk for lactose intolerance?". NICHD. 6 May 2014. Retrieved 25 October 2016.
120. Ingram, Catherine J. E.; Mulcare, Charlotte A.; Itan, Yuval; Thomas, Mark G.; Swallow, Dallas M. (2008-11-26). "Lactose digestion and the evolutionary genetics of lactase persistence". Human Genetics. 124 (6): 579–591. doi:10.1007/s00439-008-0593-6. ISSN 0340-6717.
121. Bahna SL (2002). "Cow›s milk allergy versus cow milk intolerance.". Ann Allergy Asthma Immunol (Review. Comparative Study.). 89 (6 Suppl 1): 56–60. doi:10.1016/S1081-1206(10)62124-2. PMID 12487206.
122. Savaiano DA, Levitt MD (1987). "Milk intolerance and microbe-containing dairy foods". J. Dairy Sci. 70 (2): 397–406. doi:10.3168/jds.S0022-0302(87)80023-1. PMID 3553256.
123. Mądry, E.; Krasińska, B.; Woźniewicz, M. G.; Drzymała-Czyż, S. A.; Bobkowski, W.; Torlińska, T.; Walkowiak, J. A. (2011). "Tolerance of different dairy products in subjects with symptomatic lactose malabsorption due to adult type hypolactasia". Gastroenterology Review. 5: 310–315. doi:10.5114/pg.2011.25381.
124. name="Sinden, A.A 1991 Emedicine|PED|1270|Lactose Intolerance" Guandalini S, Frye R, Rivera-Hernández D, Miller L, Borowitz S
125. Lactose intolerance~overview at eMedicine
126. Swallow DM (2003). "Genetics of lactase persistence and lactose intolerance". Annu. Rev. Genet. 37: 197–219. doi:10.1146/annurev.genet.37.110801.143820.

PMID 14616060.

127. Genetics Home Reference. “MCM6”. Genetics Home Reference.
128. Benjamin Phelan (23 October 2012). “Evolution of lactose tolerance: Why do humans keep drinking milk?”. Slate Magazine.
129. “Lactose Intolerance”. Johns Hopkins Health Library. Retrieved 2014-02-18.
130. Gibbons, Ann (2 April 2015) How Europeans evolved white skin Science, Retrieved 13 April 2015
131. Beja-Pereira A, et al. (2003). “Gene-culture coevolution between cattle milk protein genes and human lactase genes”. Nat Genet. 35: 311–313. doi:10.1038/ng1263.
132. Ingram CJ, Mulcare CA, Itan Y, Thomas MG, Swallow DM (Jan 2009). “Lactose digestion and the evolutionary genetics of lactase persistence”. Hum Genet. 124 (6): 579–91. doi:10.1007/s00439-008-0593-6.
133. Tishkoff et al. 2006.
134. Enattah NS, Sahi T, Savilahti E, Terwilliger JD, Peltonen L, Järvelä I (2002). “Identification of a variant associated with adult-type hypolactasia”. Nat. Genet. 30 (2): 233–7. doi:10.1038/ng826. PMID 11788828.
135. Swallow DM (2003). “Genetics of lactase persistence and lactose intolerance”. Annual Review of Genetics. 37: 197–219. doi:10.1146/annurev.genet.37.110801.143820. PMID 14616060.
136. “Lactose intolerance”.
137. Secundary lactase deficiency causes
138. Swagerty DL, Walling AD, Klein RM (2002). “Lactose intolerance”. Am Fam Physician. 65 (9): 1845–50. PMID 12018807.
139. Lawson, Margaret; Bentley, Donald; Lifschitz, Carlos (2002). Pediatric gastroenterology and clinical nutrition. London: Remedica. p. 109. ISBN 978-1-901346-43-5.
140. Pediatric Lactose Intolerance at eMedicine
141. Swagerty DL, Walling AD, Klein RM (2002). “Lactose intolerance”. Am Fam Physician (Review). 65 (9): 1845–50. PMID 12018807.
142. R. Bowen (December 28, 2006). “Lactose Intolerance (Lactase Non-Persistence)”. Pathophysiology of the Digestive System. Colorado State University.
143. Olivier CE, Lorena SL, Pavan CR, dos Santos RA, dos Santos Lima RP, Pinto DG, da Silva MD, de Lima Zollner R (2012). “Is it just lactose intolerance?”. Allergy and Asthma Proceedings. 33 (5): 432–6. doi:10.2500/aap.2012.33.3584. PMID 23026186.
144. “Lactose Intolerance Tests and Results”. WebMD.
145. “Lactose tolerance tests”. 3 May 2011.
146. National Digestive Diseases Information Clearinghouse (March 2006). “Lactose Intolerance — How is lactose intolerance diagnosed?”. National Institute of

Diabetes and Digestive and Kidney Diseases, National Institutes of Health.

147. "Stool Acidity Test". Jay W. Marks, M.D. Retrieved 2011-05-20.
148. Hargrove, James L.; Berdanier, Carolyn D. (1993). Nutrition and gene expression. Boca Raton: CRC Press. ISBN 0-8493-6961-4.
149. Kuokkanen M, Myllyniemi M, Vauhkonen M, Helske T, Kääriäinen I, Karesvuori S, Linnala A, Härkönen M, Järvelä I, Sipponen P (2006). "A biopsy-based quick test in the diagnosis of duodenal hypolactasia in upper gastrointestinal endoscopy". Endoscopy. 38 (7): 708–12. doi:10.1055/s-2006-925354. PMID 16761211.
150. Deng Y, Misselwitz B, Dai N, Fox M (2015). "Lactose Intolerance in Adults: Biological Mechanism and Dietary Management". Nutrients (Review). 7 (9): 8020–35. doi:10.3390/nu7095380. PMC 4586575 . PMID 26393648.
151. Enattah NS, Sahi T, Savilahti E, Terwilliger JD, Peltonen L, Järvelä I (2002). "Identification of a variant associated with adult-type hypolactasia". Nature Genetics. 30 (2): 233–7. doi:10.1038/ng826. PMID 11788828.
152. Vandenplas Y (2015). "Lactose intolerance.". Asia Pac J Clin Nutr (Review). 24 Suppl 1: S9–13. doi:10.6133/apjcn.2015.24.s1.02. PMID 26715083.
153. Levy J, Bernstein L, Silber N (Dec 2014). "Celiac disease: an immune dysregulation syndrome". Curr Probl Pediatr Adolesc Health Care (Review). 44 (11): 324–7. doi:10.1016/j.cppeds.2014.10.002. PMID 25499458. Initially, reduced levels of lactase and sucrase activities might necessitate further dietary restrictions until the villi have healed and those sugars are better tolerated.
154. Lactose Intolerance at eMedicine Roy, Barakat, Nwakakwa, Shojamanesh, Khurana, July 5, 2006
155. Szilagyi A (2015). "Adaptation to Lactose in Lactase Non Persistent People: Effects on Intolerance and the Relationship between Dairy Food Consumption and Evalution sic of Diseases". Nutrients (Review). 7 (8): 6751–79. doi:10.3390/nu7085309. PMC 4555148 . PMID 26287234.
156. http://www.efsa.europa.eu/en/efsajournal/doc/1763.pdf
157. Gary Pfalzbot (25 December 2003). "Composition of Human, Cow, and Goat Milks - Goat Milk - GOATWORLD.COM".
158. Peeva (2001). "Composition of buffalo milk. Sources of specific effects on the separate components". Bulg. J. Agric. Sci. 7: 329–35.
159. C:\JAG2\Jiang.vp
160. "Can a Lactose Intolerant Eat Some Yogurt & Aged Cheese?".
161. "Dairy Good: Home".
162. "PDO - Our Provenance, speciality fine cheese : West Country Farmhouse Cheesemakers : Handmade Westcountry Farmhouse Cheeses".
163. Reger, Combs, Coulter and Koch (February 1, 1951). "A Comparison of Dry Sweet Cream Buttermilk and Non-Fat Dry Milk Solids in Breadmaking". Journal of Dairy Science. 34 (2): 136–44. doi:10.3168/jds.S0022-0302(51)91682-7.

164. "Goat Dairy Foods".

165. "Diet for Lactose Intolerance".

166. "General guidelines for milk allergy". Oregon Health & Science University.

167. "Margarine Regulations".

168. "Enriched White Bread in Canada". The Canadian Celiac Association.

169. Riggs, Lloyd K; Beaty, Annabel; Johnson, Arnold H (December 1946). "Influence of Nonfat Dry Milk Solids on the Nutritive Value of Bread". Journal of Dairy Science. 29 (12): 821–9. doi:10.3168/jds.S0022-0302(46)92546-5.

170. "Bartek, food additive company" (PDF).

171. Montalto M, Curigliano V, Santoro L, Vastola M, Cammarota G, Manna R, Gasbarrini A, Gasbarrini G (2006). "Management and treatment of lactose malabsorption". World J. Gastroenterol. 12 (2): 187–91. PMID 16482616.

172. He M, Yang Y, Bian L, Cui H (1999). "Effect of exogenous lactase on the absorption of lactose and its intolerance symptoms". Wei Sheng Yan Jiu (in Chinese). 28 (5): 309–11. PMID 12712706.

173. O›Connell S, Walsh G (2006). "Physicochemical characteristics of commercial lactases relevant to their application in the alleviation of lactose intolerance". Appl. Biochem. Biotechnol. 134 (2): 179–91. doi:10.1385/ABAB:134:2:179. PMID 16943638.

174. Lactose intolerant? Drink more milk Steve Tally

175. Yoshida Y, Sasaki G, Goto S, Yanagiya S, Takashina K (1975). "Studies on the etiology of milk intolerance in Japanese adults". Gastroenterol. Jpn. 10 (1): 29–34. PMID 1234085.

176. "Lactose intolerance". Genetics Home Reference. Retrieved 18 November 2016.

177. Curry, Andrew (31 July 2013). "Archaeology: The milk revolution". Nature.

178. Tishkoff SA, Reed FA, Ranciaro A, Voight BF, Babbitt CC, Silverman JS, Powell K, Mortensen HM, Hirbo JB, Osman M, Ibrahim M, Omar SA, Lema G, Nyambo TB, Ghori J, Bumpstead S, Pritchard JK, Wray GA, Deloukas P (10 December 2006). "Convergent adaptation of human lactase persistence in Africa and Europe". Nature Genetics. 39 (1): 31–40. doi:10.1038/ng1946. PMC 2672153 . PMID 17159977. Retrieved 18 April 2013.

179. Wilson J (December 2005). "Milk Intolerance: Lactose Intolerance and Cow›s Milk Protein Allergy". Newborn and Infant Nursing Reviews. 5 (4): 203–7. doi:10.1053/j.nainr.2005.08.004.

180. Auricchio S, Rubino A, Landolt M, Semenza G, Prader A (1963). "Isolated intestinal lactase deficiency in the adult". Lancet. 2 (7303): 324–6. doi:10.1016/s0140-6736(63)92991-x. PMID 14044269.

181. Simoons FJ (December 1969). "Primary adult lactose intolerance and the milking habit: a problem in biological and cultural interrelations. I. Review of the medical research". Am J Dig Dis. 14 (12): 819–36. doi:10.1007/bf02233204. PMID 4902756.

182. Itan Y, Jones BL, Ingram CJ, Swallow DM, Thomas MG (2010). "A worldwide correlation of lactase persistence phenotype and genotypes". BMC Evolutionary Biology. 10: 36. doi:10.1186/1471-2148-10-36. PMC 2834688 . PMID 20144208.
183. Bayless TM, Rosensweig NS (1966). "A racial difference in incidence of lactase deficiency. A survey of milk intolerance and lactase deficiency in healthy adult males". JAMA. 197 (12): 968–72. doi:10.1001/jama.1966.03110120074017. PMID 5953213.
184. Welsh JD, Rohrer V, Knudsen KB, Paustian FF (1967). "Isolated Lactase Deficiency: Correlation of Laboratory Studies and Clinical Data.". Archives of Internal Medlit. 120 (3): 261–269. doi:10.1001/archinte.1967.00300030003003.
185. Huang SS, Bayless TM (1968). "Milk and lactose intolerance in healthy Orientals". Science. 160 (3823): 83–4. doi:10.1126/science.160.3823.83-a. PMID 5694356.
186. Cook GC, Kajubi SK (1966). "Tribal incidence of lactase deficiency in Uganda". Lancet. 1 (7440): 725–9. doi:10.1016/s0140-6736(66)90888-9. PMID 4159716.
187. Jersky J, Kinsley RH (1967). "Lactase Deficiency in the South African Bantu". South African Medical Journal. 41 (Dec): 1194–1196.
188. Bolin TD, Crane GG, Davis AE (1968). "Lactose intolerance in various ethnic groups in South-East Asia". Australas Ann Med. 17 (4): 300–6. PMID 5701921.
189. Flatz G, Saengudom C, Sanguanbhokhai T (1969). "Lactose intolerance in Thailand". Nature. 221 (5182): 758–9. doi:10.1038/221758b0. PMID 5818369.
190. Elliott RB, Maxwell GM, Vawser N (1967). "Lactose maldigestion in Australian Aboriginal children". Med. J. Aust. 1 (2): 46–9. PMID 6016903.
191. Flatz G, Rotthauwe HW (1971). "Evidence against nutritional adaption of tolerance to lactose". Humangenetik. 13 (2): 118–25. doi:10.1007/bf00295793. PMID 5114667.
192. Swallow DM (2003). "Genetics Oflactasepersistence Andlactoseintolerance". Annual Review of Genetics. 37: 197–219. doi:10.1146/annurev.genet.37.110801.143820. PMID 14616060.
193. "glycogen storage disease" at Dorland›s Medical Dictionary
194. Stegelmeier BL, Molyneux RJ, Elbein AD, James LF (May 1995). "The lesions of locoweed (Astragalus mollissimus), swainsonine, and castanospermine in rats". Veterinary Pathology. 32 (3): 289–98. doi:10.1177/030098589503200311. PMID 7604496.
195. Ludwig M, Wolfson S, Rennert O (October 1972). "Glycogen storage disease, type 8". Arch. Dis. Child. 47 (255): 830–3. doi:10.1136/adc.47.255.830. PMC 1648209 . PMID 4508182.
196. "eMedicine - Glycogen-Storage Disease Type VI : Article by Lynne Ierardi-Curto".
197. "Definition: glycogen storage disease type VIII from Online Medical Dictionary".
198. Warren MF, Hamilton PB (January 1981). "Glycogen storage disease type X caused by ochratoxin A in broiler chickens". Poult. Sci. 60 (1): 120–3. doi:10.3382/ps.0600120. PMID 6940112.

199. Huff WE, Doerr JA, Hamilton PB (January 1979). "Decreased glycogen mobilization during ochratoxicosis in broiler chickens". Appl. Environ. Microbiol. 37 (1): 122–6. PMC 243410 . PMID 760630.

200. eMedicine Specialties > Glycogen-Storage Disease Type I Author: Karl S Roth. Updated: Aug 31, 2009

201. The Association for Glycogen Storage Disease > Type I Glycogen Storage Disease Type I GSD This page was created in October 2006.

202. Ausems MG, Verbiest J, Hermans MP, et al. (September 1999). "Frequency of glycogen storage disease type II in The Netherlands: implications for diagnosis and genetic counselling". Eur. J. Hum. Genet. 7 (6): 713–6. doi:10.1038/sj.ejhg.5200367. PMID 10482961.

203. http://mcardlesdisease.org/

204. eMedicine Specialties > Pediatrics: Genetics and Metabolic Disease > Metabolic Diseases > Glycogen-Storage Disease Type VI Author: Lynne Ierardi-Curto, MD, PhD. Updated: Aug 4, 2008

205. Goldman, Lee; Schafer, Andrew (2012). Goldman›s Cecil medicine (24th ed.). Philadelphia: Elsevier/Saunders. p. 1356. ISBN 978-1-4377-1604-7.

206. "Rare Disease Database". Orpha.net. Retrieved 2015-09-20.

207. http://neuromuscular.wustl.edu/msys/glycogen.html#enolase

208. Applegarth DA, Toone JR, Lowry RB (January 2000). "Incidence of inborn errors of metabolism in British Columbia, 1969-1996". Pediatrics. 105 (1): e10. doi:10.1542/peds.105.1.e10. PMID 10617747.

CHAPTER 6

Protein Metabolism

Chapter Contents

- **Introduction**
- **Protein Biosynthesis**

Protein metabolism is a description of the physical and chemical processes that cause both the building, or synthesis, of amino acids into proteins and the breakdown, or catabolism, of proteins into amino acids. Amino acids are circulated through the blood and enter the body tissues, where they are synthesized back into protein. Balance between protein synthesis and catabolism is essential to maintain normal cell functioning.

INTRODUCTION

Protein metabolism denotes the various biochemical processes responsible for the synthesis of proteins and amino acids, and the breakdown of proteins (and other large molecules, too) by catabolism.

Dietary proteins are first broken down to individual amino acids by various enzymes and hydrochloric acid present in the gastro-intestinal tract. These amino acids are further broken down to α-keto acids which can be recycled in the body for generation of energy, and production of glucose or fat or other amino acids. This break-down of amino acids to α-keto acids occurs in the liver by a process known as transamination, which follows a bimolecular ping pong mechanism.

PROTEIN BIOSYNTHESIS

Protein synthesis is the process whereby biological cells generate new proteins; it is balanced by the loss of cellular proteins via degradation or export. Translation, the assembly of amino acids by ribosomes, is an essential part of the biosynthetic pathway, along with generation of messenger RNA (mRNA), aminoacylation of transfer RNA (tRNA), co-translational transport, and post-translational modification. Protein biosynthesis is strictly regulated at multiple steps. They are principally during transcription (phenomena of RNA synthesis from DNA template) and translation (phenomena of amino acid assembly from RNA). The cistron DNA is transcribed into the first of a series of RNA intermediates. The last version is used as a template in synthesis of a polypeptide chain. Protein will often be synthesized directly from genes by translating mRNA. However, when a protein must be available on short notice or in large quantities, a protein precursor is produced. A proprotein is an inactive protein containing one or more inhibitory peptides that can be activated when the inhibitory sequence is removed by proteolysis during posttranslational modification. A preprotein is a form that contains a signal sequence (an N-terminal signal peptide) that specifies its insertion into or through membranes, i.e., targets them for secretion. The signal peptide is cleaved off in the endoplasmic reticulum. Preproproteins have both sequences (inhibitory and signal) still present.

In protein synthesis, a succession of tRNA molecules charged with appropriate amino acids are brought together with an mRNA molecule and matched up by base-pairing through the anti-codons of the tRNA with successive codons of the mRNA. The amino acids are then linked together to extend the growing protein chain, and the tRNAs, no longer carrying amino acids, are released. This whole complex of processes is carried out by the ribosome, formed of two main chains of RNA, called ribosomal RNA (rRNA), and more than 50 different proteins. The ribosome latches onto the end of an mRNA molecule and moves along it, capturing loaded tRNA molecules and joining together their amino acids to form a new protein chain.

Protein biosynthesis, although very similar, is different for prokaryotes and eukaryotes.

In transcription an mRNA chain is generated, with one strand of the DNA double helix in the genome as a template. This strand is called the template strand. Transcription can be divided into 3 stages: initiation, elongation, and termination, each regulated by a large number of proteins such as transcription factors and coactivators that ensure that the correct gene is transcribed.

Transcription occurs in the cell nucleus, where the DNA is held. The DNA structure of the cell is made up of two helixes made up of sugar and phosphate held together by hydrogen bonds between the bases of opposite strands. The sugar and the phosphate in each strand are joined together by stronger phosphodiester covalent bonds. The DNA is "unzipped" (disruption of hydrogen bonds between different single strands) by the enzyme helicase, leaving the single nucleotide chain open to be copied. RNA polymerase reads the DNA strand from the 3-prime (3') end to the 5-prime (5') end, while it synthesizes a single strand of messenger RNA in the 5'-to-3' direction. The general RNA structure is very similar to the DNA structure, but in RNA the nucleotide uracil takes the place that thymine occupies in DNA. The single strand of mRNA leaves the nucleus through nuclear pores, and migrates into the cytoplasm.

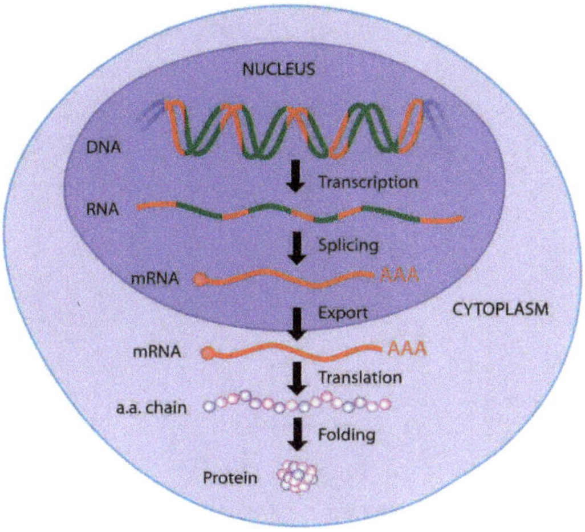

RNA is transcribed in the nucleus; once completely processed, it is transported to the cytoplasm and translated by the ribosome (shown in very pale grey behind the tRNA).

Transcription

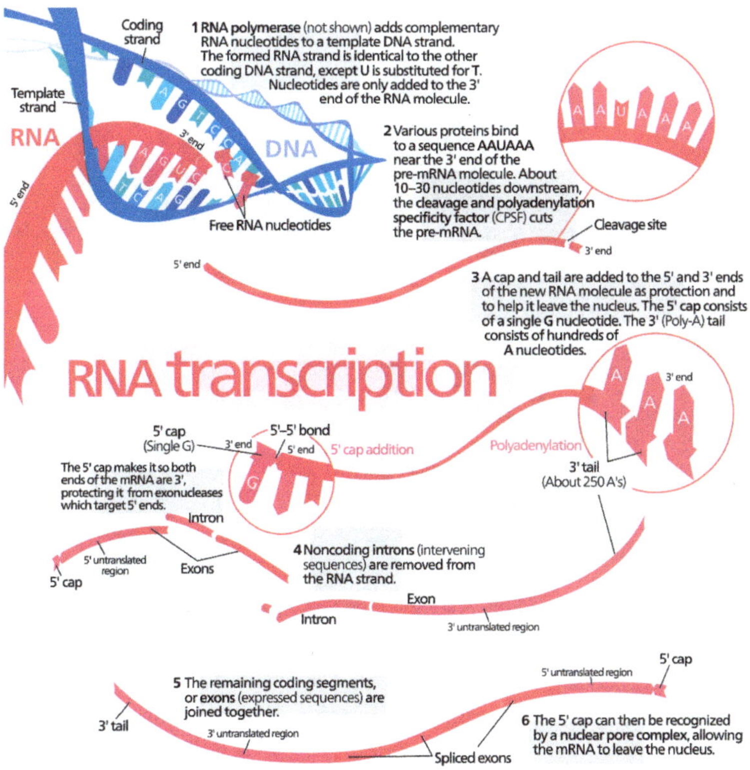

Diagram showing the process of transcription

The first product of transcription differs in prokaryotic cells from that of eukaryotic cells, as in prokaryotic cells the product is mRNA, which needs no post-transcriptional modification, whereas, in eukaryotic cells, the first product is called primary transcript, that needs post-transcriptional modification (capping with 7-methyl-guanosine, tailing with a poly A tail) to give hnRNA (heterogeneous nuclear RNA). hnRNA then undergoes splicing of introns (noncoding parts of the gene) via spliceosomes to produce the final mRNA.

Translation

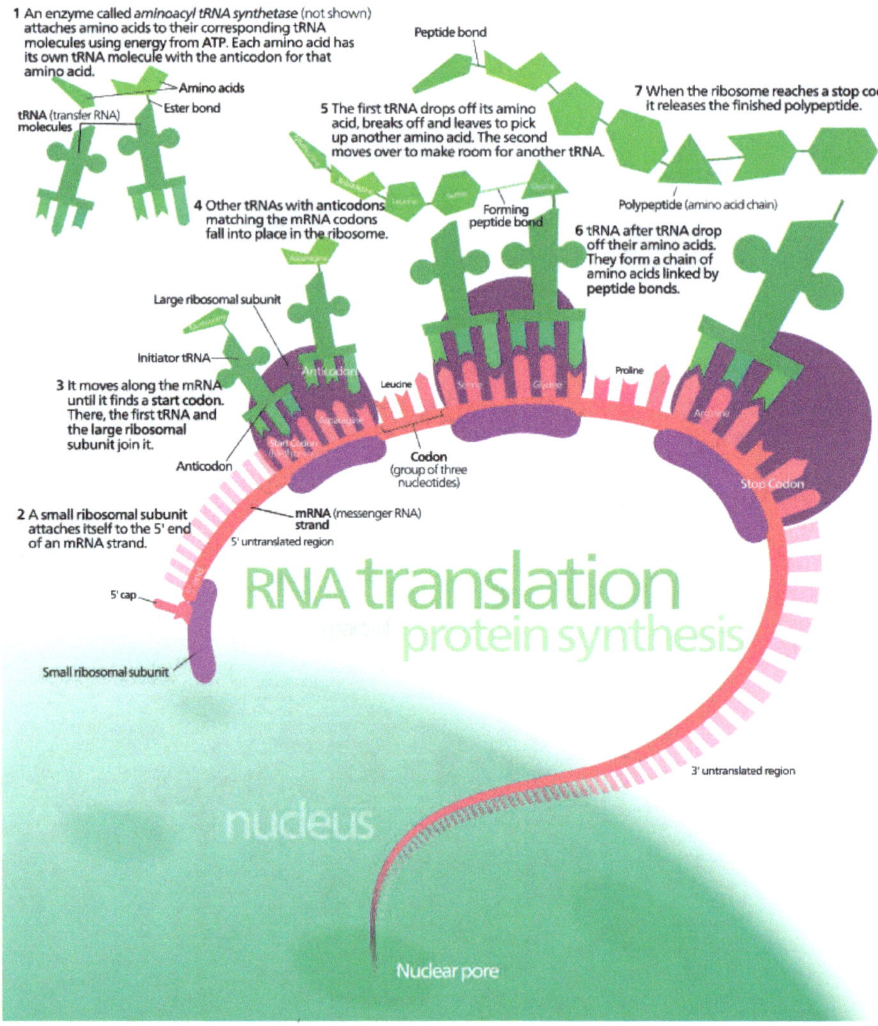

Diagram showing the process of translation

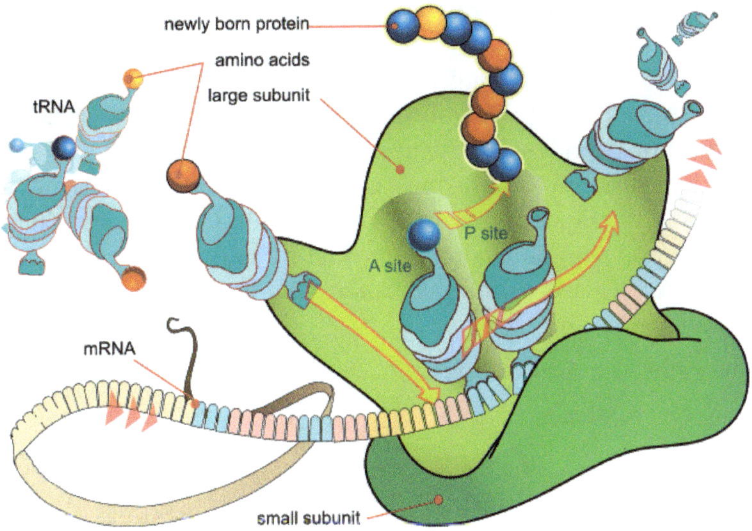

Diagram showing the translation of mRNA and the synthesis of proteins by a ribosome

The synthesis of proteins from RNA is known as translation. In eukaryotes, translation occurs in the cytoplasm, where the ribosomes are located. Ribosomes are made of a small and large subunit that surround the mRNA. In translation, messenger RNA (mRNA) is decoded to produce a specific polypeptide according to the rules specified by the trinucleotide genetic code. This uses an mRNA sequence as a template to guide the synthesis of a chain of amino acids that form a protein. Translation proceeds in four phases: activation, initiation, elongation, and termination (all describing the growth of the amino acid chain, or polypeptide that is the product of translation).

In activation, the correct amino acid (AA) is joined to the correct transfer RNA (tRNA). While this is not, in the technical sense, a step in translation, it is required for translation to proceed. The AA is joined by its carboxyl group to the 3' OH of the tRNA by an ester bond. When the tRNA has an amino acid linked to it, it is termed "charged". Initiation involves the small subunit of the ribosome binding to 5' end of mRNA with the help of initiation factors (IF), other proteins that assist the process. Elongation occurs when the next aminoacyl-tRNA (charged tRNA) in line binds to the ribosome along with GTP and an elongation factor. Termination of the polypeptide happens when the A site of the ribosome faces a stop codon (UAA, UAG, or UGA). When this happens, no tRNA can recognize it, but releasing factor can recognize nonsense codons and causes the release of the polypeptide chain. The capacity of disabling or inhibiting translation in protein biosynthesis is used by some antibiotics such as anisomycin, cycloheximide, chloramphenicol, tetracycline, streptomycin, erythromycin, puromycin, etc.

Events During or Following Protein Translation

Events that occur during or following biosynthesis include Proteolysis, post-translational modification and protein folding. Proteolysis may remove N-terminal, C-terminal or internal amino-acid residues or peptides from the polypeptide. The termini and side-chains of the polypeptide may be subjected to post-translational modification. These modifications may be required for correct cellular localisation or the natural function of the protein. During and after synthesis, polypeptide chains often fold to assume, so called, native secondary and tertiary structures. This is known as *protein folding* and is typically required for the natural function of the protein.

Protein biosynthesis relies on four processes:

- amino acid synthesis
- RNA synthesis
- transcription
- translation

Protein anabolism is the process by which protein are formed from amino acids (aka anabolic amino acid synthesis).

Protein Breakdown

Protein catabolism is the process by which proteins are broken down to their amino acids. This is also called proteolysis.

This can be followed by further amino acid degradation.

Amino Acid Metabolism

The following list contains links to information about the metabolism of individual amino acids.

- Positively charged side chains
    - Arginine
    - Histidine
    - Lysine
- Negatively charged side chains
    - Aspartic acid
    - Glutamic acid
- Polar uncharged side chains
    - Serine
    - Threonine
    - Asparagine
    - Glutamine

- Special cases
    - Cysteine
    - Selenocysteine
    - Glycine
    - Proline

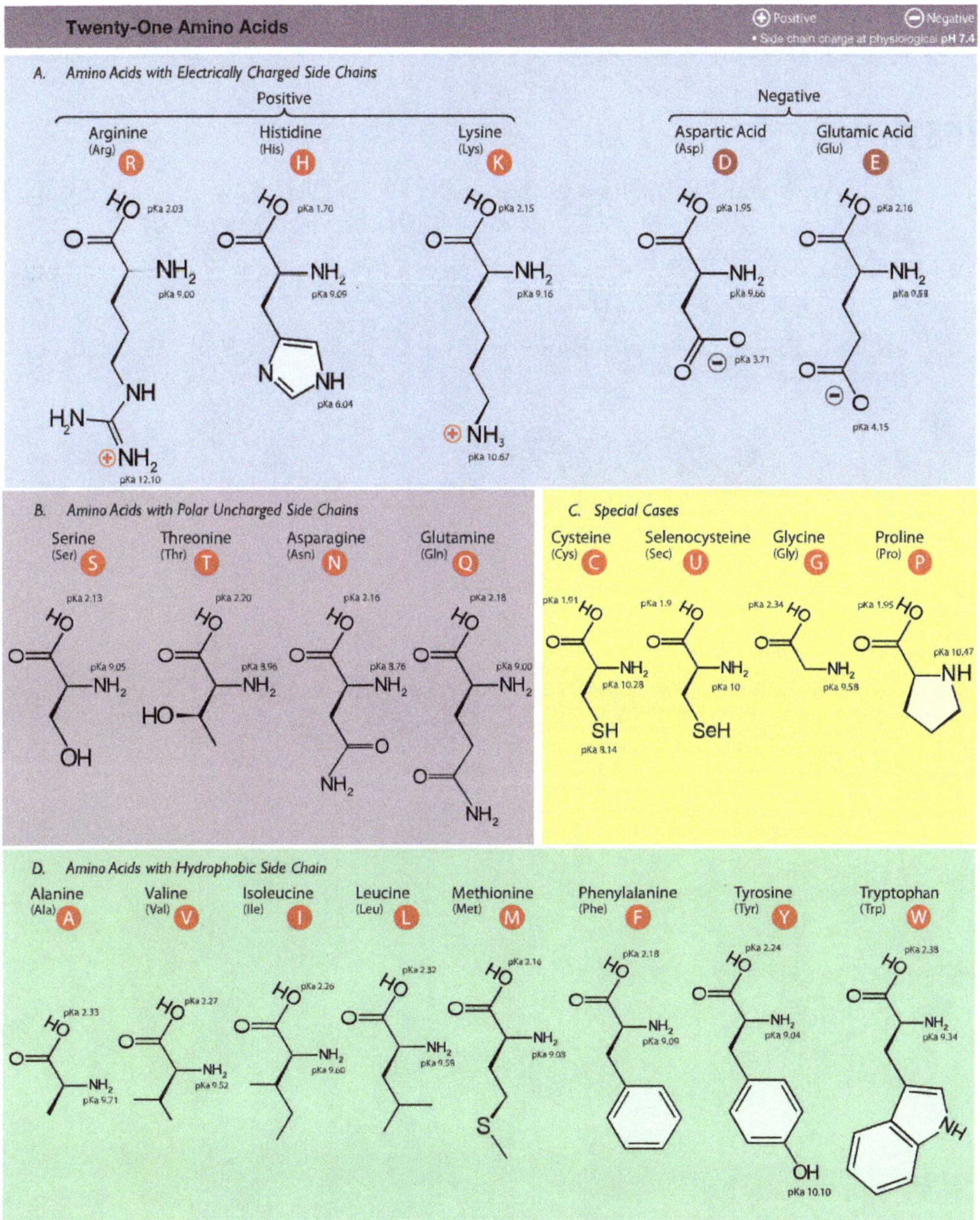

- Hydrophobic side chains
    - Alanine

- Valine
- Isoleucine
- Leucine
- Methionine
- Phenylalanine
- Tyrosine
- Tryptophan

REFERENCES

- Kafri M, Metzl-Raz E, Jona G, Barkai N. 2016. The Cost of Protein Production. Cell Rep 14:22–31. http://dx.doi.org/10.1016/j.celrep.2015.12.015
- Alberts, Bruce (2002). Molecular biology of the cell. New York: Garland Science. p. 760. ISBN 0-8153-3218-1.
- Alberts, Bruce. Molecular Biology of the Cell, 5e. New York: Garland Science, 2008.

CHAPTER 7

Lipid Metabolism

Chapter Contents

Lipid metabolism is the process by which fatty acids are digested, broken down for energy, or stored in the human body for later energy use. These fatty acids are a component of triglycerides, which make up the bulk of the fat humans eat in foods like vegetable oils and animal products. Triglycerides can be found in the blood vessels as well as stored for future energy needs in the cells of adipose tissue, better known as body fat, and in liver cells. Though the body's main source of energy is carbohydrates, when this source is exhausted, the fatty acids in triglycerides will then be broken down as a backup energy source. Examples of times the body draws energy from lipid metabolism are during exercise, when the supply of glycogen, or the stored form of the carbohydrate glucose, is used up, or when there is insufficient carbohydrate in the diet to meet the body's energy needs.

INTRODUCTION

Lipid metabolism is the synthesis and degradation of lipids in cells.

Lipid metabolism is the break down or storage of fats for energy; these fats are obtained from consuming food and absorbing them or they are synthesized by an animal's liver. Lipid metabolism does exist in plants, though the processes differ in some ways when compared to animals. Lipogenesis is the process of synthesizing these fats. Lipid metabolism often begins with hydrolysis, which occurs when a chemical breaks down as a reaction to coming in contact with water. Since lipids (fats) are hydrophobic, hydrolysis in lipid metabolism occurs in the cytoplasm which ends up creating glycerol and fatty acids. Due to the hydrophobic nature of lipids they require special transport proteins known as lipoproteins, which are hydrophilic. Lipoproteins are categorized by their density levels. The varying densities between the types of lipoproteins are characteristic to what type of fats they transport. A number of these lipoproteins are synthesized in the liver, but not all of them originate from this organ.

Lipid Metabolism Disorders are illnesses where trouble occurs in breaking down or synthesizing fats (or fat-like substances). A good deal of the time these disorders are hereditary, meaning it's a condition that is passed along from parent to child through their genes. Gaucher's Disease (Type I, Type II, and Type III), Neimann-Pick Disease, Tay-sachs Disease, and Fabry's Disease are all diseases where those afflicted can have a disorder of their body's lipid metabolism. Rarer diseases concerning a disorder of the lipid metabolism are Sitosterolemia, Wolman's Disease, Refsum's Disease, and Cerebrotendinous Xanthomatosis.

BILE ACID

Bile acids are steroid acids found predominantly in the bile of mammals and other vertebrates. Different molecular forms of bile acids can be synthesized in the liver by different species. Bile acids are conjugated with taurine or glycine in the liver, forming bile salts.

Primary bile acids are those synthesized by the liver. Secondary bile acids result from bacterial actions in the colon. In humans, taurocholic acid and glycocholic acid (derivatives of cholic acid) and taurochenodeoxycholic acid and glycochenodeoxycholic acid (derivatives of chenodeoxycholic acid) are the major bile salts in bile and are roughly equal in concentration. The conjugated salts of their 7-alpha-dehydroxylated derivatives, deoxycholic acid and lithocholic acid, are also found, with derivatives of cholic, chenodeoxycholic and deoxycholic acids accounting for over 90% of human biliary bile acids.

Bile acids comprise about 80% of the organic compounds in bile (others are phospholipids and cholesterol). An increased secretion of bile acids produces an increase in bile flow. The main function of bile acids is to allow digestion of dietary fats and oils by acting as a surfactant that emulsifies them into micelles, allowing them to be colloidally suspended in the chyme before further processing. They also have hormonal actions throughout the body, particularly through the farnesoid X receptor and GPBAR1 (also known as TGR5).

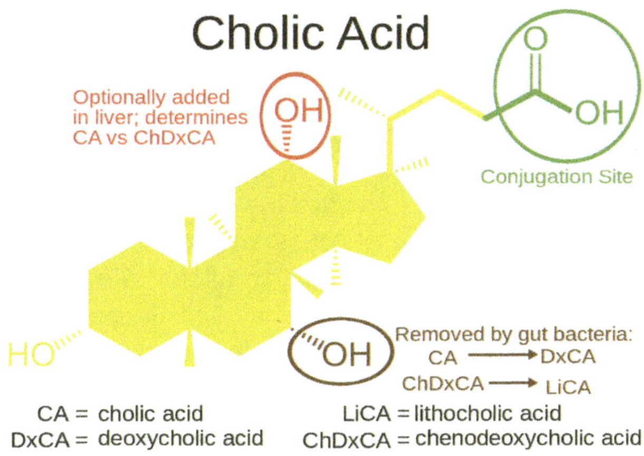

Structure of cholic acid showing relationship to other bile acids

Production

Bile acid synthesis occurs in liver cells which synthesize **primary bile acids** (cholic acid and chenodeoxycholic acid in humans) via cytochrome P450-mediated oxidation of cholesterol in a multi-step process. Approximately 600 mg of bile salts are synthesized daily to replace bile acids lost in the feces. The rate-limiting step is the addition of a hydroxyl group on position 7 of the steroid nucleus by the enzyme cholesterol 7 alpha-hydroxylase. This enzyme is down-regulated by cholic acid, up-regulated by cholesterol and is inhibited by the actions of the ileal hormone FGF15/19.

Prior to secreting any of the bile acids (primary or secondary, see below), liver cells conjugate them with one of two amino acids, glycine or taurine, to form a total of 8 possible **conjugated bile acids**. These conjugated bile acids are often referred to as **bile salts** because of their physiologically-important acid-base properties. The pKa of the unconjugated bile acids are between 5 and 6.5, and the pH of the duodenum ranges between 3 and 5, so when unconjugated bile acids are in the duodenum, they are almost always protonated (HA form), which makes them relatively insoluble in water. Conjugating bile acids with amino acids lowers the pKa of the bile-acid/amino-acid conjugate to between 1 and 4. Thus conjugated bile acids are almost always in their deprotonated (A-) form in the duodenum, which makes them much more water-soluble and much more able to fulfil their physiologic function of emulsifying fats.

When these bile salts are secreted into the lumen of the intestine, bacterial partial dehydroxylation and removal of the glycine and taurine groups forms the **secondary bile acids**, deoxycholic acid and lithocholic acid. Cholic acid is converted into deoxycholic acid and chenodeoxycholic acid into lithocholic acid. All four of these bile acids can be taken back up into the blood stream, return to the liver, and be re-secreted in a process known as enterohepatic circulation.

Functions

As amphipathic molecules with hydrophobic and hydrophilic regions, conjugated bile salts sit at the lipid/water interface and, at the right concentration, form micelles. The added solubility of conjugated bile salts aids in their function by preventing passive re-absorption in the small intestine. As a result, the concentration of bile acids/salts in the small intestine is high enough to form micelles and solubilize lipids. "Critical micellar concentration" refers to both an intrinsic property of the bile acid itself and amount of bile acid necessary to function in the spontaneous and dynamic formation of micelles. Bile acid-containing micelles aid lipases to digest lipids and bring them near the intestinal brush border membrane, which results in fat absorption.

Synthesis of bile acids is a major route of cholesterol metabolism in most species other than humans. The body produces about 800 mg of cholesterol per day and about half of that is used for bile acid synthesis producing 400–600 mg daily. Human adults secrete between 12-18 g of bile acids into the intestine each day, mostly after meals. The bile acid pool size is between 4–6 g, which means that bile acids are recycled several times each day. About 95% of bile acids are reabsorbed by active transport in the ileum and recycled back to the liver for further secretion into the biliary system and gallbladder. This enterohepatic circulation of bile acids allows a low rate of synthesis but with large amounts being secreted into the intestine.

Bile acids have other functions, including eliminating cholesterol from the body, driving the flow of bile to eliminate certain catabolites (including bilirubin), emulsifying fat-soluble vitamins to enable their absorption, and aiding in motility and the reduction of the bacteria flora found in the small intestine and biliary tract.

Bile acids have metabolic actions in the body resembling those of hormones, acting through two specific receptors, the farnesoid X receptor and G protein-coupled bile acid receptor/TGR5. They bind less specifically to some other receptors and have been reported to regulate the activity of certain enzymes and ion channels and the synthesis of diverse substances including endogenous fatty acid ethanolamides.

Structure and Synthesis

- The structures of the principal human bile acids

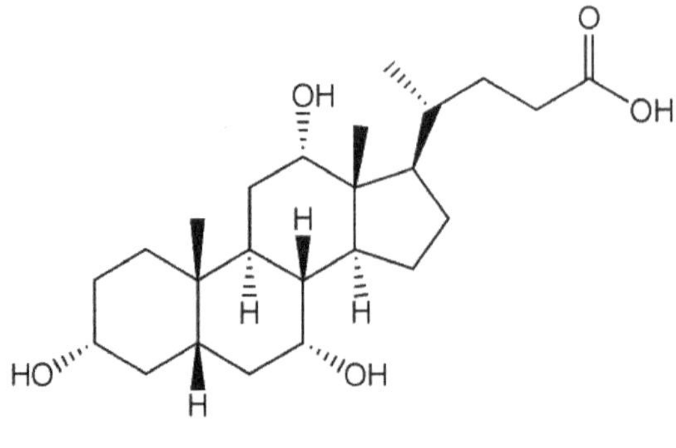

Cholic acid

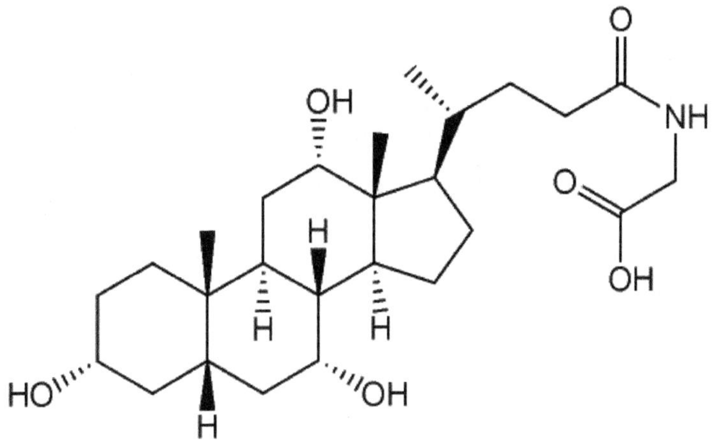

Glycocholic acid

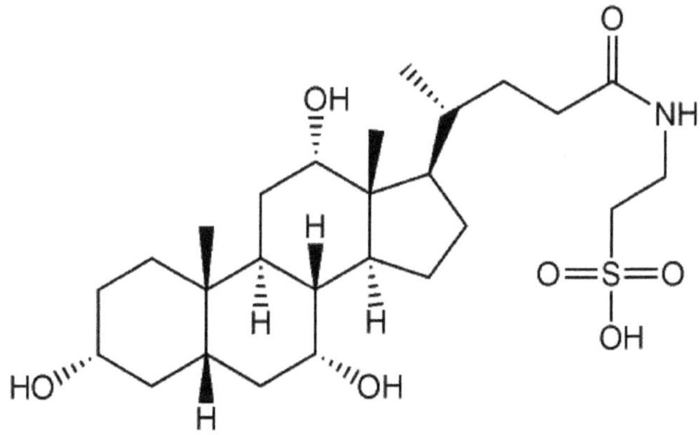

Taurocholic acid

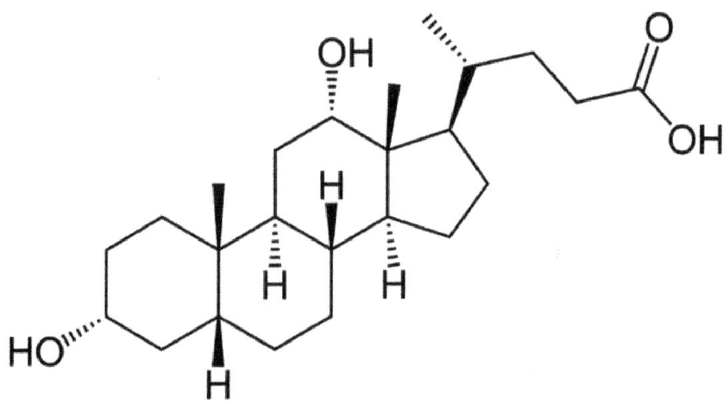

Deoxycholic acid

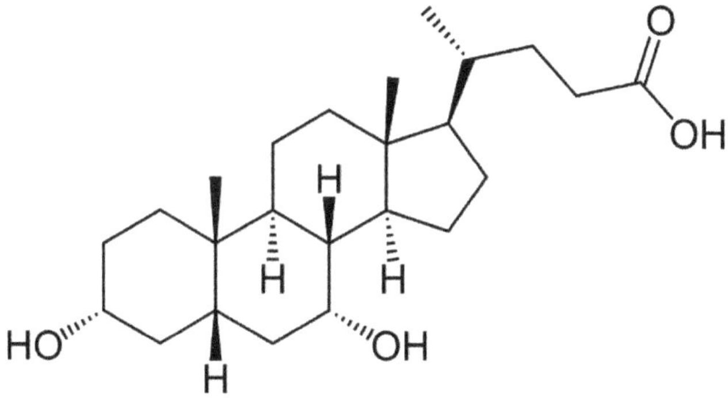

Chenodeoxycholic acid

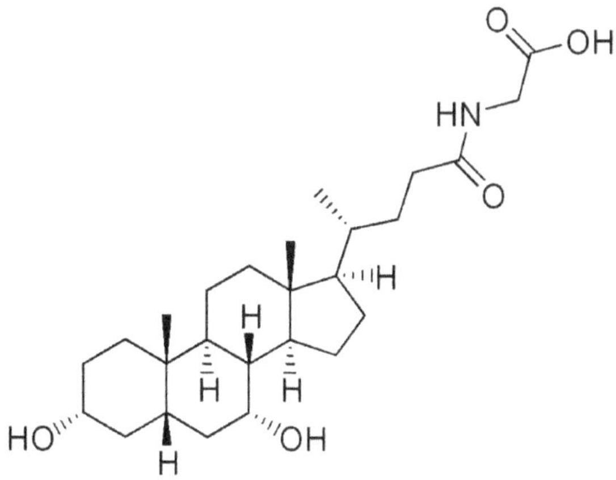

Glycochenodeoxycholic acid

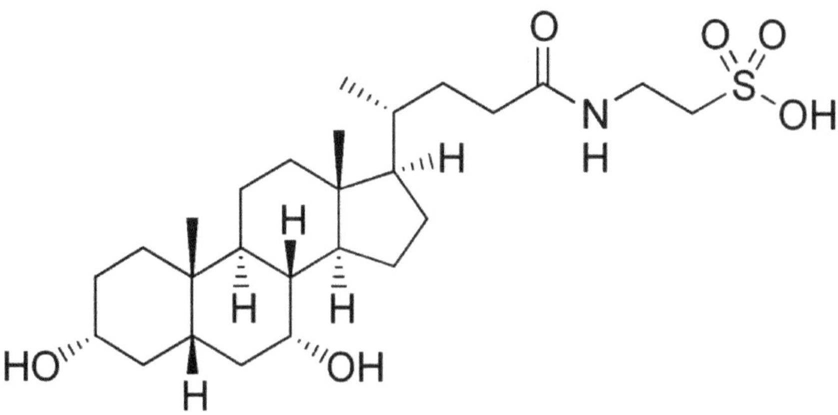

Taurochenodeoxycholic acid

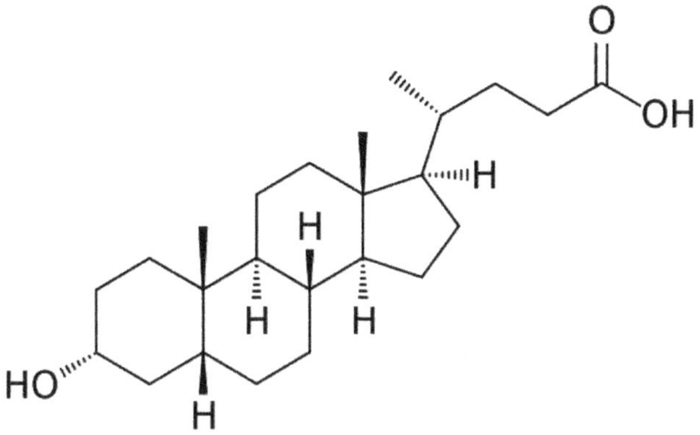

Lithocholic acid

Bile salts constitute a large family of molecules, composed of a steroid structure with four rings, a five- or eight-carbon side-chain terminating in a carboxylic acid, and several hydroxyl groups, the number and orientation of which is different among the specific bile salts. The four rings are labeled A, B, C, and D, from the farthest to the closest to the side chain with the carboxyl group. The D-ring is smaller by one carbon than the other three. The structure is commonly drawn with A at the left and D at the right. The hydroxyl groups can be in either of two configurations: either up (or out), termed beta (β; often drawn by convention as a solid line), or down, termed alpha (α; displayed as a dashed line). All bile acids have a 3-hydroxyl group, derived from the parent molecule, cholesterol, in which the 3-hydroxyl is beta.

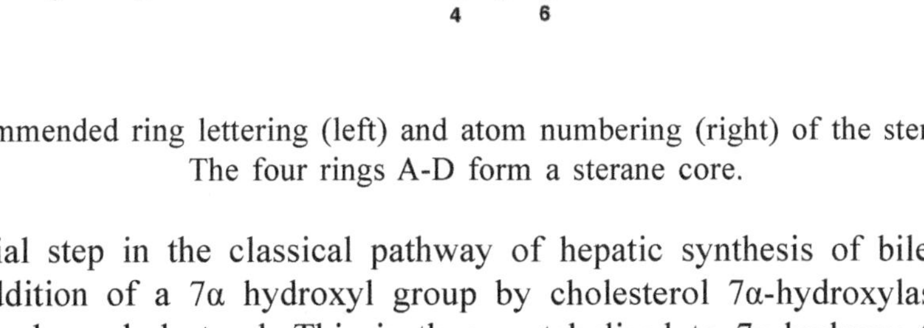

IUPAC recommended ring lettering (left) and atom numbering (right) of the steroid skeleton. The four rings A-D form a sterane core.

The initial step in the classical pathway of hepatic synthesis of bile acids is the enzymatic addition of a 7α hydroxyl group by cholesterol 7α-hydroxylase (CYP7A1) forming 7α-hydroxycholesterol. This is then metabolised to 7α-hydroxy-4-cholesten-3-one. There are multiple steps in bile acid synthesis requiring 14 enzymes in all. These result in the junction between the first two steroid rings (A and B) being altered, making the molecule bent; in this process, the 3-hydroxyl is converted to the α orientation. The simplest 24-carbon bile acid has two hydroxyl groups at positions 3α and 7α. This is 3α,7α-dihydroxy-5β-cholan-24-oic acid, or, as more usually known, chenodeoxycholic acid. This bile acid was first isolated from the domestic goose, from which the "cheno" portion of the name was derived. The 5β in the name denotes the orientation of the junction between rings A and B of the steroid nucleus (in this case, they are bent). The term "cholan" denotes a particular steroid structure of 24 carbons, and the "24-oic acid" indicates that the carboxylic acid is found at position 24, at the end of the side-chain. Chenodeoxycholic acid is made by many species, and is the prototypic functional bile acid.

An alternative (acidic) pathway of bile acid synthesis is initiated by mitochondrial sterol 27-hydroxylase (CYP27A1), expressed in liver, and also in macrophages and other tissues. CYP27A1 contributes significantly to total bile acid synthesis by catalyzing sterol side chain oxidation, after which cleavage of a three-carbon unit in the peroxisomes leads to formation of a C24 bile acid. Minor pathways initiated by 25-hydroxylase in the liver and 24-hydroxylase in the brain also may contribute to bile acid synthesis. 7α-hydroxylase (CYP7B1) generates oxysterols, which may be further converted in the liver to CDCA.

Cholic acid, 3α,7α,12α-trihydroxy-5β-cholan-24-oic acid, the most abundant bile acid in humans and many other species, was discovered before chenodeoxycholic acid. It is a tri-hydroxy-bile acid with 3 hydroxyl groups (3α, 7α and 12α). In its synthesis in the liver, 12α hydroxylation is performed by the additional action of CYP8B1. As this had already been described, the discovery of chenodeoxcholic acid (with 2 hydroxyl groups) made this new bile acid a "deoxycholic acid" in that it had one fewer hydroxyl group than cholic acid.

Deoxycholic acid is formed from cholic acid by 7-dehydroxylation, resulting in 2 hydroxyl groups (3α and 12α). This process with chenodeoxycholic acid results in a bile acid with only a 3α hydroxyl group, termed lithocholic acid (litho = stone) having been identified first in a gallstone from a calf. It is poorly water-soluble and rather toxic to cells.

Different vertebrate families have evolved to use modifications of most positions on the steroid nucleus and side-chain of the bile acid structure. To avoid the problems associated with the production of lithocholic acid, most species add a third hydroxyl group to chenodeoxycholic acid. The subsequent removal of the 7α hydroxyl group by intestinal bacteria will then result in a less toxic but still-functional dihydroxy bile acid. Over the course of vertebrate evolution, a number of positions have been chosen for placement of the third hydroxyl group. Initially, the 16α position was favored, in particular in birds. Later, this position was superseded in a large number of species selecting the 12α position. Primates (including humans) utilize 12α for their third hydroxyl group position, producing cholic acid. In mice and other rodents, 6β hydroxylation forms muricholic acids (α or β depending on the 7 hydroxyl position). Pigs have 6α hydroxylation in hyocholic acid (3α,6α,7α-trihydroxy-5β-cholanoic acid), and other species have a hydroxyl group on position 23 of the side-chain.

Ursodeoxycholic acid was first isolated from bear bile, which has been used medicinally for centuries. Its structure resembles chenodeoxycholic acid but with the 7-hydroxyl group in the β position.

Obeticholic acid, 6α-ethyl-chenodeoxycholic acid, is a semi-synthetic bile acid with greater activity as FXR agonist which is undergoing investigation as a pharmaceutical agent.

Hormonal Actions

Bile acids also act as steroid hormones, secreted from the liver, absorbed from the intestine and having various direct metabolic actions in the body through the nuclear receptor Farnesoid X receptor (FXR), also known by its gene name *NR1H4*. Another bile acid receptor is the cell membrane receptor known as G protein-coupled bile acid receptor 1 or TGR5. Many of their functions as signaling molecules in the liver and the intestines are by activating FXR, whereas TGR5 may be involved in metabolic, endocrine and neurological functions.

Regulation of Synthesis

As surfactants or detergents, bile acids are potentially toxic to cells, and so their concentrations are tightly regulated. Activation of FXR in the liver inhibits synthesis of bile acids, and is one mechanism of feedback control when bile acid levels are too high. Secondly, FXR activation by bile acids during absorption in the intestine increases transcription and synthesis of FGF19, which then inhibits bile acid synthesis in the liver.

Metabolic Functions

Emerging evidence associates FXR activation with alterations in triglyceride metabolism, glucose metabolism, and liver growth.

Other Interactions

Bile acids bind to some other proteins in addition to their hormone receptors (FXR and TGR5) and their transporters. Among these protein targets, the enzyme N-acyl phosphatidylethanolamine-specific phospholipase D (NAPE-PLD) generates bioactive lipid amides (e.g. the endogenous cannabinoid anandamide) that play important roles in several physiological pathways including stress and pain responses, appetite, and lifespan. NAPE-PLD orchestrates a direct cross-talk between lipid amide signals and bile acid physiology.

Clinical Significance

Hyperlipidemia

As bile acids are made from endogenous cholesterol, disruption of the enterohepatic circulation of bile acids will lower cholesterol. Bile acid sequestrants bind bile acids in the gut, preventing reabsorption. In so doing, more endogenous cholesterol is shunted into the production of bile acids, thereby lowering cholesterol levels. The sequestered bile acids are then excreted in the feces.

Cholestasis

Tests for bile acids are useful in both human and veterinary medicine, as they aid in the diagnosis of a number of conditions, including types of cholestasis such as intrahepatic cholestasis of pregnancy, portosystemic shunt, and hepatic microvascular dysplasia in dogs. Structural or functional abnormalities of the biliary system result in an increase in bilirubin (jaundice) and in bile acids in the blood. Bile acids are related to the itching (pruritus) which is common in cholestatic conditions such as primary biliary cirrhosis (PBC), primary sclerosing cholangitis or intrahepatic cholestasis of pregnancy. Treatment with ursodeoxycholic acid has been used for many years in these cholestatic disorders.

Gallstones

The relationship of bile acids to cholesterol saturation in bile and cholesterol precipitation to produce gallstones has been studied extensively. Gallstones may result from increased saturation of cholesterol or bilirubin, or from bile stasis. Lower concentrations of bile acids or phospholipids in bile reduce cholesterol solubility and lead to microcrystal formation. Oral therapy with chenodeoxycholic acid and/or ursodeoxycholic acid has been used to dissolve cholesterol gallstones.Stones may recur when treatment is stopped. Bile acid therapy may be of value to prevent stones is certain circumstances such as following bariatric surgery.

Bile Acid Diarrhea

Excess concentrations of bile acids in the colon are a cause of chronic diarrhea. It is commonly found when the ileum is abnormal or has been surgically removed, as in Crohn's disease, or cause a condition that resembles diarrhea-predominant irritable bowel syndrome (IBS-D). This condition of bile acid diarrhea/bile acid malabsorption can be diagnosed by the SeHCAT test and treated with bile acid sequestrants.

Bile Acids and Colon Cancer

Bile acids may have some importance in the development of colorectal cancer. Deoxycholic acid (DCA) is increased in the colonic contents of humans in response to a high fat diet. In populations with a high incidence of colorectal cancer, fecal concentrations of bile acids are higher, and this association suggests that increased colonic exposure to bile acids could play a role in the development of cancer. In one particular comparison, the fecal DCA concentrations in Native Africans in South Africa (who eat a low fat diet) compared to African Americans (who eat a higher fat diet) was 7.30 vs. 37.51 nmol/g wet weight stool.Native Africans in South Africa have a low incidence rate of colon cancer of less than 1:100,000, compared to the high incidence rate for male African Americans of 72:100,000.

Experimental studies also suggest mechanisms for bile acids in colon cancer. Exposure of colonic cells to high DCA concentrations increase formation of reactive oxygen species, causing oxidative stress, and also increase DNA damage. Mice fed a diet with added DCA mimicking colonic DCA levels in humans on a high fat diet developed colonic neoplasia, including adenomas and adenocarcinomas (cancers), unlike mice fed a control diet producing one-tenth the level of colonic DCA who had no colonic neoplasia.

The effects of ursodeoxycholic acid (UDCA) in modifying the risk of colorectal cancer has been looked at in several studies, particularly in primary sclerosing cholangitis and inflammatory bowel disease, with varying results partly related to dosage. Genetic variation in the key bile acid synthesis enzyme, CYP7A1, influenced the effectiveness of UDCA in colorectal adenoma prevention in a large trial.

Dermatology

Bile acids may be used in subcutaneous injections to remove unwanted fat (see Mesotherapy). Deoxycholic acid as an injectable has received FDA approval to dissolve submental fat. Phase III trials showed significant responses although many subjects had mild adverse reactions of bruising, swelling, pain, numbness, erythema, and firmness around the treated area.

Historical Aspects

The history of research into bile acids has been documented thoroughly in a review coauthored by Alan Hofmann, who has been instrumental in a large number of these findings.

CHOLESTEROL

Cholesterol, from the Ancient Greek chole- (bile) and stereos (solid) followed by the chemical suffix -ol for an alcohol, is an organic molecule. It is a sterol (or modified steroid), a type of lipid molecule, and is biosynthesized by all animal cells, because it is an essential structural component of all animal cell membranes; essential to maintain both membrane structural integrity and fluidity. Cholesterol enables animal cells to dispense with a cell wall (to protect membrane integrity and cell viability), thereby allowing animal cells to change shape and animals to move (unlike bacteria and plant cells, which are restricted by their cell walls).

In addition to its importance for animal cell structure, cholesterol also serves as a precursor for the biosynthesis of steroid hormones and bile acids. Cholesterol is the principal sterol synthesized by all animals. In vertebrates, hepatic cells typically produce the greatest amounts. It is absent among prokaryotes (bacteria and archaea), although there are some exceptions, such as Mycoplasma, which require cholesterol for growth.

François Poulletier de la Salle first identified cholesterol in solid form in gallstones in 1769. However, it was not until 1815 that chemist Michel Eugène Chevreul named the compound “cholesterine”.

Physiology

Since cholesterol is essential for all animal life, each cell synthesizes it by way of a complex 37-step process, beginning with the mevalonate pathway and ending with a 19-step conversion of lanosterol to cholesterol.

A human male weighing 68 kg (150 lb) normally synthesizes about 1 gram (1,000 mg) per day, and his body contains about 35 g, mostly contained within the cell membranes. Typical daily cholesterol dietary intake for a man in the United States is 307 mg (above the upper limit recommended by the Dietary Guidelines Advisory Committee).

Most ingested cholesterol is esterified, and esterified cholesterol is poorly absorbed. The body also compensates for any absorption of additional cholesterol by reducing cholesterol synthesis. For these reasons, cholesterol in food, seven to ten hours after ingestion, has little, if any effect on concentrations of cholesterol in the blood. However, during the first seven hours after ingestion of cholesterol, as absorbed fats are being distributed around the body within extracellular water by the various lipoproteins (which transport all fats in the water outside cells), the concentrations increase. It is also important to recognize, however, that the concentrations measured in the samples of blood plasma vary with the measurement methods used. Traditional, cheaper methods do not reflect (a) which lipoproteins are transporting the various fat molecules, nor (b) which cells are ingesting, burning or exporting the fat molecules being measured as totals from samples of blood plasma.

Cholesterol is recycled in the body. The liver excretes it in a non-esterified form (via bile) into the digestive tract. Typically, about 50% of the excreted cholesterol is reabsorbed by the small intestine back into the bloodstream.

Plants make cholesterol in very small amounts. Plants manufacture phytosterols (substances chemically similar to cholesterol), which can compete with cholesterol for reabsorption in the intestinal tract, thus potentially reducing cholesterol reabsorption. When intestinal lining cells absorb phytosterols, in place of cholesterol, they usually excrete the phytosterol molecules back into the GI tract, an important protective mechanism.

Function

Cholesterol, given that it composes about 30% of all animal cell membranes, is required to build and maintain membranes and modulates membrane fluidity over the range of physiological temperatures. The hydroxyl group on cholesterol interacts with the polar heads of the membrane phospholipids and sphingolipids, while the bulky steroid and the hydrocarbon chain are embedded in the membrane, alongside the nonpolar fatty-acid chain of the other lipids. Through the interaction with the phospholipid fatty-acid chains, cholesterol increases membrane packing, which both alters membrane fluidity and maintains membrane integrity so that animal cells do not need to build cell walls (like plants and most bacteria). The membrane remains stable and durable without being rigid, allowing animal cells to change shape and animals to move.

The structure of the tetracyclic ring of cholesterol contributes to the fluidity of the cell membrane, as the molecule is in a *trans* conformation making all but the side chain of cholesterol rigid and planar. In this structural role, cholesterol also reduces the permeability of the plasma membrane to neutral solutes, hydrogen ions, and sodium ions.

Within the cell membrane, cholesterol also functions in intracellular transport, cell signaling and nerve conduction. Cholesterol is essential for the structure and function of invaginated caveolae and clathrin-coated pits, including caveola-dependent and clathrin-dependent endocytosis. The role of cholesterol in endocytosis of these types can be investigated by using methyl beta cyclodextrin (MβCD) to remove cholesterol from the plasma membrane. Recent studies show that cholesterol is also implicated in cell signaling processes, assisting in the formation of lipid rafts in the plasma membrane, which brings receptor proteins in close proximity with high concentrations of second messenger molecules. In multiple layers, cholesterol and phospholipids, both electrical insulators, can facilitate speed of transmission of electrical impulses along nerve tissue. For many neuron fibers, a myelin sheath, rich in cholesterol since it is derived from compacted layers of Schwann cell membrane, provides insulation for more efficient conduction of impulses. Demyelination (loss of some of these Schwann cells) is believed to be part of the basis for multiple sclerosis.

Within cells, cholesterol is also a precursor molecule for several biochemical pathways. For example, it is the precursor molecule for the synthesis of vitamin D and all steroid hormones, including the adrenal gland hormones cortisol and aldosterone, as well as the sex hormones progesterone, estrogens, and testosterone, and their derivatives.

The liver excretes cholesterol into biliary fluids, which is then stored in the gallbladder. Bile contains bile salts, which solubilize fats in the digestive tract and aid in the intestinal absorption of fat molecules as well as the fat-soluble vitamins, A, D, E, and K.

Dietary Sources

Animal fats are complex mixtures of triglycerides (stored energy, see: *"Introduction to Energy Storage".*), with lesser amounts of both the phospholipids and cholesterol molecules from which all animal (and human) cell membranes are constructed. Since all animal cells manufacture cholesterol, all animal-based foods contain cholesterol in varying amounts. Major dietary sources of cholesterol include cheese, egg yolks, beef, pork, poultry, fish, and shrimp. Human breast milk also contains significant quantities of cholesterol.

From a dietary perspective, because plant cells do not manufacture cholesterol, it is not found in plant-based foods. Some plant-based products, such as avocado, flax seeds and peanuts, contain cholesterol-like compounds called phytosterols, which are believed to compete with cholesterol for absorption in the intestines, reducing the absorption of both dietary and bile cholesterol.

Phytosterols can be supplemented through the use of phytosterol-containing functional foods or nutraceuticals that are recognized as having LDL-cholesterol (more relevant LDL-P responses not studied) lowering efficacy. This data does not reflect actual changes in LDL particle concentrations and has not been evaluated for cardiovascular disease outcomes. Some supplemental guidelines have recommended doses of phytosterols in the 1.6-3.0 grams per day range (Health Canada, EFSA, ATP III, FDA) with a recent meta-analysis demonstrating an 8.8% reduction in LDL-cholesterol at a mean dose of 2.15 grams per day. However, the benefits of a diet supplemented with phytosterol have been questioned, and evidence exists that absorbed plant phytosterols are much more atherogenic than animal cholesterol.

The fraction of cholesterol in the intestines which is absorbed varies from 15% to 75%, and group averages are about 50%, with the remainder excreted in the feces. Free cholesterol is much more likely to be absorbed than esterified cholesterol, and the proportion of free versus esterified cholesterol varies between different food sources. In February 2015, reversing decades-long recommendations, the USDA Dietary Guidelines Advisory Committee recommended repealing the guideline that Americans limit cholesterol intake, because dietary cholesterol intake has never correlated well with serum cholesterol levels. The committee looked for and found evidence that replacing saturated fat with unsaturated fat could lower LDL-cholesterol levels, and that low-fat diets which replaced saturated fat with carbohydrates could lower both LDL-cholesterol (LDL-P not evaluated) and HDL-cholesterol (HDL-P not evaluated) concentrations. Trans fats have been shown to reduce levels of HDL while increasing levels of LDL. Based on such evidence and evidence implicating low HDL-C and high LDL-C levels in cardiovascular disease (see Hypercholesterolemia), many health authorities advocate reducing LDL-cholesterol through changes in diet in addition to other lifestyle modifications. However, LDL-C is a calculated estimate rather than a measurement of the LDL particles. Similarly, HDL-C is not a measured HDL-P. Outcome data has always tracked particle concentrations rather than cholesterol values.

Increased dietary intake of industrial trans fats is associated with an increased risk in all-cause mortality, cardiovascular diseases and type 2 diabetes.

Biosynthesis

All animal cells manufacture cholesterol, for both membrane structure and other uses, with relative production rates varying by cell type and organ function. About 20% of total daily cholesterol production occurs in the liver; other sites of higher synthesis rates include the intestines, adrenal glands, and reproductive organs.

Synthesis within the body starts with the mevalonate pathway where two molecules of acetyl CoA condense to form acetoacetyl-CoA. This is followed by a second condensation between acetyl CoA and acetoacetyl-CoA to form 3-hydroxy-3-methylglutaryl CoA (HMG-CoA).

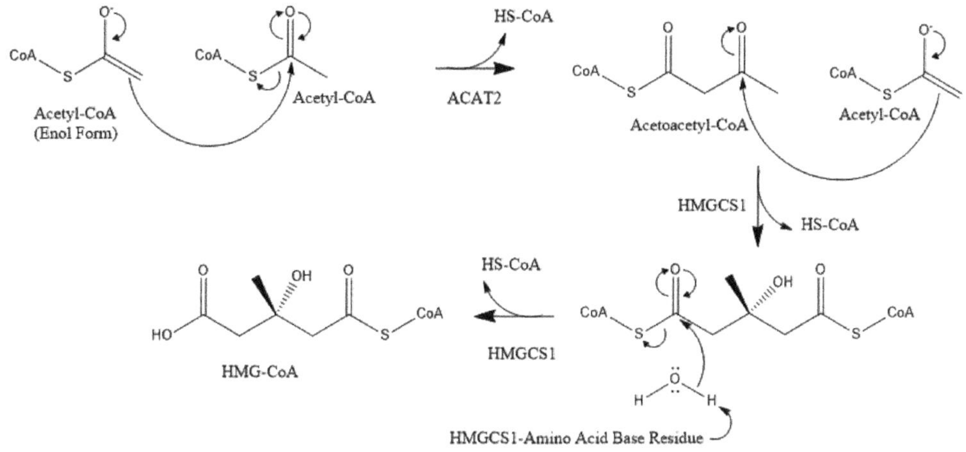

This molecule is then reduced to mevalonate by the enzyme HMG-CoA reductase. Production of mevalonate is the rate-limiting and irreversible step in cholesterol synthesis and is the site of action for statins (a class of cholesterol lowering drugs).

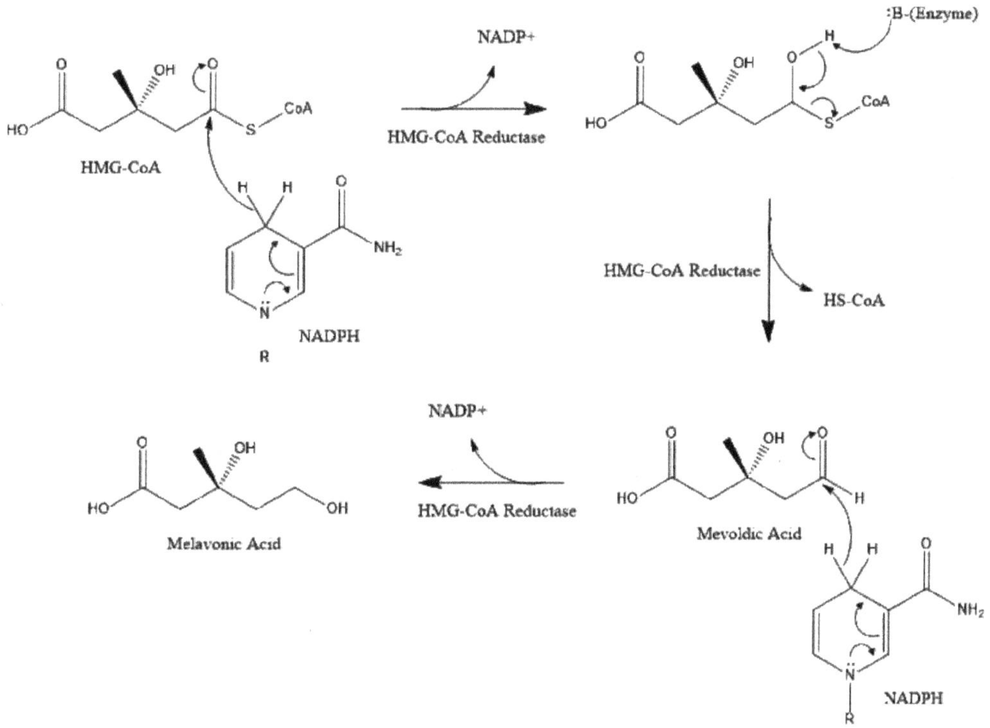

Mevalonate is finally converted to isopentenyl pyrophosphate (IPP) through two phosphorylation steps and one decarboxylation step that requires ATP.

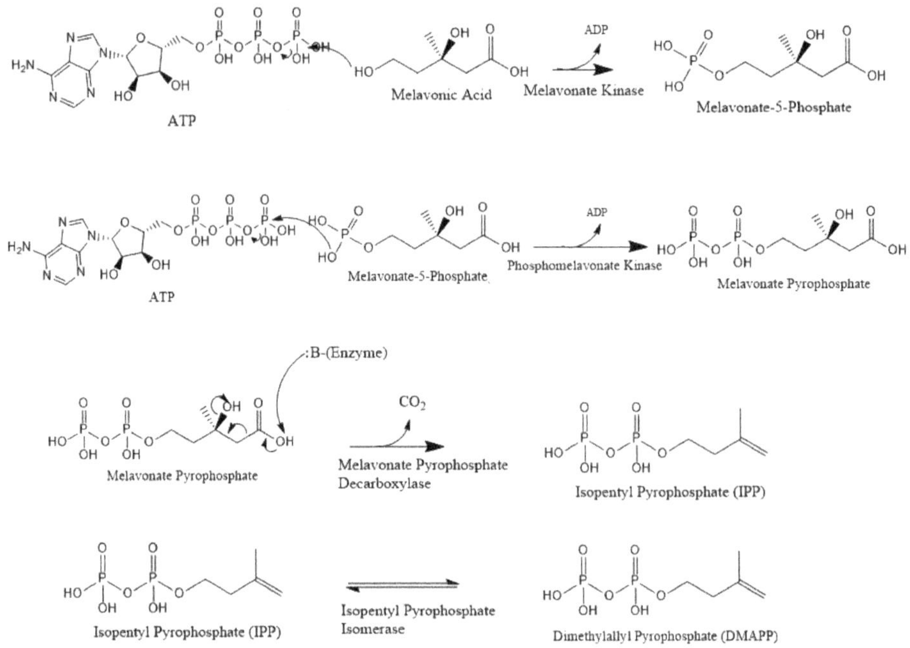

Three molecules of isopentenyl pyrophosphate condense to form farnesyl pyrophosphate through the action of geranyl transferase.

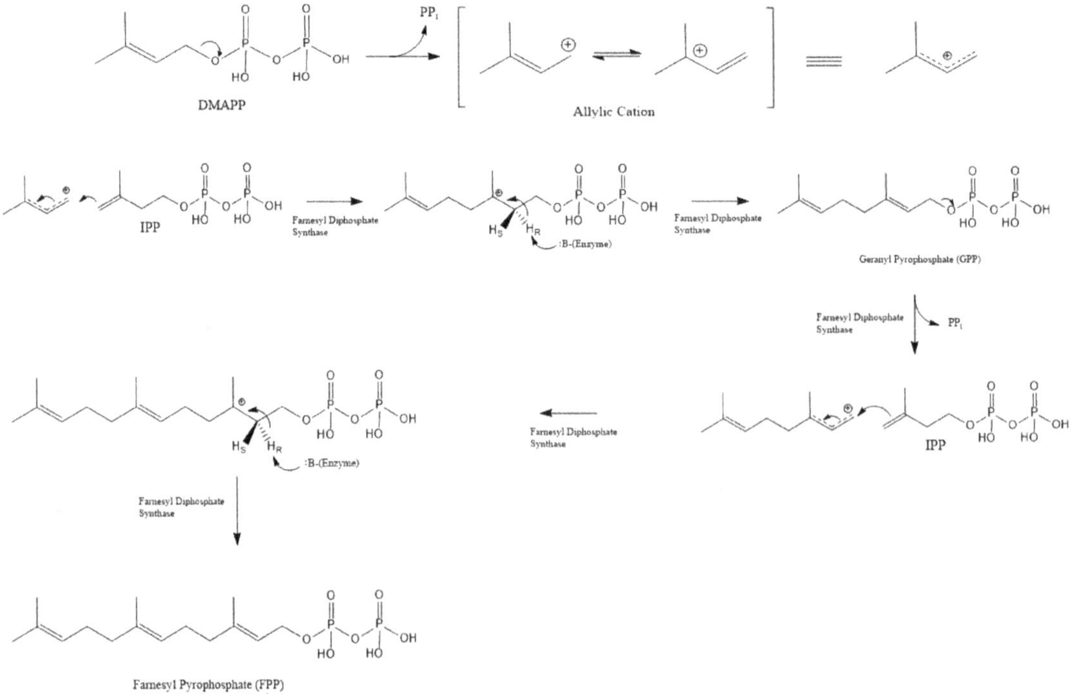

Two molecules of farnesyl pyrophosphate then condense to form squalene by the action of squalene synthase in the endoplasmic reticulum.

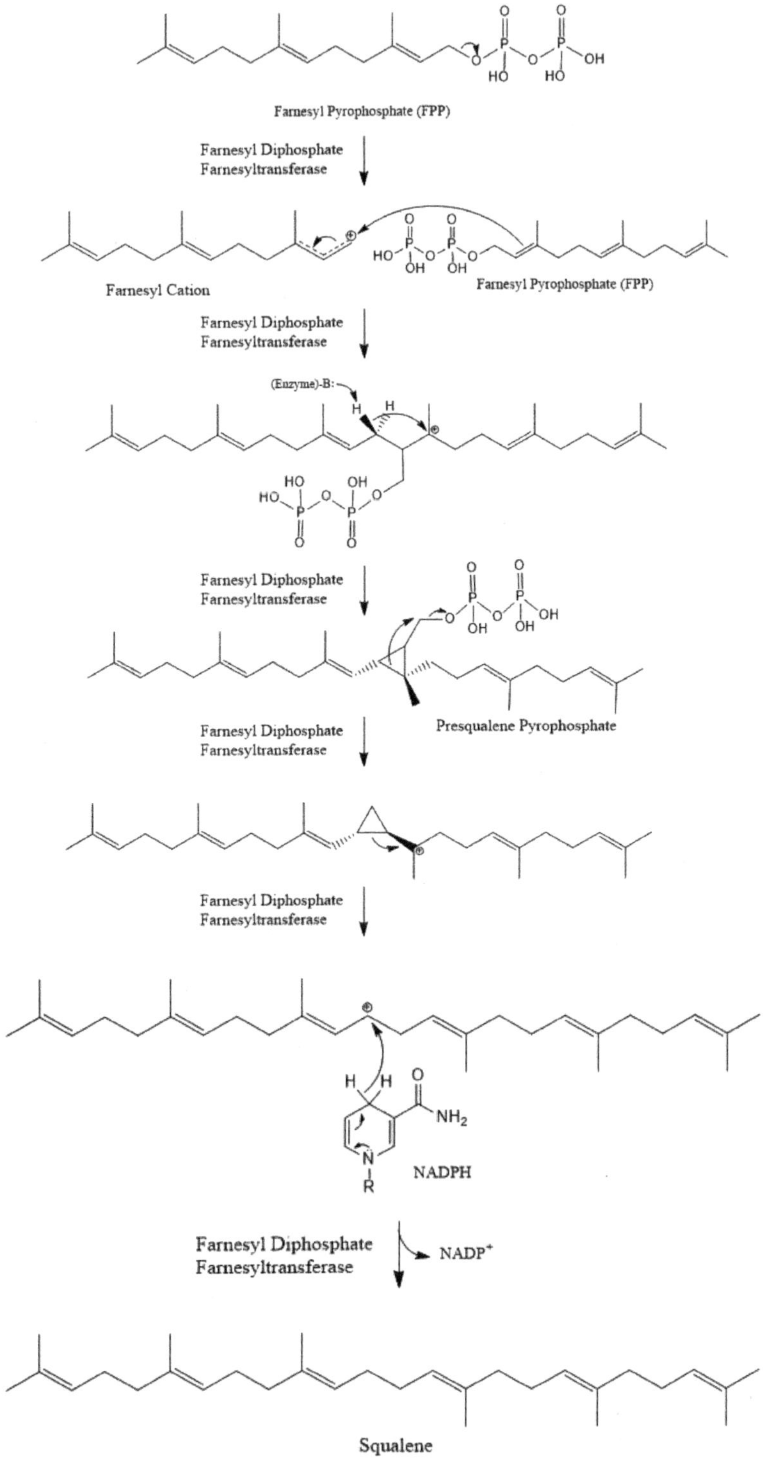

Oxidosqualene cyclase then cyclizes squalene to form lanosterol. Finally, lanosterol is converted to cholesterol through a 19-step process.

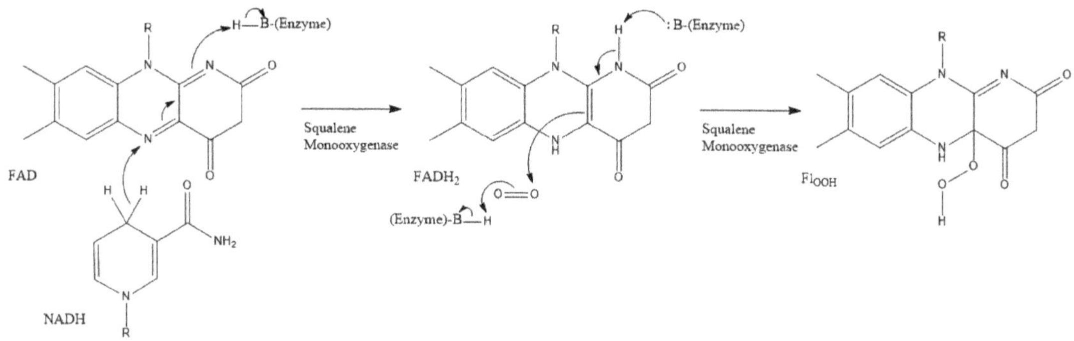

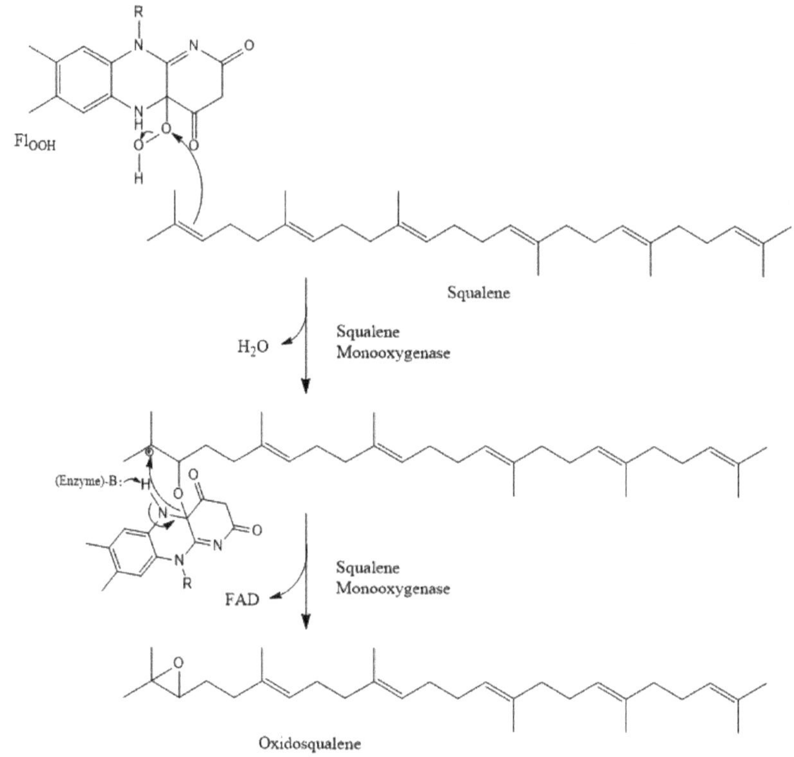

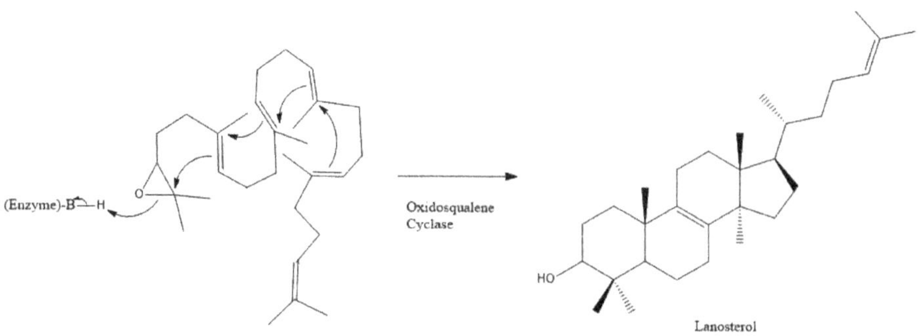

The final 19 steps to cholesterol contain NADPH and Oxygen to help oxidize methyl groups for removal of carbons, mutases to move alkene groups, and NADH to help reduce ketones.

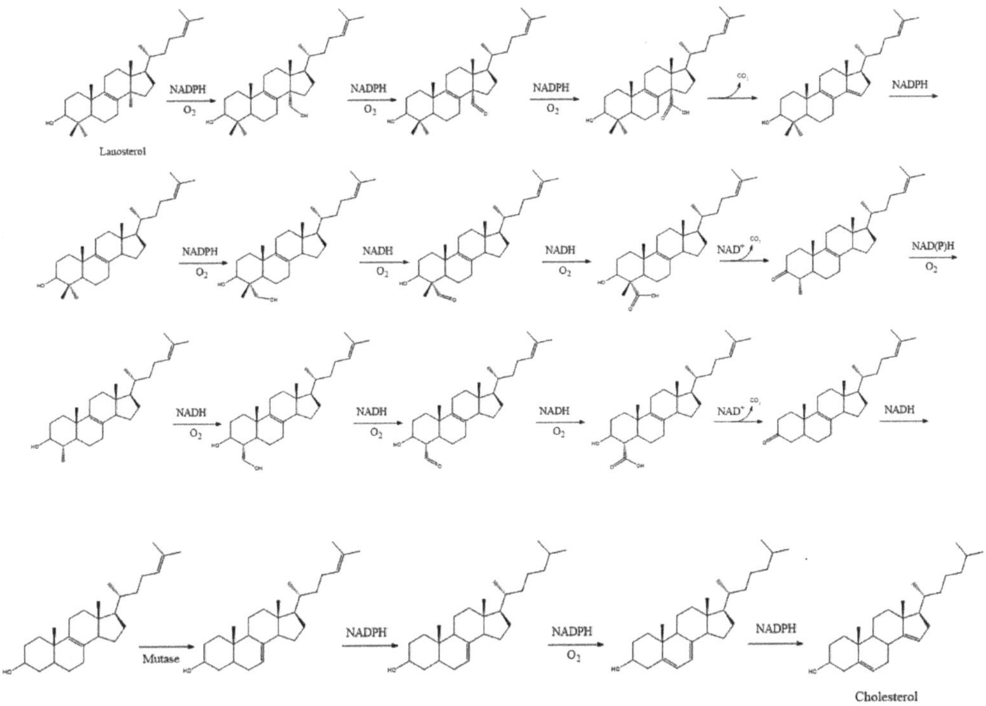

Konrad Bloch and Feodor Lynen shared the Nobel Prize in Physiology or Medicine in 1964 for their discoveries concerning some of the mechanisms and methods of regulation of cholesterol and fatty acid metabolism, though lots of complexities remain to be sorted out.

Regulation of Cholesterol Synthesis

Biosynthesis of cholesterol is directly regulated by the cholesterol levels present, though the homeostatic mechanisms involved are only partly understood. A higher intake from food leads to a net decrease in endogenous production, whereas lower intake from food has the opposite effect. The main regulatory mechanism is the sensing of intracellular cholesterol in the endoplasmic reticulum by the protein SREBP (sterol regulatory element-binding protein 1 and 2). In the presence of cholesterol, SREBP is bound to two other proteins: SCAP (SREBP cleavage-activating protein) and INSIG-1. When cholesterol levels fall, INSIG-1 dissociates from the SREBP-SCAP complex, which allows the complex to migrate to the Golgi apparatus. Here SREBP is cleaved by S1P and S2P (site-1 protease and site-2 protease), two enzymes that are activated by SCAP when cholesterol levels are low.

The cleaved SREBP then migrates to the nucleus, and acts as a transcription factor to bind to the sterol regulatory element (SRE), which stimulates the transcription of many genes. Among these are the low-density lipoprotein (LDL) receptor and HMG-CoA reductase. The LDL receptor scavenges circulating LDL from the bloodstream, whereas HMG-CoA reductase leads to an increase of endogenous production of cholesterol. A large part of this signaling pathway was clarified by Dr. Michael S. Brown and Dr. Joseph L.

Goldstein in the 1970s. In 1985, they received the Nobel Prize in Physiology or Medicine for their work. Their subsequent work shows how the SREBP pathway regulates expression of many genes that control lipid formation and metabolism and body fuel allocation.

Cholesterol synthesis can also be turned off when cholesterol levels are high. HMG-CoA reductase contains both a cytosolic domain (responsible for its catalytic function) and a membrane domain. The membrane domain senses signals for its degradation. Increasing concentrations of cholesterol (and other sterols) cause a change in this domain's oligomerization state, which makes it more susceptible to destruction by the proteosome. This enzyme's activity can also be reduced by phosphorylation by an AMP-activated protein kinase. Because this kinase is activated by AMP, which is produced when ATP is hydrolyzed, it follows that cholesterol synthesis is halted when ATP levels are low.

Plasma Transport and Regulation of Absorption

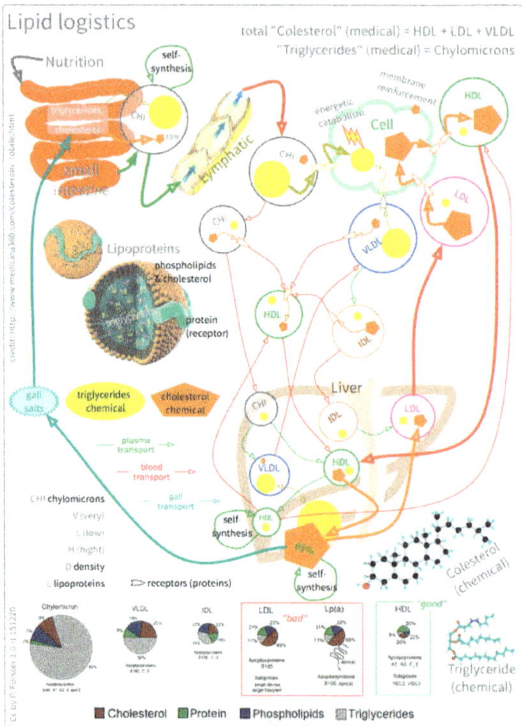

Lipid logistics: transport of triglycerides and cholesterol in organisms in form of lipoproteins as chylomicrons, VLDL, LDL, IDL, HDL.

As an isolated molecule, cholesterol is only minimally soluble in water; it dissolves into the (water-based) bloodstream only at exceedingly small concentrations. Instead, cholesterol is transported within lipoproteins, complex discoidal particles with exterior amphiphilic proteins and lipids, whose outward-facing surfaces are water-soluble and inward-facing surfaces are lipid-soluble; i.e. transport via emulsification. Triglycerides and cholesterol esters are carried internally. Phospholipids and cholesterol, being amphipathic, are transported in the monolayer surface of the lipoprotein particle.

There are several types of lipoproteins in the blood. In order of increasing density, they are chylomicrons, very-low-density lipoprotein (VLDL), intermediate-density lipoprotein (IDL), low-density lipoprotein (LDL), and high-density lipoprotein (HDL). Lower protein/lipid ratios make for less dense lipoproteins. Cholesterol within different lipoproteins is identical, although some is carried as its native "free" alcohol form (the cholesterol-OH group facing the water surrounding the particles), while others as fatty acyl esters, known also as cholesterol esters, within the particles.

Lipoprotein particles are organized by complex apolipoproteins, typically 80-100 different proteins per particle, which can be recognized and bound by specific receptors on cell membranes, directing their lipid payload into specific cells and tissues currently ingesting these fat transport particles. Lipoprotein particles thus include a molecular addresses which play key roles in distribution and delivery of fats around the body in the water outside cells.

Chylomicrons, the least dense cholesterol transport molecules, contain apolipoprotein B-48, apolipoprotein C, and apolipoprotein E (the principal cholesterol carrier in the brain) in their shells. Chylomicrons carry fats from the intestine to muscle and other tissues in need of fatty acids for energy or fat production. Unused cholesterol remains in more cholesterol-rich chylomicron remnants, and taken up from here to the bloodstream by the liver.

VLDL molecules are produced by the liver from triacylglycerol and cholesterol which was not used in the synthesis of bile acids. These molecules contain apolipoprotein B100 and apolipoprotein E in their shells, and are degraded by lipoprotein lipase on the blood vessel wall to IDL.

Blood vessels cleave and absorb triacylglycerol from IDL molecules, increasing the concentration of cholesterol. IDL molecules are then consumed in two processes: half is metabolized by HTGL and taken up by the LDL receptor on the liver cell surfaces, while the other half continues to lose triacylglycerols in the bloodstream until they become LDL molecules, with the highest concentration of cholesterol within them.

LDL particles are the major blood cholesterol carriers. Each one contains approximately 1,500 molecules of cholesterol ester. LDL molecule shells contain just one molecule of apolipoprotein B100, recognized by LDL receptors in peripheral tissues. Upon binding of apolipoprotein B100, many LDL receptors concentrate in clathrin-coated pits. Both LDL and its receptor form vesicles within a cell via endocytosis. These vesicles then fuse with a lysosome, where the lysosomal acid lipase enzyme hydrolyzes the cholesterol esters. The cholesterol can then be used for membrane biosynthesis or esterified and stored within the cell, so as to not interfere with the cell membranes.

LDL receptors are used up during cholesterol absorption, and its synthesis is regulated by SREBP, the same protein that controls the synthesis of cholesterol *de novo*, according to its presence inside the cell. A cell with abundant cholesterol will have its LDL receptor synthesis blocked, to prevent new cholesterol in LDL molecules from being taken up. Conversely, LDL receptor synthesis proceeds when a cell is deficient in cholesterol.

When this process becomes unregulated, LDL molecules without receptors begin to appear in the blood. These LDL molecules are oxidized and taken up by macrophages, which become engorged and form foam cells. These foam cells often become trapped in the walls of blood vessels and contribute to atherosclerotic plaque formation. Differences in cholesterol homeostasis affect the development of early atherosclerosis (carotid intima-media thickness). These plaques are the main causes of heart attacks, strokes, and other serious medical problems, leading to the association of so-called LDL cholesterol (actually a lipoprotein) with "bad" cholesterol.

HDL particles are thought to transport cholesterol back to the liver, either for excretion or for other tissues that synthesize hormones, in a process known as reverse cholesterol transport (RCT). Large numbers of HDL particles correlates with better health outcomes., whereas low numbers of HDL particles is associated with atheromatous disease progression in the arteries.

Metabolism, Recycling and Excretion

Cholesterol is susceptible to oxidation and easily forms oxygenated derivatives known as oxysterols. Three different mechanisms can form these; autoxidation, secondary oxidation to lipid peroxidation, and cholesterol-metabolizing enzyme oxidation. A great interest in oxysterols arose when they were shown to exert inhibitory actions on cholesterol biosynthesis. This finding became known as the "oxysterol hypothesis". Additional roles for oxysterols in human physiology include their: participation in bile acid biosynthesis, function as transport forms of cholesterol, and regulation of gene transcription.

In biochemical experiments radiolabelled forms of cholesterol, such as tritiated-cholesterol are used. These derivatives undergo degradation upon storage and it is essential to purify cholesterol prior to use. Cholesterol can be purified using small Sephadex LH-20 columns.

Cholesterol is oxidized by the liver into a variety of bile acids. These, in turn, are conjugated with glycine, taurine, glucuronic acid, or sulfate. A mixture of conjugated and nonconjugated bile acids, along with cholesterol itself, is excreted from the liver into the bile. Approximately 95% of the bile acids are reabsorbed from the intestines, and the remainder are lost in the feces. The excretion and reabsorption of bile acids forms the basis of the enterohepatic circulation, which is essential for the digestion and absorption of dietary fats. Under certain circumstances, when more concentrated, as in the gallbladder, cholesterol crystallises and is the major constituent of most gallstones. Although, lecithin and bilirubin gallstones also occur, but less frequently. Every day, up to 1 g of cholesterol enters the colon. This cholesterol originates from the diet, bile, and desquamated intestinal cells, and can be metabolized by the colonic bacteria. Cholesterol is converted mainly into coprostanol, a nonabsorbable sterol that is excreted in the feces. A cholesterol-reducing bacterium origin has been isolated from human feces.

Although cholesterol is a steroid generally associated with mammals, the human pathogen *Mycobacterium tuberculosis* is able to completely degrade this molecule and contains a large number of genes that are regulated by its presence. Many of these cholesterol-regulated genes are homologues of fatty acid β-oxidation genes, but have evolved in such a way as to bind large steroid substrates like cholesterol.

Research

Cholesterol binds to and affects the gating of a number of ion channels such as the nicotinic acetylcholine receptor, $GABA_A$ receptor, and the inward-rectifier potassium ion channel. Cholesterol also activates the estrogen-related receptor alpha, and may be the endogenous ligand for the receptor.

Clinical Significance

Hypercholesterolemia

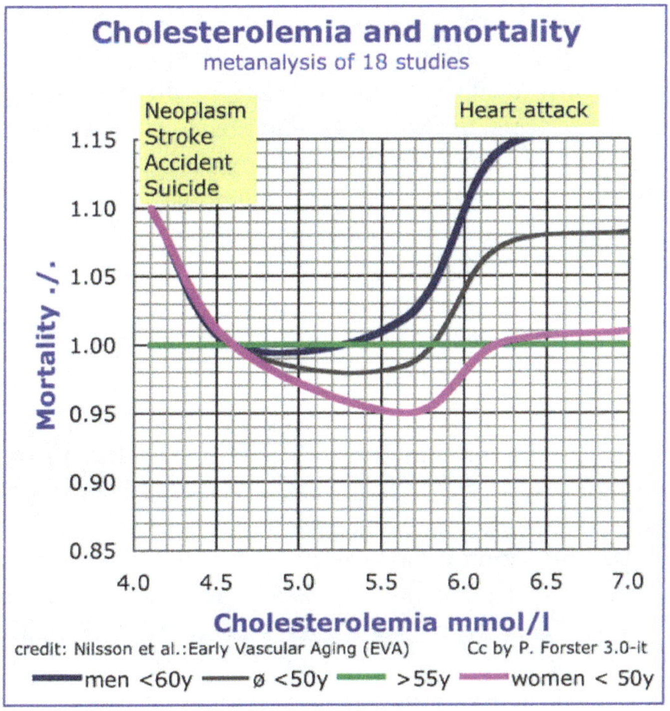

Cholesterolemia and mortality for men and women <50 years and >60 years

According to the lipid hypothesis, since cholesterol (like all fat molecules) is transported around the body (in the water outside cells) inside lipoprotein particles, elevated cholesterol concentrations (hypercholesterolemia) — potentially offers a lower cost way to estimate concentrations of LDL particles; possibly even low concentrations of functional HDL particles — both variations strongly associated with cardiovascular disease because LDL particles promote atheroma development in arteries (atherosclerosis).

The problem with this hypothesis is that a single LDL-particle typically carries 3,000 to 6,000 fat molecules and the percentage which are cholesterol (vs. all other fat molecules) is: (a) highly variable, (b) not measured (only guessed at) by lipid tests,

(c) correlates better only when cholesterol concentrations are very high, over 350 mg/dL, and (d) the majority of individuals who suffer heart attacks, strokes and peripheral arterial disease complications have "normal" cholesterol values, i.e. values <200 mg/dL.

This atherosclerotic disease process, over decades, leads to myocardial infarction (heart attack), stroke, and peripheral vascular disease. Since higher blood LDL, especially higher LDL particle concentrations and smaller LDL particle size, contribute to this process more than the cholesterol content of the HDL particles, LDL particles are often termed "bad cholesterol" because they have been linked to atheroma formation. On the other hand, high concentrations of functional HDL, which can remove cholesterol from cells and atheroma, offer protection and are sometimes referred to as "good cholesterol". These balances are mostly genetically determined, but can be changed by body build, medications, food choices, and other factors.

Conditions with elevated concentrations of oxidized LDL particles, especially "small dense LDL" (sdLDL) particles, are associated with atheroma formation in the walls of arteries, a condition known as atherosclerosis, which is the principal cause of coronary heart disease and other forms of cardiovascular disease. In contrast, HDL particles (especially large HDL) have been identified as a mechanism by which cholesterol and inflammatory mediators can be removed from atheroma. Increased concentrations of HDL correlate with lower rates of atheroma progressions and even regression. A 2007 study pooling data on almost 900,000 subjects in 61 cohorts demonstrated that blood total cholesterol levels have an exponential effect on cardiovascular and total mortality, with the association more pronounced in younger subjects. Still, because cardiovascular disease is relatively rare in the younger population, the impact of high cholesterol on health is still larger in older people.

Elevated levels of the lipoprotein fractions, LDL, IDL and VLDL are regarded as atherogenic (prone to cause atherosclerosis). Levels of these fractions, rather than the total cholesterol level, correlate with the extent and progress of atherosclerosis. Conversely, the total cholesterol can be within normal limits, yet be made up primarily of small LDL and small HDL particles, under which conditions atheroma growth rates would still be high. Recently, a *post hoc* analysis of the IDEAL and the EPIC prospective studies found an association between high levels of HDL cholesterol (adjusted for apolipoprotein A-I and apolipoprotein B) and increased risk of cardiovascular disease, casting doubt on the cardioprotective role of "good cholesterol".

Elevated cholesterol levels are treated with a strict diet consisting of low saturated fat, trans fat-free, low cholesterol foods, often followed by one of various hypolipidemic agents, such as statins, fibrates, cholesterol absorption inhibitors, nicotinic acid derivatives or bile acid sequestrants. Extreme cases have previously been treated with partial ileal bypass surgery, which has now been superseded by medication. Apheresis-based treatments are still used for very severe hyperlipidemias that are either unresponsive to treatment or require rapid lowering of blood lipids. There are several international guidelines on the treatment of hypercholesterolaemia.

Multiple human trials using HMG-CoA reductase inhibitors, known as statins, have repeatedly confirmed that changing lipoprotein transport patterns from unhealthy to healthier patterns significantly lowers cardiovascular disease event rates, even for people with cholesterol values currently considered low for adults. Studies have also found that statins reduce atheroma progression. As a result, people with a history of cardiovascular disease may derive benefit from statins irrespective of their cholesterol levels, and in men without cardiovascular disease, there is benefit from lowering abnormally high cholesterol levels ("primary prevention"). Primary prevention in women was originally practiced only by extension of the findings in studies on men, since, in women, none of the large statin trials conducted prior to 2007 demonstrated a statistically significant reduction in overall mortality or in cardiovascular endpoints. In 2008, a large clinical trial reported that, in apparently healthy adults with increased levels of the inflammatory biomarker high-sensitivity C-reactive protein but with low initial LDL, 20 mg/day of rosuvastatin for 1.9 years resulted in a 44% reduction in the incidence of cardiovascular events and a 20% reduction in all-cause mortality; the effect was statistically significant for both genders. Though this result was met with some skepticism, later studies and meta-analyses likewise demonstrated statistically significant (but smaller) reductions in all-cause and cardiovascular mortality, without significant heterogeneity by gender.

Level mg/dL	**Level** mmol/L	**Interpretation**
< 200	< 5.2	Desirable level corresponding to lower risk for heart disease
200–240	5.2–6.2	Borderline high risk
> 240	> 6.2	High risk

The 1987 report of National Cholesterol Education Program, Adult Treatment Panels suggests the total blood cholesterol level should be: < 200 mg/dL normal blood cholesterol, 200–239 mg/dL borderline-high, > 240 mg/dL high cholesterol. The American Heart Association provides a similar set of guidelines for total (fasting) blood cholesterol levels and risk for heart disease: However, as today's testing methods determine LDL ("bad") and HDL ("good") cholesterol separately, this simplistic view has become somewhat outdated. The desirable LDL level is considered to be less than 130 mg/dL (2.6 mmol/L), although a newer upper limit of 70 mg/dL (1.8 mmol/L) can be considered in higher-risk individuals based on some of the above-mentioned trials. A ratio of total cholesterol to HDL—another useful measure—of far less than 5:1 is thought to be healthier.

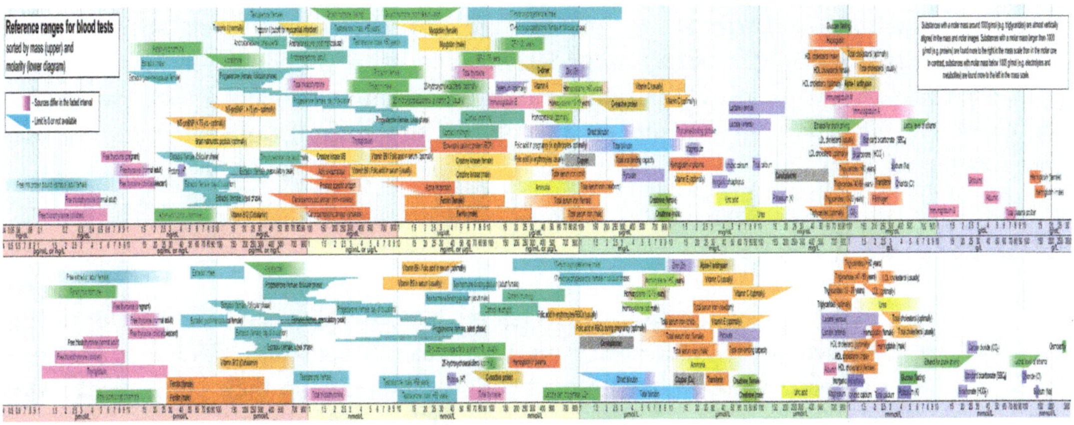

Reference ranges for blood tests, showing usual, as well as optimal, levels of HDL, LDL and total cholesterol in mass and molar concentrations, is found in orange color at right, that is, among the blood constituents with the highest concentration.

Total cholesterol is defined as the sum of HDL, LDL, and VLDL. Usually, only the total, HDL, and triglycerides are measured. For cost reasons, the VLDL is usually estimated as one-fifth of the triglycerides and the LDL is estimated using the Friedewald formula (or a variant): estimated LDL = [total cholesterol] − [total HDL] − [estimated VLDL]. VLDL can be calculated by dividing total triglycerides by five. Direct LDL measures are used when triglycerides exceed 400 mg/dL. The estimated VLDL and LDL have more error when triglycerides are above 400 mg/dL.

Given the well-recognized role of cholesterol in cardiovascular disease, some studies have shown an inverse correlation between cholesterol levels and mortality. A 2009 study of patients with acute coronary syndromes found an association of hypercholesterolemia with better mortality outcomes. In the Framingham Heart Study, in subjects over 50 years of age, they found an 11% increase overall and 14% increase in cardiovascular disease mortality per 1 mg/dL per year drop in total cholesterol levels. The researchers attributed this phenomenon to the fact that people with severe chronic diseases or cancer tend to have below-normal cholesterol levels. This explanation is not supported by the Vorarlberg Health Monitoring and Promotion Programme, in which men of all ages and women over 50 with very low cholesterol were likely to die of cancer, liver diseases, and mental diseases. This result indicates the low-cholesterol effect occurs even among younger respondents, contradicting the previous assessment among cohorts of older people that this is a proxy or marker for frailty occurring with age.

Although the vast majority of doctors and medical scientists consider that there is a link between cholesterol and atherosclerosis as discussed above, a 2014 meta-analysis of over 500,000 patients concluded there is insufficient evidence to support the recommendation of high consumption of polyunsaturated fatty acids and low consumption of total saturated fats for cardiovascular health.

Hypocholesterolemia

Abnormally low levels of cholesterol are termed *hypocholesterolemia*. Research into the causes of this state is relatively limited, but some studies suggest a link with depression, cancer, and cerebral hemorrhage. In general, the low cholesterol levels seem to be a consequence, rather than a cause, of an underlying illness. A genetic defect in cholesterol synthesis causes Smith-Lemli-Opitz syndrome, which is often associated with low plasma cholesterol levels. Hyperthyroidism, or any other endocrine disturbance which causes upregulation of the LDL receptor, may result in hypocholesterolemia.

Cholesterol Testing

The American Heart Association recommends testing cholesterol every 4–6 years for people aged 20 years or older. A separate set of American Heart Association guidelines issued in 2013 indicates that patients taking statin medications should have their cholesterol tested 4–12 weeks after their first dose and then every 3–12 months thereafter.

A blood sample after 12-hour fasting is taken by a doctor, or a home cholesterol-monitoring device is used to determine a lipoprotein profile. This measures total cholesterol, LDL (bad) cholesterol, HDL (good) cholesterol, and triglycerides. It is recommended to test cholesterol at least every five years if a person has total cholesterol of 5.2 mmol/L or more (200+ mg/dL), or if a man over age 45 or a woman over age 50 has HDL (good) cholesterol less than 1 mmol/L (40 mg/dL), or there are other risk factors for heart disease and stroke. Other risk factors for heart disease include Diabetes, Hypertension (or use of anti-hypertensive medications), low HDL, family history of CAD and hypercholesterolemia, and cigarette smoking.

Cholesteric Liquid Crystals

Some cholesterol derivatives (among other simple cholesteric lipids) are known to generate the liquid crystalline "cholesteric phase". The cholesteric phase is, in fact, a chiral nematic phase, and it changes colour when its temperature changes. This makes cholesterol derivatives useful for indicating temperature in liquid crystal display thermometers and in temperature-sensitive paints.

Stereoisomers

Cholesterol has 256 stereoisomers that arise from its 8 stereocenters, although only two of the stereoisomers are of biochemical significance (*nat*-cholesterol and *ent*-cholesterol, for *natural* and *enantiomer*, respectively), and only one occurs naturally (*nat*-cholesterol).

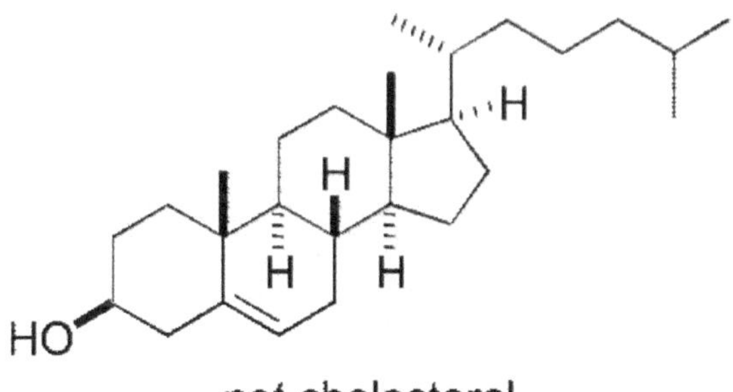

nat-cholesterol

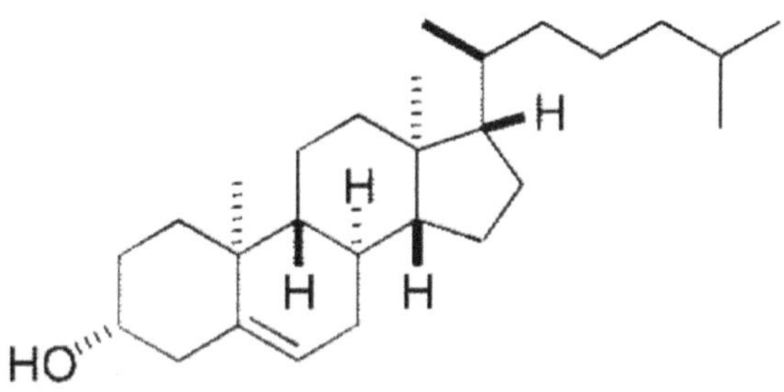

ent-cholesterol

EICOSANOID

Eicosanoids are signaling molecules made by the enzymatic or non-enzymatic oxidation of arachidonic acid or other polyunsaturated fatty acids (PUFAs) that are, like arachidonic acid, 20 carbon units in length. They are a sub-category of oxylipins, i.e. oxidized fatty acids of diverse carbon units in length but are further distinguished from other oxylipins by their overwhelming importance as cell signaling molecules. Eicosanoids function in diverse physiological and pathological systems including those: mounting or inhibiting inflammation, allergy, fever and other immune responses; influencing the abortion of pregnancy and normal childbirth; contributing to the perception of pain; regulating cell growth; controlling blood pressure; and modulating the regional flow of blood to tissues. In performing these tasks, eicosanoids most often act as autocrine signaling agents to impact their cells of origin or as paracrine signaling agents to impact cells near to their cells of origin. However, they can also act as endocrine agents to control the function of distant cells.

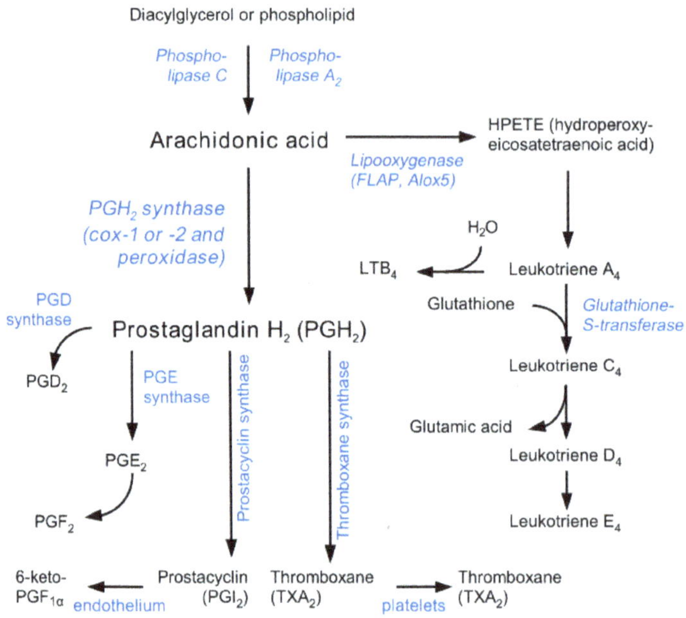

Pathways in biosynthesis of eicosanoids from arachidonic acid: there are parallel paths from EPA & DGLA.

There are multiple subfamilies of eicosanoids, including most prominently the prostaglandins, thromboxanes, leukotrienes, lipoxins, resolvins, and eoxins but also others as noted in the following Nomenclature section. For each subfamily, there is the potential to have at least 5 separate series of metabolites, two series derived from ω-6 PUFAs (arachidonic and dihomo-gamma-linolenic acids), one series derived from the ω-3 PUFA (eicosapentaenoic acid), and one series derived from the ω-9 PUFA (mead acid). This subfamily distinction is important. Mammals, including humans, are unable to convert ω-6 into ω-3 PUFA. In consequence, tissue levels of the ω-6 and ω-3 PUFAs and their corresponding eicosanoid metabolites link directly to the amount of dietary ω-6 versus ω-3 PUFAs consumed. Since certain of the ω-6 and ω-3 PUFA series of metabolites have almost diametrically opposing physiological and pathological activities, it has often been suggested that the deleterious consequences associated with the consumption of ω-6 PUFA-rich diets reflects excessive production and activities of ω-6 PUFA-derived eicosanoids while the beneficial effects associated with the consumption of ω-3 PUFA-rich diets reflect the excessive production and activities of ω-3 PUFA-derived eicosanoids. In this view, the opposing effects of ω-6 PUFA-derived and ω-3 PUFA-derived eicosanoids on key target cells underlie the detrimental and beneficial effects of ω-6 and ω-3 PUFA-rich diets on inflammation and allergy reactions, atherosclerosis, hypertension, cancer growth, and a host of other processes.

Nomenclature

Fatty Acid Sources

"Eicosanoid" (*eicosa-*, Greek for "twenty"; *see icosahedron*) is the collective term for straight-chain polyunsaturated fatty acids (PUFAs) of 20 carbon units in length that have been metabolized or otherwise converted to oxygen-containing products. The PUFA precursors to the eicosanoids include:

- Arachidonic acid (**AA**), i.e. 5*Z*, 8*Z*,11*Z*,14*Z*-eicosatetraenoic acid is ω-6 fatty acid, with four double bonds in the cis configuration (see Cis–trans isomerism) each located between carbons 5-6, 8-9, 11,-12, and 14-15.
- Adrenic acid (**AdA**), 7,10,13,16-docosatetraenoic acid, is an ω-6 fatty acid with four cis double bounds, each located between carbons 7-8, 10-11, 13-14, and 17-18.
- Eicosapentaenoic acid (**EPA**), i.e.i.e. 5*Z*, 8*Z*,11*Z*,14*Z*,17*Z*-eicosapentaenoic acid is an ω-3 fatty acid with five cis double bonds, each located between carbons 5-8, 8-9, 11,-12, 14-15, and 17-18.
- Dihomo-gamma-linolenic acid (**DGLA**), 8*Z*, 11*Z*,14*Z*-eicosatrienoic acid is an ω-6 fatty acid with three cis double bonds, each located between carbons 8-9, 11,-12, and 14-15.
- Mead acid, i.e. 5*Z*,8*Z*,11*Z*-eicosatrienoic acid, is an ω-9 fatty acid containing three cis double bonds, each located between carbons 5-6, 8-9, and 11,-12.

Abbreviation

A particular eicosanoid is denoted by a four-character abbreviation, composed of:

- its two-letter abbreviation (**LT**, **EX** or **PG**, as described above),
- one A-B-C sequence-letter,
- A subscript or plain script number following the designated eicosanoid's trivial name indicates the number of its double bonds. Examples are:
- The EPA-derived prostanoids have three double bonds (e.g. PGG_3 or PGG3) while leukotrienes derived from EPA have five double bonds (e.g. LTB_5 or LTB5).
- The AA-derived prostanoids have two double bonds (e.g. PGG_2 or PGG2) while their AA-derived leukotrienes have four double bonds (e.g. LTB_4 or LTB4).

- Hydroperoxy-, hydroxyl-, and oxo-eicosanoids possess a hydroperoxy (-OOH), hydroxy (-OH), or oxygen atom (=O) substituents link to a PUFA carbon by a single (-) or double (=) bond. Their trivial names indicate the substituent as: Hp or HP for a hydroperoxy residue (e.g. 5-hydrperooxy-eicosatraenoic acid or 5-*Hp*ETE or 5-*HP*ETE); H for a hydroxy residue (e.g. 5-hydroxy-eicosatetraenoic acid or 5-*H*ETE); and oxo- for an oxo residue (e.g. 5-oxo-eicosatetraenioic acid or 5-*oxo*-ETE or 5-*oxo*ETE). The number of their double bounds is indicated by their full and trivial names: AA-derived hydroxy metabolites have four (i.e. 'tetra' or 'T') double bonds (e.g. 5-hydroxy-eicosa*tetra*enoic acid or 5-HE*T*E; EPA-derived hydroxy metabolites have five ('penta' or 'P') double bonds (e.g. 5-hydroxy-eicosa*penta*enoic acid or 5-HE*P*E); and DGLA-derived hydroxy metabolites have three ('tri' or 'Tr') double bonds (e.g. 5-hydroxy-eicosa*tri*enoic acid or 5-HE*Tr*E).

The stereochemistry of the eicosanoid products formed may differ among the pathways. For prostaglandins, this is often indicated by Greek letters (e.g. $PGF_{2\alpha}$ versus $PGF_{2\beta}$). For hydroperoxy and hydroxy eicosanoids an *S* or *R* designates the chirality of their substituents (e.g. 5*S*-hydroxy-eicosateteraenoic acid is given the trivial names of 5*S*-HETE, 5(*S*)-HETE, 5S-HETE, or 5(S)-HETE). Since eicosanoid-forming enzymes commonly make *S* isomer products either with marked preference or essentially exclusively, the use of *S*/*R* designations has often been dropped (e.g. 5*S*-HETE is 5-HETE). Nonetheless, certain eicosanoid-forming pathways do form R isomers and their *S* versus *R* isomeric products can exhibit dramatically different biological activities. Failing to specify *S*/*R* isomers can be misleading. Here, all hydroperoxy and hydroxy substituents have the *S* configuration unless noted otherwise.

Classic Eicosanoids

Current usage limits the term eicosanoid to:

- ω-6 Series eicosanoids derived from arachidonic acid:
- Hydroxyeicosatetraenoic acids (**HETE**) include the following metabolites of arachidonic acid:
- 5-HETE, 12-HETE, 15-Hydroxyeicosatetraenoic acid (i.e. 15-HETE), 20-Hydroxyeicosatetraenoic acid (i.e. 20-HETE), and 19-HETE (see 20-Hydroxyeicosatetraenoic acid).
- Leukotrienes (**LT**) include the following metabolites of arachidonic acid:
- LTA4, LTB4, LTC4, LTD4, and LTE4.
- Eoxins (**EX**) include the following metabolites of arachidnoic acid:
- EXA4, EXC4, EXD4, and EXE4.
- Prostanoids consisting of several different types:
- Prostaglandins (**PG**) include the following metabolites of arachidonic acid:
- PGG2, PGH2, PGE2, PGD2, PGF2alpha, PGA2, PGB2, (see Prostanoid and Specialized pro-resolving mediators#Prostaglandins and Isoprostanes).
- Prostacyclins include:

- PGI2 (see prostacyclin).
- Thromboxanes (**TX**) include the following metabolites of aracidonic acid:
- TXA2 and TXB2.
- Cyclopentenone prostaglandins include the following metabolites of arachidonic acid:
- PGA1, PGA2 (see 'prostanoid, PGJ2, Δ12-PGJ2, and 15-deoxy-Δ12,14-PGJ2.
- ω-6 Series eicosanoids derived from dihomo-gamma-linolenic acid. These metabolites are analogs of arachidonic acid-derived eicosanoids but lack a double bound between carbons 5 and 6 and therefore have 1 less double bound than their arachidonic acid-derived analogs. They the following:
- PGA1, PGE1, and TXA1.
- ω-3 Series eicosanoids:
- Resolvins of the E series (**RvE**) (D series resolvins (RvD's are metabolites of the 22-carbon ω-6 fatty acid docosahexaenoic acid; see Specialized pro-resolving mediators#DHA-derived Resolvins). RvE's include the following metabolites of eicosapentaenoic acid:
- RvE1, 18S-RvE1, RvE2, and RvE3.
- Other ω-3 series eicosapentaenoic acid-derived eicosanoids are analogs of ω-6 fatty acid-derived metabolites but contain a double bond between carbon 17 and 18 and therefore have one more double bound than their arachidonic acid-derived analogs. They include (HEPE is hydroxy-eicsapentaenoic acid):
- 5-HEPE (see Arachidonate 5-lipoxygenase#Eicosapentaenoic acid), 12-HEPE, 15-HEPE, and 20-HETE; LTA5, LTB5 (see Essential fatty acid interactions#counteractions), LTC5, LTD5, and LTE5 (see Arachidonate 5-lipoxygenase#eicosapentaenoic acid);PGE3, PGD3, PGF3α, and Δ(17)-6-keto PGF1α; PGI3 (see Essential fatty acid interactions#counteraction); and TXA3 and TXB3 (see Essential fatty acid interactions#nomenclature).
- ω-9 Series eicosanoids
- Hydroxy are derived form mead acid, is metabolized to the 3 double bond-containing analog of 5-HETE viz., 5-HETrE (see arachidonate 5-lipoxygenase#mead acid).

Hydroxyeicosatetraenoic acids, leukotrienes, eoxins and prostanoids are sometimes termed "classic eicosanoids"

Nonclassic Eicosanoids

In contrast to the classic eicosanoids, several other classes of PUFA metabolites have been termed 'novel', 'eicosanoid-like' or 'nonclassic eicosanoids'. These included the following classes:

- Oxoeicosanoids (**oxo-ETE**) include the following metabolites:
- 5-oxo-eicosatetraenoic acid (5-oxo-ETE), 12-oxo-ETE (see 12-HETE#Further metabolism), and 15-oxo-ETE, which are metabolites of arachidonic acid (see

15-Hydroxyeicosatetraenoic acid) and 5-oxo-ETrE which is a metabolite of mead acid (see arachidonate 5-lipoxygenase#mead acid).

- Hepoxilins (**Hx**) include the following arachidonic acid metabolites:
- HxA3 and HxB3 (see Hepoxilins).
- Lipoxins (**Lx**) include the following metabolites of arachidonic acid:
- LxA4 and LxB4(see Specialized pro-resolving mediators).
- Epi-lipoxins (**epi-Lx**) include the following metabolites of arachidonic acid:
- 15-epi-LxA4 (also termed AT-LxA4) and 15-epi-LxB4 (also termed AT-LxB4) (see Specialized pro-resolving mediators).
- Epoxyeicosatrienoic acids (**EET**) include the following metabolites of arachidonic acid:
- 5,6-EET, 8,9-EET, 11,12-EET, and 14,15-EET (see epoxyeicosatrienoic acid).
- Epoxyeicosatetraenoic acid (*EEQ*) include the following metabolites of eicosapentaenoic acid:
- 5,6-EEQ, 8,9-EEQ, 11,12-EEQ, 14,15-EEQ, and 15,16-EEQ (see epoxyeicosatetraenoic acid).
- Isoprostanes (**isoP**) are non-enzymatically formed derivatives of polyunsaturated fatty acids studied as markers of oxidative stress; they include the following arachidonic acid-derived isoP's which are named based on their structural similarities to PGs:
- D2-isoPs, E2-isoPs, A2-isoPs, and J2-isoPs; and two epoxide-containing isoPs, 5,6-epoxyisoprostane E2 and 5,6-epoxyisoprostane A2. Some of these isoPs have been shown to possess anti-inflammatory activity(see Specialized pro-resolving mediators#Prostaglandins and Isoprostanes).
- Isofurans are non-enzymatically formed dervatives of polyunsaturated fatty acids that possess a Furan ring structure; they are studied as markers of oxidative stress. There are 256 potentially different furan ring-containing isomers that can be derived from arachidonic acid.
- Endocannabinoids are certain glycerolipids or dopamine that are esterified to polyunsaturated fatty acids that activate cannabinoid receptors. They include the following arachidonic acid-esterified agents:
- Arachidonoylethanolamine, 2-Arachidonoylglycerol, 2-Arachidonyl glyceryl ether, O-arachidonoyl-ethanolamine, and N-Arachidonoyl dopamine.

Metabolism of eicosapentaenoic acid to HEPEs, leukotrienes, prostanoids, and epoxyeicosatetraenoic acids as well as the metabolism of dihomo-gamma-linolenic acid to prostanoids and mead acid to 5(S)-hydroxy-6E,8Z,11Z-eicosatrienoic acid (5-HETrE), 5-oxo-6,8,11-eicosatrienoic acid (5-oxo-ETrE), LTA3, and LTC3 involve the same enzymatic pathways that make their arachidonic acid-derived analogs.

Biosyntheses

Eicosanoids typically are not stored within cells but rather synthesized as required. They derive from the fatty acids that make up the cell membrane and nuclear membrane. These fatty acids must be released from their membrane sites and then metabolized initially to products which most often are further metabolized through various pathways to make the large array of products we recognize as bioactive eicosanoids.

Fatty Acid Mobilization

Eicosanoid biosynthesis begins when a cell is activated by mechanical trauma, ischemia, other physical perturbations, attack by pathogens, or stimuli made by nearby cells, tissues, or pathogens such as chemotactic factors, cytokines, growth factors, and even certain eicosanoids. The activated cells then mobilize enzymes, termed phospholipase A_2's (PLA_2s), capable of releasing ω-6 and ω-3 fatty acids from membrane storage. These fatty acids are bound in ester linkage to the SN2 position of membrane phospholipids; PLA_2s act as esterases to release the fatty. There are several classes of PLA_2s with type IV cytosolic PLA_2s ($cPLA_2$s) appearing to be responsible for releasing the fatty acids under many conditions of cell activation. The $cPLA_2$s act specifically on phospholipids that contain AA, EPA or GPLA at their SN2 position. Interestingly, $cPLA_2$ may also release the lysophospholipid that becomes platelet-activating factor.

Peroxidation and Reactive Oxygen Species

Next, the free fatty acid is oxygenated along any of several pathways; see the *Pathways* table. The eicosanoid pathways (*via* lipoxygenase or COX) add molecular oxygen (O_2). Although the fatty acid is symmetric, the resulting eicosanoids are chiral; the oxidations proceed with high stereoselectivity (enzymatic oxidations are considered practically stereospecific).

Four families of enzymes initiate or contribute to the initiation of the catalysis of fatty acids to eicosanoids:

- Cyclooxygenases (COXs): COX-1 and COX-2 initiate the metabolism of arachidonic acid to prostanoids that contain two double bonds, i.e. the prostaglandins (e.g PGE2), prostacyclin (i.e. PGI2), and thromboxanes (e.g. TXA2). The two COX enzymes likewise initiate the metabolism of: **a)** eicosapentaenoic acid, which has 5 double bonds compared to the 4 double bonds of arachidonic acid, to prostanoid, prostacyclin, and thromboxane products that have three double bonds, e.g. PGE3, PGI3, and TXA3 and **b)** Dihomo-γ-linolenic acid acid, which has three double bonds, to prostanoid, prostacyclin, and thromboxane products that have only one double bond, e.g. PGE1, PGI1, and TXA1.
- Lipoxygenases (LOXs): 5-Lipoxygenase (5-LOX or ALOX5) initiates the metabolism of arachidonic acid to 5-hydroperoxyeicosatetraenoic acid (5-HpETE) which then may be rapidly reduced to 5-hydroxyeicosatetraenoic acid (5-HETE) or further metabolized to the leukotrienes (e.g. LTB4 and LTC4); 5-HETE may be oxidized to 5-oxo-eicosatetraenoic acid (5-oxo-ETE).

In similar fashions, 15-lipoxygenase (15-lipoxygenase 1, 15-LOX, 15-LOX1, or ALOX15) initiates the metabolism of arachidonic acid to 15-HpETE, 15-HETE, eoxins, 8,15-dihydroxyeicosapentaenoic acid (i.e. 8,15-DiHETE), and 15-oxo-ETE and 12-lipoxygenase (12-LOX or ALOX12) initiates the metabolism of arachidonic acid to 12-HpETE, 12-HETE, hepoxilins, and 12-oxo-ETE. These enzymes also initiate the metabolism of; **a)** eicosatetraenoic acid to analogs of the arachidonic acid metabolites that contain 5 rather than four double bonds, e.g. 5-hydroxy-eicosapentaenoic acid (5-HEPE), LTB5, LTC5, 5-oxo-EPE, 15-HEPE, and 12-HEPE; **b)** the three double bond-containing dihomo-γ-linolenic acid to products that contain 3 double bonds, e.g. 8-hydroxy-eicosatrienoic acid (8-HETrE), 12-HETrE, and 15-HETrE (this fatty acid cannot be converted to leukotrienes); and the three double bond-containing mead acid (by ALOX5) to 5-hydroperoxy-eicosatrienoic acid (5-HpETrE), 5-HETrE, and 5-oxo-HETrE. In the most studied of these pathways, ALOX5 metabolizes eicosapentaenoic acid to 5-hydroperoxyeicosapentaenoic acid (5-HpEPE), 5-HEPE, and LTB5, and 5-oxo-EPE, all of which are less active than there arachidonic acid analogs. Since eicosapentaenoic acid competes with arachidonic acid for ALOX5, production of the eicosapentaenoate metabolites leads to a reduction in the eicosatetraenoate metabolites and therefore reduction in the latter metabolites' signaling. The initial mono-hydroperoxy and mono-hydroxy products made by the aforementioned lipoxygenases have their hydroperosy and hydroxyl residues positioned in the *S* chiral configuration and are more properly termed 5*S*-HpETE, 5*S*-HETE, 12*S*-HpETE, 12*S*-HETE, 15*S*-HpETE and, 15*S*-HETE. ALOX12B (i.e. arachidonate 12-lipoxygenase, 12R type) forms *R* chirality products, i.e. 12*R*-HpETE and 12*R*-HETE. Similarly, ALOXE3 (i.e. epidermis-type lipoxygenase 3 or eLOX3) metabolizes arachidonic acid to 12*R*-HpETE and 12*R*-HETE; however these are minor products that this enzyme forms only under a limited set of conditions. ALOXE3 preferentially metabolizes arachidonic acid to hepoxilins.

- Epoxygenases: these are cytochrome P450 enzymes which generate nonclassic eicosanoid epoxides derived from: **a)** arachidonic acid viz., 5,6-epoxy-eicsattrienoic acid (5,6-EET), 8,9-EET, 11,12-EET, and 14,15-EET (see Epoxyeicosatrienoic acid); **b)** eicosapentaenoic acid viz., 5,6,-epoxy-eicosatetraenoic acid (5,6-EEQ), 8,9-EEQ, 11,12-EEQ, 14,15-EEQ, and 17,18-EEQ (see Epoxyeicosatetraenoic acid); **c)** di-homo-γ-linolenic acid viz., 8,9-epoxy-eicosadienoic acid (8,9-EpEDE), 11,12-EpEDE, and 14,15-EpEDE; and **d)** adrenic acid viz., 7,8-epox-eicosatrienoic acid (7,8-EpETrR), 10,11-EpTrE, 13,14-EpTrE, and 16,17-EpETrE. All of these epoxides are converted, sometimes rapidly, to their dihydroxy metabolites, by various cells and tissues. For example, 5,6-EET is converted to 5,6-dihydroxy-eicosatrienoic acid (5,6-DiHETrE), 8,9-EEQ to 8,9-dihydroxy-eicosatetraenoic acid (8,9-DiHETE, 11,12-EpEDE to 11,12-dihydroxy-eicosadienoic acid (11,12DiHEDE), and 16,17-EpETrE to 16,17-dihydroxy-eicosatrienoic acid (16,17-DiETrE

- Cytochrome P450 microsome ω-hydroxylases: CYP4A11, CYP4A22, CYP4F2, and CYP4F3 metabolize arachidonic acid primarily to 20-Hydroxyeicosatetraenoic acid (20-HETE) but also to 16-HETE, 17-HETE, 18-HETE, and 19-HETE; they also metabolize eicosapentaenoic acid primarily to 20-hydroxy-eicosapentaenoic acid (20-HEPE) but also to 19-HEPE.

Two different enzymes may act in series on a PUFA to form more complex metabolites. For example, ALOX5 acts with ALOX12 or aspirin-treated COX-2 to metabolize arachidonic acid to lipoxins and with cytochrome P450 monooxygenase(s), bacterial cytochrome P450 (in infected tissues), or aspirin-treated COX2 to metabolize eicosapentaenoic acid to the E series resolvins (RvEs) (see Specialized pro-resolving mediators). When this occurs with enzymes located in different cell types and involves the transfer of one enzyme›s product to a cell which uses the second enzyme to make the final product it is referred to as transcellular metabolism or transcellular biosynthesis.

The oxidation of lipids is hazardous to cells, particularly when close to the nucleus. There are elaborate mechanisms to prevent unwanted oxidation. COX, the lipoxygenases, and the phospholipases are tightly controlled—there are at least eight proteins activated to coordinate generation of leukotrienes. Several of these exist in multiple isoforms.

Oxidation by either COX or lipoxygenase releases reactive oxygen species (ROS) and the initial products in eicosanoid generation are themselves highly reactive peroxides. LTA_4 can form adducts with tissue DNA. Other reactions of lipoxygenases generate cellular damage; murine models implicate 15-lipoxygenase in the pathogenesis of atherosclerosis. The oxidation in eicosanoid generation is compartmentalized; this limits the peroxides' damage. The enzymes that are biosynthetic for eicosanoids (e.g., glutathione-S-transferases, epoxide hydrolases, and carrier proteins) belong to families whose functions are involved largely with cellular detoxification. This suggests that eicosanoid signaling might have evolved from the detoxification of ROS.

The cell must realize some benefit from generating lipid hydroperoxides close-by its nucleus. PGs and LTs may signal or regulate DNA-transcription there; LTB_4 is ligand for PPARα. *(See diagram at PPAR).*

Structures of Selected Eicosanoids

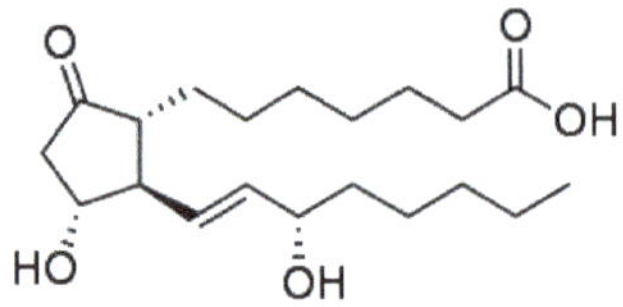

Prostaglandin E_1. The 5-member ring is characteristic of the class.

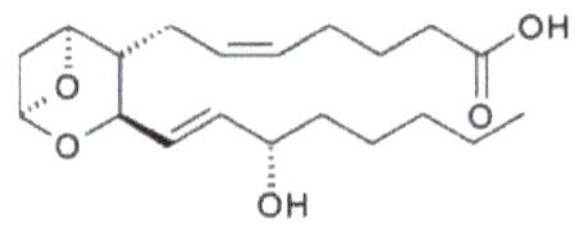

Thromboxane A_2. Oxygens have moved into the ring.

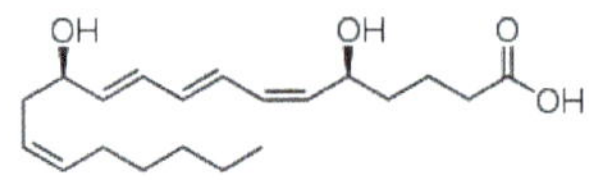

Leukotriene B_4. Note the 3 conjugated double bonds.

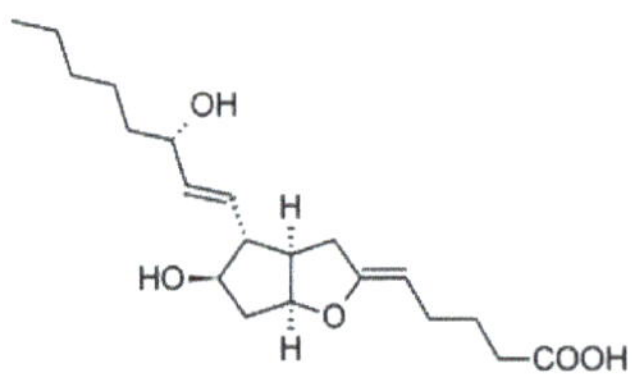

Prostacyclin I_2. The second ring distinguishes it from the prostaglandins.

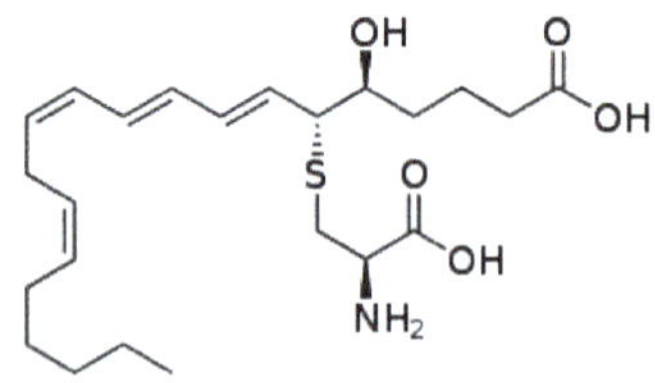

Leukotriene E_4, an example of a cysteinyl leukotriene.

Prostanoid Pathways

Both COX1 and COX2 (also termed prostaglandin-endoperoxide synthase-1 (PTGS1) and PTGS2, respectively) metabolize arachidonic acid by adding molecular O_2 between carbons 9 and 11 to form an endoperoxide bridge between these two carbons, adding molecular O_2 to carbon 15 to yield a 15-hydroperoxy product, creating a carbon-carbon bond between carbons 8 and 12 to create a cyclopentane ring in the middle of the fatty acid, and in the process making PGG2, a product that has two fewer double bonds than arachidonic acid. The 15-hydrpperoxy residue of PGG2 is then reduced to a 15-hydroxyl residue thereby forming PGH2. PGH2 is the parent prostanoid to all other postanoids. It is metabolized by (see diagram in Prostanoids: **a)** the Prostaglandin E synthase pathway in which any one of three isozymes, PTGES, PTGES2, or PTGES3, convert PGH2 to PGE2 (subsequent products of this pathway include PGA2 and PGB2 (see Prostanoid#Biosynthesis); **b)** PGF synthase which converts PGH2 to PGF2α; **c)** Prostaglandin D2 synthase which converts PGH2 to PGD2 (subsequent products in this pathway include 15-dPGJ2 (see Cyclopentenone prostaglandin); **d)** thromboxane synthase which converts PGH2 to TXA2 (subsequent products in this pathway include TXB2); and **e)** Prostacyclin synthase which converts PGH2 to PGI2 (subsequent products in this pathway include 6-keto-PGFα. These pathways have been shown or in some cases presumed to metabolize eicosapentaenoic acid to eicosanoid analogs of the sited products that have three rather than two double bonds and therefore contain the number 3 in place of 2 attached to their names (e.g. PGE3 instead of PGE2).

The PGE2, PGE1, and PGD2 products formed in the pathways just cited can undergo a spontaneous dehydration reaction to form PGA2, PGA1, and PGJ2, respectively; PGJ2 may then undergo a spontaneous isomerization followed by a dehydration reaction to form in series Δ12-PGJ2 and 15-deoxy-Δ12,14-PGJ2.

PGH2 has a 5-carbon ring bridged by molecular oxygen. Its derived PGS have lost this oxygen bridge and contain a single, unsaturated 5-carbon ring with the exception of thromboxane A2 which posseses a 6-member ring consisting of one oxygen and 5 carbon atoms. The 5-carbon ring of prostacyclin is conjoined to a second ring consisting of 4 carbon and one oxygen atom. And, the 5 member ring of the cyclopentenone prostaglandins possesses an unsaturated bond in a conjugated system with a carbonyl group that causes these PGs to form bonds with a diverse range of bioactive proteins (for more see the diagrams at Prostanoid).

Hydroxyeicosatetraenoate (HETE) and Leukotriene (LT) Pathways

The enzyme 5-lipoxygenase (5-LO or ALOX5) converts arachidonic acid into 5-hydroperoxyeicosatetraenoic acid (5-HPETE), which may be released and rapidly reduced to 5-hydroxyeicosatetraenoic acid (5-HETE) by ubiquitous cellular glutathione-dependent peroxidases.Alternately, ALOX5 uses its LTA synthase activity to act convert 5-HPETE to leukotriene A_4 (LTA_4). LTA4 is then metabolized either to LTB_4 by Leukotriene A4 hydrolase or Leukotriene C4 (LTC4) by either LTC4 synthase or microsomal glutathione S-transferase 2 (MGST2). Either of the latter two enzymes act to attach the sulfur of cysteine's thio- (i.e. SH) group in the tripeptide glutamate-cysteine-glycine to carbon 6 of LTA4 thereby forming LTC4. After release from its parent cell, the glutamate and glycine residues of LTC4 are removed step-wise by gamma-glutamyltransferase and a dipeptidase to form sequentially LTD4 and LTE4. The decision to form LTB4 versus LTC4 depends on the relative content of LTA4 hydrolase versus LTC4 synthase (or glutathione S=transferase in cells; Eosinophils, mast cells, and alveolar macrophages possess relatively high levels of LTC4 synthase and accordingly form LTC4 rather than or to a far greater extent than LTB4. 5-LOX may also work in series with cytochrome P450 oxygenases or aspirin-treated COX2 to form Resolvins RvE1, RvE2, and 18S-RvE1 (see Specialized pro-resolving mediators#EPA-derived resolvins).

The enzyme arachidonate 12-lipoxygenase (12-LO or ALOX12) metabolizes arachidonic acid to the *S* stereoisomer of 12-hydroperoxyeicosatetraenoic acid (5-HPETE) which is rapidly reduced by cellular peroxidases to the *S* stereoisomer of 12-hydroxyeicosatetraenoic acid (12-HETE) or further metabolized to hepoxilins (Hx) such as HxA3 and HxB.

The enzymes 15-lipoxygenase-1 (15-LO-1 or ALOX15) and 15-lipoxygenase-2 (15-LO-2, ALOX15B) metabolize arachidonic acid to the *S* stereoisomer of 15-Hydroperoxyeicosatetraenoic acid (15(S)-HPETE) which is rapidly reduced by cellular peroxidases to the *S* stereoisomer of 15-Hydroxyicosatetraenoic acid (15(S)-HETE). The 15-lipoxygenases (particularly ALOX15) may also act in series with 5-lipoxygenase, 12-lipoxygenase, or aspirin-treated COX2 to form the lipoxins and epi-lipoxins or with P450 oxygenases or aspirin-treated COX2 to form Resolvin E3 (see Specialized pro-resolving mediators#EPA-derived resolvins.

A subset of Cytochrome P450 (CYP450) microsome-bound ω-hydroxylases (see 20-Hydroxyeicosatetraenoic acid) metabolize arachidonic acid to 20-Hydroxyeicosatetraenoic acid (20-HETE) and 19-hydroxyeicosatetraenoic acid by an omega oxidation reaction.

Epoxyeicosanoid Pathway

The human cytochrome P450 (CYP) epoxygenases, CYP1A1, CYP1A2, CYP2C8, CYP2C9, CYP2C18, CYP2C19, CYP2E1, CYP2J2, and CYP2S1 metabolize arachidonic acid to the non-classic Epoxyeicosatrienoic acids (EETs) by coverting one of the fatty acid's double bonds to its epoxide to form one or more of the following EETs, 14,15-ETE, 11,12-EET, 8,9-ETE, and 4,5-ETE. 14,15-EET and 11,12-EET are the major EETs produced by mammalian, including human, tissues. The same CYPs but also CYP4A1, CYP4F8, and CYP4F12 metabolize eicosapentaenoic acid to five epoxide epoxyeicosatetraenoic acids (EEQs) viz., 17,18-EEQ, 14,15-EEQ, 11,12-EEQ. 8,9-EEQ, and 5,6-EEQ (see epoxyeicosatetraenoic acid).

Function, Pharmacology, and Clinical Significance

The following table lists a sampling of the major eicosanoids that possess clinically relevant biological activity, the cellular receptors (see Cell surface receptor) that they stimulate or, where noted, antagonize to attain this activity, some of the major functions which they regulate (either promote or inhibit) in humans and mouse models, and some of their relevancies to human diseases.

Eicosanoid	Targeted receptors	Functions regulated	Clinical relevancy
PGE2	PTGER1, PTGER2, PTGER3, PTGER4	inflammation; fever; pain perception; allodynia; Partuition	NSAIDs inhibit its production to reduce inflammation, fever, and pain; used to promote labor in childbirth; an Abortifacient
PGD2	Prostaglandin DP1 receptor 1, Prostaglandin DP2 receptor	allergy reactions; allodynia; hair growth	NSAIDs may target it to inhibit allodynia and male-pattern hair loss
TXA2	Thromboxane receptor α and β	blood platelet aggregation; blood clotting; allergic reactions	NSAIDs inhibit its production to reduce incidence of strokes and heart attacks
PGI2	Prostacyclin receptor	platelet aggregation, vascular smooth muscle contraction	PGI2 analogs used to treat vascular disorders like pulmonary hypertension, Raynaud's syndrome, and Buerger's disease
15-d-Δ12,14-PGJ2	PPARγ, Prostaglandin DP2 receptor	inhibits inflammation and cell growth	Inhibits diverse inflammatory responses in animal models; structural model for developing anti-inflammatory agents
20-HETE	?	vasoconstriction, inhibits platelets	inactivating mutations in the 20-HETE-forming enzyme, CYP2U1, associated with Hereditary spastic paraplegia
5-Oxo-ETE	OXER1	chemotactic factor for and activator of eosinophils	studies needed to determine if inhibiting its production or action inhibits allergic reactons
LTB4	LTB4R, LTB4R2	chemotactic factor for and activator of leukocytes; inflammation	studies to date shown no clear benefits of LTB4 receptor antagonists for human inflammatory diseases
LTC4	CYSLTR1, CYSLTR2, GPR17	vascular permeability; vascular smooth muscle contraction; allergy	antagonists of CYSLTR1 used in asthma as well as other allergic and allergic-like reactions

LTD4	CYSLTR1, CYSLTR2, GPR17	vascular permeability; vascular smooth muscle contraction; allergy	antagonists of CYSLTR1 used in asthma as well as other allergic and allergic-like reactions
LTE4	GPR99	increases vascular permeability and airway mucin secretion	thought to contribute to asthma as well as other allergic and allergic-like reactions
LxA4	?	inhibits functions of pro-inflammatory cells	Specialized pro-resolving mediators class of inflammatory reaction suppressors
LxB4	FPR2, GPR32, AHR	inhibits functions of pro-inflammatory cells	Specialized pro-resolving mediators class of inflammatory reaction suppressors
RvE1	CMKLR1, inhibits BLT, TRPV1, TRPV3, NMDAR, TNFR	inhibits functions of pro-inflammatory cells	Specialized pro-resolving mediators class of inflammatory reaction suppressors; also suppresses pain perception
RvE2	CMKLR1, receptor antagonist of BLT	inhibits functions of pro-inflammatory cells	Specialized pro-resolving mediators class of inflammatory reaction suppressors
14,15-EET	?	vasodilation, inhibits platelets and pro-inflammatory cells	role(s) in human disease not yet proven

Prostanoids

Many of the prostanoids are know to mediate local symptoms of inflammation: vasoconstriction or vasodilation, coagulation, pain, and fever. Inhibition of COX-1 and/or the inducible COX-2 isoforms, is the hallmark of NSAIDs (non-steroidal anti-inflammatory drugs), such as aspirin. Prostanoids also activate the $PPAR_{\gamma}$ members of the steroid/thyroid family of nuclear hormone receptors, and directly influence gene transcription. Prostanoids have numerous other relevancies to clinical medicine as evidence by the their use, the use of their more stable pharmacological analogs, of the use of their receptor antagonists as indicated in the following chart.

Medicine	Type	Medical condition or use	Medicine	Type	Medical condition or use
Alprostadil	PGE1	Erectile dysfunction, maintaining a patent ductus arteriosus in the fetus	Beraprost	PGI1 analog	Pulmonary hypertension, avoiding reperfusion injury
Bimatoprost	PGF2α analog	Glaucoma, ocular hypertension	Carboprost	PGF2α analog	Labor induction, abortifacient in early pregnancy
Dinoprostone	PGE2	labor induction	Iloprost	PGI2 analog	pulmonary artery hypertension
Latanoprost	PGF2α analog	Glaucoma, ocular hypertension	Misoprostol	PGE1 analog	stomach ulcers labor induction, abortifacient
Travoprost	PGF2α analog	Glaucoma, ocular hypertension	U46619	Longer lived TX analog Longer lived TX analog	Research only

Cyclopentenone Prostaglandins

PGA1, PGA2, PGJ2, Δ12-PGJ2, and 15-deox-Δ12,14-PGJ2 exhibit a wide range of anti-inflammatory and inflammation-resolving actions in diverse animal models. They therefore appear to function in a manner similar to Specialized pro-resolving mediators although one of their mechanisms of action, forming covalent bonds with key signaling proteins, differs from those of the specialized pro-resolving mediators.

HETEs and oxo-ETEs

As indicated in their individual Wikipedia pages, 5-hydroxyeicosatetraenoic acid (which, like 5-oxo-eicosatetraenoic acid, acts through the OXER1 receptor), 5-oxo-eicosatetraenoic acid, 12-Hydroxyeicosatetraenoic acid, 15-Hydroxyeicosatetraenoic acid, and 20-Hydroxyeicosatetraenoic acid show numerous activities in animal and human cells as well as in animal models that are related to, for example, inflammation, allergic reactions, cancer cell growth, blood flow to tissues, and/or blood pressure. However, their function and relevancy to human physiology and pathology have not as yet been shown.

leukotrienes

The three cysteinyl leukotrienes, LTC4, LTD4, and LTE4, are potent bronchoconstrictors, increasers of vascular permeability in postcapillary venules, and stimulators of mucus secretion that are released from the lung tissue of asthmatic subjects exposed to specific allergens. They play a pathophysiological role in diverse types of immediate hypersensitivity reactions. Drugs that block their activation of the CYSLTR1 receptor viz., montelukast, zafirlukast, and pranlukast, are used clinically as maintenance treatment for allergen-induced asthma and rhinitis; nonsteroidal anti-inflammatory drug-induced asthma and rhinitis (see Aspirin-induced asthma); exercise- and cold-air induced asthma (see Exercise-induced bronchoconstriction); and childhood sleep apnea due to adenotonsillar hypertrophy (see Acquired non-inflammatory myopathy#Diet and Trauma Induced Myopathy). When combined with antihistamine drug therapy, they also appear useful for treating urticarial diseases such as hives.

Lipoxins and Epi-Lipoxins

LxA4, LxB4, 15-epi-LxA4, and 15-epi-LXB4, like other members of the Specialized pro-resolving mediators) class of eicosanoids, possess anti-inflammatory and inflammation resolving activity. In a randomized controlled trial, AT-LXA4 and a comparatively stable analog of LXB4, 15*R/S*-methyl-LXB4, reduced the severity of eczema in a study of 60 infants and, in another study, inhaled LXA4 decreased LTC4-initiated bronchoprovocation in patients with asthma.

Eoxins

The eoxins (EXC4, EXD4, EXE5) are newly described. They stimulate vascular permeability in an ex vivo human vascular endothelial model system, and in a small study of 32 volunteers EXC4 production by eosinophils isolated from severe and aspirin-intolerant asthmatics was greater than that from healthy volunteers and mild asthmatic patients; these findings have been suggested to indicate that the eoxins have pro-inflammatory actions and therefore potentially involved in various allergic reactions. Production of eoxins by Reed-Sternburg cells has also led to suggestion that they are involve in Hodgkins disease. However, the clinical significance of eoxins has not yet been demonstrated.

Resolvin Metabolites of Eicosapentaenoic Acid

RvE1, 18S-RvE1, RvE2, and RvE3, like other members of the Specialized pro-resolving mediators) class of eicosanoids, possess anti-inflammatory and inflammation resolving activity. A synthetic analog of ReV1 is in clinical phase III testing (see Phases of clinical research) for the treatment of the inflammation-based dry eyesyndrome; along with this study, other clinical trials (NCT01639846, NCT01675570, NCT00799552 and NCT02329743) using an RvE1 analogue to treat various ocular conditions are underway. RvE1 is also in clinical development studies for the treatment of neurodegenerative diseases and hearing loss.

Other Metabolites of Eicosapentaenoic Acid

The metabolites of eicosapentaenoic acid that are analogs of their arachidonic acid-derived prostanoid, HETE, and LT counterparts include: the 3-series prostanoids (e.g. PGE3, PGD3, PGF3α, PGI3, and TXA3), the hydroxyeicosapentaenoic acids (e.g. 5-HEPE, 12-HEPE, 15-HEPE, and 20-HEPE), and the 5-series LTs (e.g. LTB5, LTC5, LTD5, and LTE5). Many of the 3-series prostanoids, the hydroxyeicosapentaenoic acids, and the 5-series LT have been shown or though to be weaker stimulators of their target cells and tissues than their arachidonic acid-derived analogs. They are proposed to reduce the actions of their aracidonate-derived analogs by replacing their production with weaker analogs. Eicosapentaenoic acid-derived counterparts of the Eoxins have not been described.

Epoxyeicosanoids

The epoxy eicostrienoic acids (or EETs) — and, presumably, the epoxy eicosatetraenoic acids — have vasodilating actions on heart, kidney, and other blood vessels as well as on the kidney's reabsorption of sodium and water, and act to reduce blood pressure and ischemic and other injuries to the heart, brain, and other tissues; they may also act to reduce inflammation, promote the growth and metastasis of certain tumors, promote the growth of new blood vessels, in the central nervous system regulate the release of neuropeptide hormones, and in the peripheral nervous system inhibit or reduce pain perception.

Mechanisms of ω-3 Action

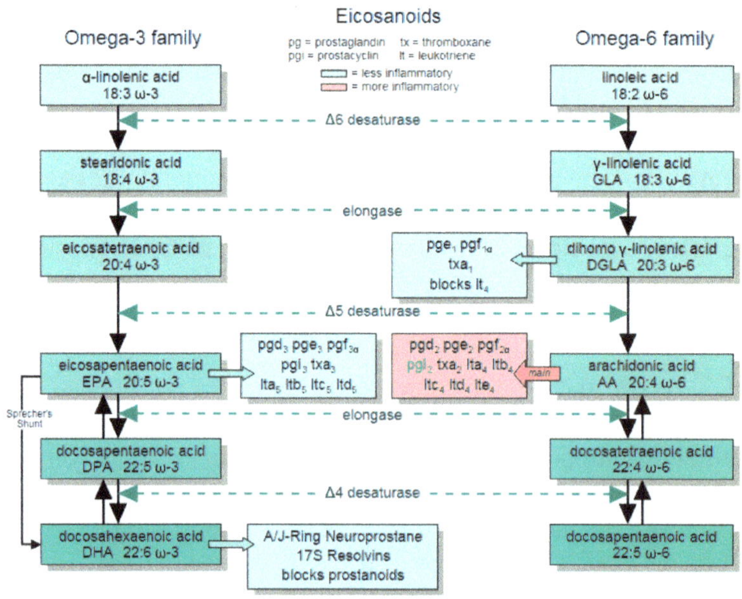

EFA sources: Essential fatty acid production and metabolism to form eicosanoids. At each step, the ω-3 and ω-6 cascades compete for the enzymes.

In general, the eicosanoids derived from AA promote inflammation, and those from EPA and from GLA (*via* DGLA) are less inflammatory, or inactive, or even anti-inflammatory and pro-resolving.

The figure shows the ω-3 and -6 synthesis chains, along with the major eicosanoids from AA, EPA, and DGLA.

Dietary ω-3 and GLA counter the inflammatory effects of AA›s eicosanoids in three ways, along the eicosanoid pathways:

- *Displacement*—Dietary ω-3 decreases tissue concentrations of AA, so there is less to form ω-6 eicosanoids.
- *Competitive inhibition*—DGLA and EPA compete with AA for access to the cyclooxygenase and lipoxygenase enzymes. So the presence of DGLA and EPA in tissues lowers the output of AA's eicosanoids.
- *Counteraction*—Some DGLA and EPA derived eicosanoids counteract their AA derived counterparts.

Role in Inflammation

Since antiquity, the cardinal signs of inflammation have been known as: calor (warmth), dolor (pain), tumor (swelling), and rubor (redness). The eicosanoids are involved with each of these signs.

Redness—An insect's sting will trigger the classic inflammatory response. Short acting vasoconstrictors — TXA_2—are released quickly after the injury. The site may momentarily turn pale. Then TXA_2 mediates the release of the vasodilators PGE_2 and LTB_4. The blood vessels engorge and the injury reddens.

Swelling—LTB_4 makes the blood vessels more permeable. Plasma leaks out into the connective tissues, and they swell. The process also loses pro-inflammatory cytokines. *Pain*—The cytokines increase COX-2 activity. This elevates levels of PGE_2, sensitizing pain neurons. *Heat*—PGE_2 is also a potent pyretic agent. Aspirin and NSAIDS—drugs that block the COX pathways and stop prostanoid synthesis—limit fever or the heat of localized inflammation.

GLYCOLIPID

Glycolipids are lipids with a carbohydrate attached by a glycosidic bond. Their role is to maintain stability of the membrane and to facilitate cellular recognition. The carbohydrates are found on the outer surface of all eukaryotic cell membranes. They extend from the phospholipid bilayer into the aqueous environment outside the cell where it acts as a recognition site for specific chemicals as well as helping to maintain the stability of the membrane and attaching cells to one another to form tissues

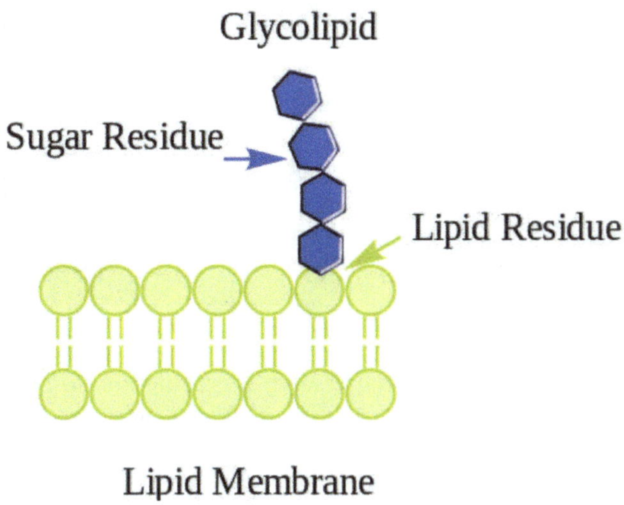

Glycolipid

Structure

The basic structure of a glycolipid is the presence of a carbohydrate monosaccharide or oligosaccharide bound to a lipid moiety. The lipid complex is most often composed of either a glycerol or sphingosine backbone, which gives rise to the two main categories of glycolipids, glyceroglycolipids and sphingolipids. Lipids are non-polar molecules, providing them the capability of interacting with the lipid-bilayer of the cell membrane and anchoring the glycolipid to the surface of the cell. Carbohydrates are used as the ligand component of glycolipids and their structure varies depending on the structure of the molecule it binds to. The carbohydrate contains polar groups that enable the molecule to be soluble in the aqueous environment surrounding the cell. The two molecular groups form a glycoconjugate through a covalent bond referred to as a glycosidic bond. The anomeric carbon of the sugar binds to the hydroxyl group present on the lipid.

Metabolism

Glycosyltransferases

Glycolipids formation is dependent on the activity of glycosyltransferases. Glycoslytransferases are the enzymes responsible for catalyzing the reaction of the covalent bond formation linking the carbohydrate complex to the lipid molecule. It also functions to form the correct oligosaccharide that will be present in the complete structure to act as the receptor for cell signaling. The glycolipid is assembled in the golgi-apparatus and transported to the membrane via vesicles where the lipid remains embedded in the membrane and the carbohydrate is on the outer surface of the cell.

Glycoside Hydrolases

Glycoside hydrolases catalyze the breakage of glycosidic bonds. They are used to modify the glycan after it has been added onto the lipid to represent the final oligosaccharide structure. It is also involved in the natural degradation of glycolipids into their non-conjugated forms. The lipids and carbohydrates will then assume their common uses as energy in the body.

Defects in Metabolism

Sphingolipidoses can be associated with defects in metabolism. Sphingolipidoses are a category of diseases that can be associated with the accumulation of sphingolipids from failure to degrade compounds correctly. Sphingolipidoses are typically inherited and have varying effects among the various types of diseases. One notable example is Niemann–Pick disease which can cause pain to, damage to neural networks, and, in severe cases, death.

Function

Cell–Cell Interactions

The main function of glycolipids in the body is to serve as recognition sites for cell–cell interactions. The sugar moiety of the glycolipid will bind to a specific complementary carbohydrate or lectin, type of cell-surface protein, of a neighboring cell. The interaction of these cell surface markers initiates cellular responses that contribute to activities such as cell recognition, regulation, growth, and apoptosis. Sphingolipidoses can be associated with defects in metabolism.

Immune Responses

An example of how glycolipids function within the body is the interaction between leukocytes and endothelial cells during inflammation. Selectins on the surface of leukocytes and endothelial cells will bind to the carbohydrates attached to glycolipids to initiate the immune response. This binding allows for leukocytes to leave circulation and congregate near the site of inflammation. This is the initial binding mechanism, after which it is followed by expression of integrins which form stronger bonds and allow leukocytes to migrate toward the specific site of inflammation.Glycolipipds are also responsible for other immune responses, notably the recognition of viruses within the body.

Blood Types

Blood type are an example of how glycolipids on cell membranes mediate cell interactions with the surrounding environment. There are four different blood types present in humans (A, B, AB, O) that are determined by the sugar moiety attached to a specific glycolipid on blood cells. Blood type A individuals have an N-acetylgalactosamine sugar attachment as the main determining structure, blood type B has a galactose, and Blood type O has no extra addition to the oligosaccharide. Erythroctes have the specific glycolipid for that individuals blood type covering their surface (with AB individuals have both types of antigens). Antibodies are produced in the body and bind to a specific blood type's glycolipids. Blood type A individuals produce antibodies that bind to the B antigen and so forth, so that any cells possessing the corresponding antigen will be targeted by the antibodies.

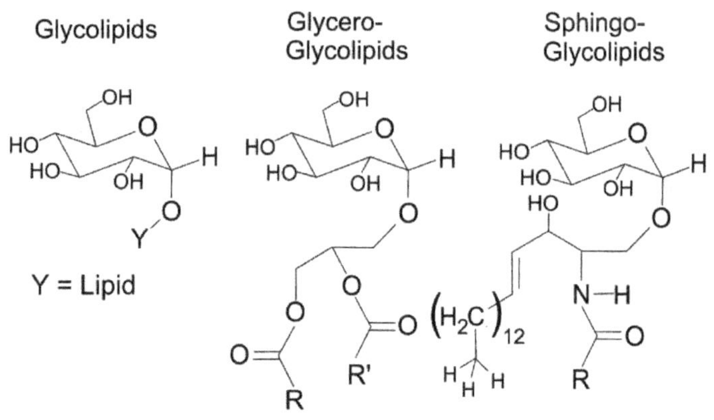

Chemical structure of glycolipids

Types of Glycolipids

The following is an incomplete listing of glycolipid types.

This list is incomplete; you can help by expanding it.

- Glyceroglycolipids: Glyceroglycolipids are a sub-group of glycolipids characterized by an acetylated or non-acetylated glycerol with at least one fatty acid as the lipid complex. Glyceroglycolipids are often associated with photosynthetic membranes and the functions within them. Smaller sub-branches exist within this category of glycolipids depending upon the carbohydrate attached.
- Galactolipids: Galactolipids are defined by a galactose sugar attached to glycerol lipid molecule. They are found in chloroplast membranes and are associated with photosynthetic properties.
- Sulfolipids (SQDG): Sulfolipids possess a sulfur-containing functional group in the sugar moiety attached to a lipid and can be associated with the sulfur cycle in plants.
- Glycosphingolipids: Glycosphingolipids are a sub-group of glycolipids characterized by a sphingosine as the lipid complex. A sphingosine is a long carbon chain with an amine and alcohol functional groups. Glycosphingolipids are mostly located in nervous tissue and are responsible for cell signaling.
- Cerebrosides: Cerebrosides are a group glycosphingolipids involved in nerve cell membranes.
- Galactocerebrosides: Galactocerebrosides are types of cerebroseides with a galactose group and specifically involved in neural tissue and other tissues respectively
- Glucocerebrosides: Glucocerebrosides are a classified as a glycolipid with a cerebroside lipid base with glucose as the carbohydrate head group and are often found in non-neural tissue.
- Sulfatides: Sulfatides are a class of glycolipids containing a sulfate group in the carbohydrate with a ceramide lipid backbone. They are involved in numerous biological functions ranging from immune response to nervous system signaling.
- Gangliosides: Gangliosides are the most complex animal glycolipids; contain negatively charged oligosacchrides with one or more sialic acid residues; more than 200 different gangliosides have been identified; they are most abundant in nerve cells)
- Globosides: Globosides are glycosphingolipids with more than one sugar as part of the carbohydrate complex. They have a variety of functions and failure of degradation of these molecules leads to Fabry's disease.
- Glycophosphosphingolipids: Glycophosphosphingolipid are complex glycophospholipids from fungi, including yeasts, and in plants, where they were originally called "phytoglycolipids" by Herbert Carter, et al., may comprise as complicated a set of compounds as the negatively charged gangliosides in animals. The head group of a glycolipid is composed of sugars.

- Glycophosphatidylinositols: Glycophosphatidylinositols are a sub-group of glycolipids defined by a phosphatidylinositol lipid moiety bound to a carbohydrate complex. Glycosylphosphatidylinositols can be bound to the C-terminus of a protein and have various functions associated with the different proteins they can be bound to.

REFERENCES

1. "Overview of Lipid Metabolism". Merck Manuals Professional Edition. Retrieved 2016-11-01.
2. "Reviewed Work: Plant Lipid Biochemistry.". The New Phytologist. 71. May 1972.
3. "Hydrolysis - Chemistry Encyclopedia - structure, reaction, water, proteins, examples, salt, molecule". www.chemistryexplained.com. Retrieved 2016-11-01.
4. Freifelder, David (1987). Molecular Biology, 2nd edition. Boston: Jones and Bartlett.
5. "Lipid Metabolism Summary". chemistry.elmhurst.edu. Retrieved 2016-11-01.
6. Ophardt, Charles (2003). "Virtual Chembook Elmhurst College". http://chemistry.elmhurst.edu/vchembook/622overview.html. External link in |website= (help)
7. "Lipid Metabolism Disorders: MedlinePlus". Retrieved 2016-11-20.
8. "Disorders of Lipid Metabolism". Merck Manuals Consumer Version. Retrieved 2016-11-20.
9. Hofmann AF, Hagey LR, Krasowski MD (February 2010). "Bile salts of vertebrates: structural variation and possible evolutionary significance". J. Lipid Res. 51 (2): 226–46. doi:10.1194/jlr.R000042. PMC 2803226 . PMID 19638645.
10. Russell DW (2003). "The enzymes, regulation, and genetics of bile acid synthesis". Annu. Rev. Biochem. 72: 137–74. doi:10.1146/annurev.biochem.72.121801.161712. PMID 12543708.
11. Chiang JY (October 2009). "Bile acids: regulation of synthesis". J. Lipid Res. 50 (10): 1955–66. doi:10.1194/jlr.R900010-JLR200. PMC 2739756 . PMID 19346330.
12. Carey, MC.; Small, DM. (Oct 1972). "Micelle formation by bile salts. Physical-chemical and thermodynamic considerations.". Arch Intern Med. 130 (4): 506–27. doi:10.1001/archinte.1972.03650040040005. PMID 4562149.
13. Hofmann AF (1999). "The continuing importance of bile acids in liver and intestinal disease". Arch. Intern. Med. 159 (22): 2647–58. doi:10.1001/archinte.159.22.2647. PMID 10597755.
14. Hofmann AF, Borgström B (February 1964). "The intraluminal phase of fat digestion in man: the lipid content of the micellar and oil phases of intestinal content obtained during fat digestion and absorption". J. Clin. Invest. 43: 247–57. doi:10.1172/JCI104909. PMC 289518 . PMID 14162533.
15. Fiorucci S, Mencarelli A, Palladino G, Cipriani S (November 2009). "Bile-

acid-activated receptors: targeting TGR5 and farnesoid-X-receptor in lipid and glucose disorders". Trends Pharmacol. Sci. 30 (11): 570–80. doi:10.1016/j.tips.2009.08.001. PMID 19758712.

16. 'Essentials of Medical Biochemistry, Lieberman, Marks and Smith, eds, p432, 2007'
17. Hofmann AF (October 1963). "The function of bile salts in fat absorption. The solvent properties of dilute micellar solutions of conjugated bile salts". Biochem. J. 89: 57–68. PMC 1202272 . PMID 14097367.
18. Li T, Chiang JY (2014). "Bile acid signaling in metabolic disease and drug therapy". Pharmacol. Rev. 66 (4): 948–83. doi:10.1124/pr.113.008201. PMID 25073467.
19. Nagahashi M, Takabe K, Liu R, Peng K, Wang X, Wang Y, Hait NC, Wang X, Allegood JC, Yamada A, Aoyagi T, Liang J, Pandak WM, Spiegel S, Hylemon PB, Zhou H (2015). "Conjugated bile acid-activated S1P receptor 2 is a key regulator of sphingosine kinase 2 and hepatic gene expression". Hepatology. 61 (4): 1216–26. doi:10.1002/hep.27592. PMID 25363242.
20. Wiemuth D, Sahin H, Falkenburger BH, Lefevre CM, Wasmuth HE, Grunder S (2012). "BASIC--a bile acid-sensitive ion channel highly expressed in bile ducts". FASEB J. 26 (10): 4122–30. doi:10.1096/fj.12-207043. PMID 22735174.
21. ^ Jump up to:a b Magotti P, Bauer I, Igarashi M, Babagoli M, Marotta R, Piomelli D, Garau G (2014). "Structure of Human N-Acylphosphatidylethanolamine-Hydrolyzing Phospholipase D: Regulation of Fatty Acid Ethanolamide Biosynthesis by Bile Acids". Structure. 24 (3): 598–604. doi:10.1016/j.str.2014.12.018. PMC 4351732 . PMID 25684574.
22. Makishima M, Okamoto AY, Repa JJ, et al. (May 1999). "Identification of a nuclear receptor for bile acids". Science. 284 (5418): 1362–5. doi:10.1126/science.284.5418.1362. PMID 10334992.
23. Parks DJ, Blanchard SG, Bledsoe RK, et al. (May 1999). "Bile acids: natural ligands for an orphan nuclear receptor". Science. 284 (5418): 1365–8. doi:10.1126/science.284.5418.1365. PMID 10334993.
24. Wang H, Chen J, Hollister K, Sowers LC, Forman BM (May 1999). "Endogenous bile acids are ligands for the nuclear receptor FXR/BAR". Mol. Cell. 3 (5): 543–53. doi:10.1016/s1097-2765(00)80348-2. PMID 10360171.
25. Kim, I; Ahn, SH; Inagaki, T; Choi, M; Ito, S; Guo, GL; Kliewer, SA; Gonzalez, FJ (2007). "Differential regulation of bile acid homeostasis by the farnesoid X receptor in liver and intestine". Journal of lipid research. 48 (12): 2664–72. doi:10.1194/jlr.M700330-JLR200. PMID 17720959.
26. Davidson MH (2011). "A systematic review of bile acid sequestrant therapy in children with familial hypercholesterolemia". J Clin Lipidol. 5 (2): 76–81. doi:10.1016/j.jacl.2011.01.005. PMID 21392720.
27. Allen L, Stobie D, Mauldin GN, Baer KE (January 1999). "Clinicopathologic features of dogs with hepatic microvascular dysplasia with and without portosystemic shunts: 42 cases (1991-1996)". J. Am. Vet. Med. Assoc. 214

(2): 218–20. PMID 9926012.

28. Pusl T, Beuers U (2007). "Intrahepatic cholestasis of pregnancy". Orphanet J Rare Dis. 2: 26. doi:10.1186/1750-1172-2-26. PMC 1891276 . PMID 17535422.
29. Poupon RE, Balkau B, Eschwège E, Poupon R (May 1991). "A multicenter, controlled trial of ursodiol for the treatment of primary biliary cirrhosis. UDCA-PBC Study Group". N. Engl. J. Med. 324 (22): 1548–54. doi:10.1056/NEJM199105303242204. PMID 1674105.
30. Glantz A, Marschall HU, Lammert F, Mattsson LA (December 2005). "Intrahepatic cholestasis of pregnancy: a randomized controlled trial comparing dexamethasone and ursodeoxycholic acid". Hepatology. 42 (6): 1399–405. doi:10.1002/hep.20952. PMID 16317669.
31. Danzinger RG, Hofmann AF, Schoenfield LJ, Thistle JL (January 1972). "Dissolution of cholesterol gallstones by chenodeoxycholic acid". N. Engl. J. Med. 286 (1): 1–8. doi:10.1056/NEJM197201062860101. PMID 5006919.
32. Thistle JL, Hofmann AF (September 1973). "Efficacy and specificity of chenodeoxycholic acid therapy for dissolving gallstones". N. Engl. J. Med. 289 (13): 655–9. doi:10.1056/NEJM197309272891303. PMID 4580472.
33. Petroni ML, Jazrawi RP, Pazzi P, et al. (January 2001). "Ursodeoxycholic acid alone or with chenodeoxycholic acid for dissolution of cholesterol gallstones: a randomized multicentre trial. The British-Italian Gallstone Study group". Aliment. Pharmacol. Ther. 15 (1): 123–8. doi:10.1046/j.1365-2036.2001.00853.x. PMID 11136285.
34. Uy MC, Talingdan-Te MC, Espinosa WZ, Daez ML, Ong JP (December 2008). "Ursodeoxycholic acid in the prevention of gallstone formation after bariatric surgery: a meta-analysis". Obes Surg. 18 (12): 1532–8. doi:10.1007/s11695-008-9587-7. PMID 18574646.
35. Pattni, S; Walters, JR (2009). "Recent advances in the understanding of bile acid malabsorption". British medical bulletin. 92: 79–93. doi:10.1093/bmb/ldp032. PMID 19900947.
36. Degirolamo C, Modica S, Palasciano G, Moschetta A (2011). "Bile acids and colon cancer: Solving the puzzle with nuclear receptors". Trends Mol Med. 17 (10): 564–72. doi:10.1016/j.molmed.2011.05.010. PMID 21724466.
37. Reddy BS, Hanson D, Mangat S, et al. (September 1980). "Effect of high-fat, high-beef diet and of mode of cooking of beef in the diet on fecal bacterial enzymes and fecal bile acids and neutral sterols". J. Nutr. 110 (9): 1880–7. PMID 7411244.
38. Hill MJ (May 1990). "Bile flow and colon cancer". Mutat. Res. 238 (3): 313–20. doi:10.1016/0165-1110(90)90023-5. PMID 2188127.
39. Cheah PY (1990). "Hypotheses for the etiology of colorectal cancer--an overview". Nutr Cancer. 14 (1): 5–13. doi:10.1080/01635589009514073. PMID 2195469.
40. Ou J, DeLany JP, Zhang M, Sharma S, O'Keefe SJ (2012). "Association between low colonic short-chain fatty acids and high bile acids in high colon cancer

risk populations". Nutr Cancer. 64 (1): 34–40. doi:10.1080/01635581.2012.630164. PMID 22136517.

41. O'Keefe SJ, Kidd M, Espitalier-Noel G, Owira P (May 1999). "Rarity of colon cancer in Africans is associated with low animal product consumption, not fiber". Am. J. Gastroenterol. 94 (5): 1373–80. doi:10.1111/j.1572-0241.1999.01089.x. PMID 10235221.
42. American Cancer Society. Cancer Facts and Figures 2009. http://www.cancer.org/Research/CancerFactsFigures/cancer-facts-figures-2009
43. Bernstein H, Bernstein C, Payne CM, Dvorak K (July 2009). "Bile acids as endogenous etiologic agents in gastrointestinal cancer". World J. Gastroenterol. 15 (27): 3329–40. doi:10.3748/wjg.15.3329. PMC 2712893 . PMID 19610133.
44. Bernstein C, Holubec H, Bhattacharyya AK, et al. (August 2011). "Carcinogenicity of deoxycholate, a secondary bile acid". Arch. Toxicol. 85 (8): 863–71. doi:10.1007/s00204-011-0648-7. PMC 3149672 . PMID 21267546.
45. Prasad AR, Prasad S, Nguyen H, Facista A, Lewis C, Zaitlin B, Bernstein H, Bernstein C. Novel diet-related mouse model of colon cancer parallels human colon cancer. World J Gastrointest Oncol. 2014 Jul 15;6(7):225-43. doi: 10.4251/wjgo.v6.i7.225. PMID 25024814
46. Singh S, Khanna S, Pardi DS, Loftus EV, Talwalkar JA (2013). "Effect of ursodeoxycholic acid use on the risk of colorectal neoplasia in patients with primary sclerosing cholangitis and inflammatory bowel disease: a systematic review and meta-analysis". Inflamm. Bowel Dis. 19 (8): 1631–8. doi:10.1097/MIB.0b013e318286fa61. PMID 23665966.
47. Eaton JE, Silveira MG, Pardi DS, Sinakos E, Kowdley KV, Luketic VA, Harrison ME, McCashland T, Befeler AS, Harnois D, Jorgensen R, Petz J, Lindor KD (2011). "High-dose ursodeoxycholic acid is associated with the development of colorectal neoplasia in patients with ulcerative colitis and primary sclerosing cholangitis". Am. J. Gastroenterol. 106 (9): 1638–45. doi:10.1038/ajg.2011.156. PMC 3168684 . PMID 21556038.
48. Wertheim BC, Smith JW, Fang C, Alberts DS, Lance P, Thompson PA (2012). "Risk modification of colorectal adenoma by CYP7A1 polymorphisms and the role of bile acid metabolism in carcinogenesis". Cancer Prev Res (Phila). 5 (2): 197–204. doi:10.1158/1940-6207.CAPR-11-0320. PMC 3400261 . PMID 22058145.
49. "Deoxycholic acid injection". Medline plus. Retrieved 26 August 2015.
50. Ascher B, Hoffmann K, Walker P, Lippert S, Wollina U, Havlickova B (2014). "Efficacy, patient-reported outcomes and safety profile of ATX-101 (deoxycholic acid), an injectable drug for the reduction of unwanted submental fat: results from a phase III, randomized, placebo-controlled study.". J Eur Acad Dermatol Venereol. 28 (12): 1707–15. doi:10.1111/jdv.12377. PMC 4263247 . PMID 24605812.
51. Wollina U, Goldman A (2015). "ATX-101 for reduction of submental fat.". Expert Opin Pharmacother. 16 (5): 755–62. doi:10.1517/14656566.2015.1019

465. PMID 25724831.

52. Hofmann AF, Hagey LR (May 2014). "Bile Acid Chemistry, Biology, and Therapeutics During the Last 80 Years: Historical Aspects". J. Lipid Res. 55: 1553–1595. doi:10.1194/jlr.R049437. PMID 24838141.
53. Hofmann AF (May 2009). "Bile acids: trying to understand their chemistry and biology with the hope of helping patients". Hepatology. 49 (5): 1403–18. doi:10.1002/hep.22789. PMID 19296471.
54. "Substance Data for 57-88-5".
55. "Safety (MSDS) data for cholesterol". Retrieved 2007-10-20.
56. http://www.pnas.org/content/70/8/2313.full.pdf
57. Cholesterol at the US National Library of Medicine Medical Subject Headings (MeSH)
58. Hanukoglu I (Dec 1992). "Steroidogenic enzymes: structure, function, and role in regulation of steroid hormone biosynthesis.". J Steroid Biochem Mol Biol. 43 (8): 779–804. doi:10.1016/0960-0760(92)90307-5. PMID 22217824.
59. Razin S, Tully JG (May 1970). "Cholesterol Requirement of Mycoplasmas". Journal of Bacteriology. 102 (2): 306–310. PMC 247552 . PMID 4911537.
60. Chevreul (1816) "Recherches chimiques sur les corps gras, et particulièrement sur leurs combinaisons avec les alcalis. Sixième mémoire. Examen des graisses d'homme, de mouton, de boeuf, de jaguar et d'oie" (Chemical researches on fatty substances, and particularly on their combinations o filippos ine kapios with alkalis. Sixth memoir. Study of human, sheep, beef, jaguar and goose fat), Annales de Chimie et de Physique, 2 : 339-372. From page 346 : "Je nommerai cholesterine, de χολη, bile, et στερεος, solide, la substance cristallisée des calculs biliares humains, ... " (I will name cholesterine — from χολη (bile) and στερεος (solid) — the crystalized substance from human gallstones ...)
61. Olson RE (February 1998). "Discovery of the lipoproteins, their role in fat transport and their significance as risk factors". J. Nutr. 128 (2 Suppl): 439S–443S. PMID 9478044.
62. "National Health and Nutrition Examination Survey" (PDF). United States Center for Disease Control. Retrieved 2012-01-28.
63. Lecerf JM, de Lorgeril M (2011). "Dietary cholesterol: from physiology to cardiovascular risk". Br J Nutr. 106 (1): 6–14. doi:10.1017/S0007114511000237. PMID 21385506.
64. Dubois C, Armand M, Mekki N, Portugal H, Pauli AM, Bernard PM, Lafont H, Lairon D (1994). "Effects of increasing amounts of dietary cholesterol on postprandial lipemia and lipoproteins in human subjects". Journal of LIPID Research. 35 (1994): 1993–2007. PMID 7868978.
65. Behrman EJ, Gopalan V (2005). Scovell WM, ed. "Cholesterol and Plants" (PDF). Journal of Chemical Education. 82 (12): 1791. Bibcode:2005JChEd..82.1791B. doi:10.1021/ed082p1791.
66. John S, Sorokin AV, Thompson PD (February 2007). "Phytosterols and vascular

disease". Curr. Opin. Lipidol. 18 (1): 35–40. doi:10.1097/MOL.0b013e328011e9e3. PMID 17218830.

67. Sadava D, Hillis DM, Heller HC, Berenbaum MR (2011). Life: The Science of Biology 9th Edition. San Francisco: Freeman. pp. 105–114. ISBN 1-4292-4646-4.
68. Ohvo-Rekilä H, Ramstedt B, Leppimäki P, Slotte JP (January 2002). "Cholesterol interactions with phospholipids in membranes". Prog. Lipid Res. 41 (1): 66–97. doi:10.1016/S0163-7827(01)00020-0. PMID 11694269.
69. Yeagle PL (October 1991). "Modulation of membrane function by cholesterol". Biochimie. 73 (10): 1303–10. doi:10.1016/0300-9084(91)90093-G. PMID 1664240.
70. Haines TH (July 2001). "Do sterols reduce proton and sodium leaks through lipid bilayers?". Prog. Lipid Res. 40 (4): 299–324. doi:10.1016/S0163-7827(01)00009-1. PMID 11412894.
71. Incardona JP, Eaton S (April 2000). "Cholesterol in signal transduction". Curr. Opin. Cell Biol. 12 (2): 193–203. doi:10.1016/S0955-0674(99)00076-9. PMID 10712926.
72. Pawlina W, Ross MW (2006). Histology: a text and atlas: with correlated cell and molecular biology. Philadelphia: Lippincott Wiliams & Wilkins. p. 230. ISBN 0-7817-5056-3.
73. Payne AH, Hales DB (2004). "Overview of steroidogenic enzymes in the pathway from cholesterol to active steroid hormones". Endocrine Reviews. 25 (6): 947–70. doi:10.1210/er.2003-0030. PMID 15583024.
74. William W C (2003). Lipid analysis: isolation, separation, identification, and structural analysis of lipids. Ayr, Scotland: Oily Press. ISBN 0-9531949-5-7.
75. "USDA National Nutrient Database for Standard Reference, Release 21" (PDF). United States Department of Agriculture. Retrieved 2008-10-24.
76. Jensen RG, Hagerty MM, McMahon KE (1 June 1978). "Lipids of human milk and infant formulas: a review" (PDF). Am J Clin Nutr. 31 (6): 990–1016. PMID 352132.
77. Behrman EJ, Gopalan V (December 2005). "Cholesterol and Plants". J. Chem. Educ. 82 (12): 1791. Bibcode:2005JChEd..82.1791B. doi:10.1021/ed082p1791.
78. http://www.whfoods.com/genpage.php?tname=foodspice&dbid=5
79. Ostlund RE, Racette SB, Stenson WF (2003). "Inhibition of cholesterol absorption by phytosterol-replete wheat germ compared with phytosterol-depleted wheat germ". Am J Clin Nutr. 77 (6): 1385–1589. PMID 12791614.
80. European Food Safety Authority, Journal (2010). "Scientific opinion on the substantiation of health claims related to plant sterols and plant stanols and maintenance of normal blood cholesterol concentrations".
81. Demonty I, Ras RT, van der Knaap HC, Duchateau GS, Meijer L, Zock PL, Geleijnse JM, Trautwein EA (February 2009). "Continuous dose-response relationship of the LDL-cholesterol-lowering effect of phytosterol intake". J. Nutr. 139 (2): 271–84. doi:10.3945/jn.108.095125. PMID 19091798.

82. Weingärtner O, Ulrich C, Lütjohann D, Ismail K, Schirmer SH, Vanmierlo T, Böhm M, Laufs U (February 2011). "Differential effects on inhibition of cholesterol absorption by plant stanol and plant sterol esters in apoE-/- mice". Cardiovasc Res. 90 (3): 484–92. doi:10.1093/cvr/cvr020. PMC 3096304 . PMID 21257611.

83. Weingärtner O, Böhm M, Laufs U (February 2009). "Controversial role of plant sterol esters in the management of hypercholesterolaemia". Eur. Heart J. 30 (4): 404–9. doi:10.1093/eurheartj/ehn580. PMC 2642922 . PMID 19158117.

84. Cohn, Jeffrey S. et. al. (February 2010). "Dietary Phospholipids and Intestinal Cholesterol Absorption". Nutrients. 2 (2): 116–127. doi:10.3390/nu2020116.

85. Wilson, Martha D. "Review of cholesterol absorption with emphasis on dietary and biliary cholesterol". Retrieved 2015-05-11.

86. http://www.health.gov/dietaryguidelines/2015-scientific-report/PDFs/Scientific-Report-of-the-2015-Dictary-Guidelines-Advisory-Committee.pdf

87. Ascherio A, Willett WC (October 1997). "Health effects of trans fatty acids". Am. J. Clin. Nutr. 66 (4 Suppl): 1006S–1010S. PMID 9322581.

88. "High cholesterol levels by NHS". National Health Service. Retrieved 2010-09-14.

89. de Souza RJ, Mente A, Maroleanu A, Cozma AI, Ha V, Kishibe T, Uleryk E, Budylowski P, Schünemann H, Beyene J, Anand SS (August 2015). "Intake of saturated and trans unsaturated fatty acids and risk of all cause mortality, cardiovascular disease, and type 2 diabetes: systematic review and meta-analysis of observational studies". British Medical Association. 351: h3978. doi:10.1136/bmj.h3978. PMC 4532752 . PMID 26268692.

90. "Biosynthesis and Regulation of Cholesterol (with Animation)". PharmaXChange.info.

91. Berg J (2002). Biochemistry. New York: WH Freeman. ISBN 0-7167-3051-0.

92. Rhodes CM, Stryer L, Tasker R (1995). Biochemistry (4th ed.). San Francisco: W.H. Freeman. pp. 280, 703. ISBN 0-7167-2009-4.

93. Espenshade PJ, Hughes AL (2007). "Regulation of sterol synthesis in eukaryotes". Annu. Rev. Genet. 41: 401–27. doi:10.1146/annurev.genet.41.110306.130315. PMID 17666007.

94. Brown MS, Goldstein JL (1997). "The SREBP pathway: regulation of cholesterol metabolism by proteolysis of a membrane-bound transcription factor". Cell. 89 (3): 331–40. doi:10.1016/S0092-8674(00)80213-5. PMID 9150132.

95. Tymoczko JL, Berg T, Stryer L, Berg JM (2002). Biochemistry. San Francisco: W.H. Freeman. pp. 726–727. ISBN 0-7167-4955-6.

96. Mahley, R. W. (2016). "Apolipoprotein E: From cardiovascular disease to neurodegenerative disorders". Journal of Molecular Medicine. 94 (7): 739–46. doi:10.1007/s00109-016-1427-y. PMC 4921111 . PMID 27277824.

97. Weingärtner O, Pinsdorf T, Rogacev KS, Blömer L, Grenner Y, Gräber S, Ulrich C, Girndt M, Böhm M, Fliser D, Laufs U, Lütjohann D, Heine GH (2010). Federici M, ed. "The relationships of markers of cholesterol homeostasis with carotid intima-media thickness". PLoS ONE. 5 (10): e13467. Bibcode:2010PLoSO...513467W.

doi:10.1371/journal.pone.0013467. PMC 2956704 . PMID 20976107.

98. Lewis GF, Rader DJ (June 2005). "New insights into the regulation of HDL metabolism and reverse cholesterol transport". Circ. Res. 96 (12): 1221–32. doi:10.1161/01.RES.0000170946.56981.5c. PMID 15976321.
99. Gordon DJ, Probstfield JL, Garrison RJ, Neaton JD, Castelli WP, Knoke JD, Jacobs DR, Bangdiwala S, Tyroler HA (January 1989). "High-density lipoprotein cholesterol and cardiovascular disease. Four prospective American studies". Circulation. 79 (1): 8–15. doi:10.1161/01.CIR.79.1.8. PMID 2642759.
100. Kandutsch AA, Chen HW, Heiniger HJ (August 1978). "Biological activity of some oxygenated sterols". Science. 201 (4355): 498–501. Bibcode:1978Sci...201..498K. doi:10.1126/science.663671. PMID 663671.
101. Russell DW (December 2000). "Oxysterol biosynthetic enzymes". Biochim. Biophys. Acta. 1529 (1–3): 126–35. doi:10.1016/S1388-1981(00)00142-6. PMID 11111082.
102. Hanukoglu I, Jefcoate CR (1980). "Pregnenolone separation from cholesterol using Sephadex LH-20 mini-columns". Journal of Chromatography A. 190 (1): 256–262. doi:10.1016/S0021-9673(00)85545-4.
103. Javitt NB (December 1994). "Bile acid synthesis from cholesterol: regulatory and auxiliary pathways". FASEB J. 8 (15): 1308–11. PMID 8001744.
104. Wolkoff AW, Cohen DE (February 2003). "Bile acid regulation of hepatic physiology: I. Hepatocyte transport of bile acids". Am. J. Physiol. Gastrointest. Liver Physiol. 284 (2): G175–9. doi:10.1152/ajpgi.00409.2002 (inactive 2015-01-01). PMID 12529265.
105. Marschall HU, Einarsson C (June 2007). "Gallstone disease". J. Intern. Med. 261 (6): 529–42. doi:10.1111/j.1365-2796.2007.01783.x. PMID 17547709.
106. Gérard P, Lepercq P, Leclerc M, Gavini F, Raibaud P, Juste C (September 2007). "Bacteroides sp. strain D8, the first cholesterol-reducing bacterium isolated from human feces". Appl. Environ. Microbiol. 73 (18): 5742–9. doi:10.1128/AEM.02806-06. PMC 2074900 . PMID 17616613.
107. Wipperman MF, Sampson NS, Thomas ST (2014). "Pathogen roid rage: Cholesterol utilization by Mycobacterium tuberculosis". Crit. Rev. Biochem. Mol. Biol. 49 (4): 269–93. doi:10.3109/10409238.2014.895700. PMID 24611808.
108. Thomas ST, Sampson NS (2013). "Mycobacterium tuberculosis utilizes a unique heterotetrameric structure for dehydrogenation of the cholesterol side chain". Biochemistry. 52 (17): 2895–2904. doi:10.1021/bi4002979. PMC 3726044 . PMID 23560677.
109. Wipperman MF, Yang M, Thomas ST, Sampson NS (2013). "Shrinking the FadE Proteome of Mycobacterium tuberculosis: Insights into Cholesterol Metabolism through Identification of an α2β2Heterotetrameric Acyl Coenzyme A Dehydrogenase Family". J. Bacteriol. 195 (19): 4331–4341. doi:10.1128/JB.00502-13. PMC 3807453 . PMID 23836861.
110. Levitan I, Singh DK, Rosenhouse-Dantsker A (2014). "Cholesterol binding to

ion channels". Frontiers in Physiology. 5: 65. doi:10.3389/fphys.2014.00065. PMC 3935357 . PMID 24616704.

111. Wei W, Schwaid AG, Wang X, Wang X, Chen S, Chu Q, Saghatelian A, Wan Y (March 2016). "Ligand Activation of ERRα by Cholesterol Mediates Statin and Bisphosphonate Effects". Cell Metabolism. 23 (3): 479–91. doi:10.1016/j.cmet.2015.12.010. PMID 26777690.

112. Brunzell JD, Davidson M, Furberg CD, Goldberg RB, Howard BV, Stein JH, Witztum JL (April 2008). "Lipoprotein management in patients with cardiometabolic risk: consensus statement from the American Diabetes Association and the American College of Cardiology Foundation". Diabetes Care. 31 (4): 811–22. doi:10.2337/dc08-9018. PMID 18375431.

113. Department of Health (UK), NHS Choices, "More evidence for Mediterranean diet". 8 March 2011. Access date: Nov 11, 2015

114. Durrington P (August 2003). "Dyslipidaemia". Lancet. 362 (9385): 717 31. doi:10.1016/S0140-6736(03)14234-1. PMID 12957096.

115. Lewington S, Whitlock G, Clarke R, Sherliker P, Emberson J, Halsey J, Qizilbash N, Peto R, Collins R (December 2007). "Blood cholesterol and vascular mortality by age, sex, and blood pressure: a meta-analysis of individual data from 61 prospective studies with 55,000 vascular deaths". Lancet. 370 (9602): 1829–39. doi:10.1016/S0140-6736(07)61778-4. PMID 18061058.

116. "Detection, Evaluation and Treatment of High Blood Cholesterol in Adults (Adult Treatment Panel III) Final Report" (PDF). National Institutes of Health. National Heart, Lung and Blood Institute. Retrieved 2008-10-27.

117. van der Steeg WA, Holme I, Boekholdt SM, Larsen ML, Lindahl C, Stroes ES, Tikkanen MJ, Wareham NJ, Faergeman O, Olsson AG, Pedersen TR, Khaw KT, Kastelein JJ (February 2008). "High-density lipoprotein cholesterol, high-density lipoprotein particle size, and apolipoprotein A-I: significance for cardiovascular risk: the IDEAL and EPIC-Norfolk studies". J. Am. Coll. Cardiol. 51 (6): 634–42. doi:10.1016/j.jacc.2007.09.060. PMID 18261682.

118. Robinson JG, Wang S, Jacobson TA (2012). "Meta-analysis of comparison of effectiveness of lowering apolipoprotein B versus low-density lipoprotein cholesterol and nonhigh-density lipoprotein cholesterol for cardiovascular risk reduction in randomized trials". The American Journal of Cardiology. 110 (10): 1468–76. doi:10.1016/j.amjcard.2012.07.007. PMID 22906895.

119. "How Can I Lower High Cholesterol" (PDF). American Heart Association. Retrieved 2011-04-03.

120. "Diseases and Conditions. High cholesterol: Olive oil, Foods with added plant sterols or stanols, Other changes to your diet". Mayo Clinic. 2012. Retrieved 11 November 2015.

121. National Institute for Health and Clinical Excellence. Clinical guideline 67: Lipid modification. London, 2008.

122. Matthew Lui, Ross Garberich, Craig Strauss, Thomas Davin, and Thomas Knickelbine, Usefulness of Lipid Apheresis in the Treatment of Familial

Hypercholesterolemia Journal of Lipids, vol. 2014, Article ID 864317, 6 pages, 2014. doi:10.1155/2014/864317

123. Mannu GS, Zaman MJ, Gupta A, Rehman HU, Myint PK (2012). "Update on guidelines for management of hypercholesterolemia". Expert Review of Cardiovascular Therapy. 10 (10): 1239–49. doi:10.1586/erc.12.94. PMID 23190064.

124. Kizer JR, Madias C, Wilner B, Vaughan CJ, Mushlin AI, Trushin P, Gotto AM, Pasternak RC (May 1, 2010). "Relation of different measures of low-density lipoprotein cholesterol to risk of coronary artery disease and death in a meta-regression analysis of large-scale trials of statin therapy.". The American journal of cardiology. 105 (9): 1289–96. doi:10.1016/j.amjcard.2009.12.051. PMC 2917836 . PMID 20403481.

125. Nicholls SJ (August 2008). "Rosuvastatin and progression of atherosclerosis". Expert Rev Cardiovasc Ther. 6 (7): 925–33. doi:10.1586/14779072.6.7.925. PMID 18666843.

126. "MRC/BHF Heart Protection Study of cholesterol lowering with simvastatin in 20,536 high-risk individuals: a randomised placebo-controlled trial". Lancet. 360 (9326): 7–22. July 2002. doi:10.1016/S0140-6736(02)09327-3. PMID 12114036.

127. Shepherd J, Cobbe SM, Ford I, Isles CG, Lorimer AR, MacFarlane PW, McKillop JH, Packard CJ (November 1995). "Prevention of coronary heart disease with pravastatin in men with hypercholesterolemia. West of Scotland Coronary Prevention Study Group". N. Engl. J. Med. 333 (20): 1301–7. doi:10.1056/NEJM199511163332001. PMID 7566020.

128. Grundy SM (May 2007). "Should women be offered cholesterol lowering drugs to prevent cardiovascular disease? Yes". BMJ. 334 (7601): 982–982. doi:10.1136/bmj.39202.399942.AD. PMC 1867899 . PMID 17494017.

129. Kendrick M (May 2007). "Should women be offered cholesterol lowering drugs to prevent cardiovascular disease? No". BMJ. 334 (7601): 983–983. doi:10.1136/bmj.39202.397488.AD. PMC 1867901 . PMID 17494018.

130. JUPITER Study Group (2008). "Rosuvastatin to Prevent Vascular Events in Men and Women with Elevated C-Reactive Protein". N Engl J Med. 359: 2195–2207. doi:10.1056/nejmoa0807646. PMID 18997196.

131. Brugts JJ, Yetgin T, Hoeks SE, Gotto AM, Shepherd J, Westendorp RG, de Craen AJ, Knopp RH, Nakamura H, Ridker P, van Domburg R, Deckers JW (2009). "The benefits of statins in people without established cardiovascular disease but with cardiovascular risk factors: meta-analysis of randomised controlled trials". BMJ. 338: b2376. doi:10.1136/bmj.b2376. PMC 2714690 . PMID 19567909.

132. "Report of the National Cholesterol Education Program Expert Panel on Detection, Evaluation, and Treatment of High Blood Cholesterol in Adults. The Expert Panel". Arch. Intern. Med. 148 (1): 36–69. January 1988. doi:10.1001/archinte.148.1.36. PMID 3422148.

133. "Cholesterol". American Heart Association. 17 November 2008. Retrieved 2009-02-21.

134. "About cholesterol". American Heart Association. Archived from the original on 3 October 2001.

135. Warnick GR, Knopp RH, Fitzpatrick V, Branson L (January 1990). "Estimating low-density lipoprotein cholesterol by the Friedewald equation is adequate for classifying patients on the basis of nationally recommended cutpoints". Clin. Chem. 36 (1): 15–9. PMID 2297909.

136. Wang TY, Newby LK, Chen AY, Mulgund J, Roe MT, Sonel AF, Bhatt DL, DeLong ER, Ohman EM, Gibler WB, Peterson ED (September 2009). "Hypercholesterolemia paradox in relation to mortality in acute coronary syndrome". Clin Cardiol. 32 (9): E22–8. doi:10.1002/clc.20518. PMID 19645040.

137. Anderson KM, Castelli WP, Levy D (April 1987). "Cholesterol and mortality. 30 years of follow-up from the Framingham study". JAMA. 257 (16): 2176–80. doi:10.1001/jama.257.16.2176. PMID 3560398.

138. Ulmer H, Kelleher C, Diem G, Concin H (2004). "Why Eve is not Adam: prospective follow-up in 149650 women and men of cholesterol and other risk factors related to cardiovascular and all-cause mortality". J Women's Health (Larchmt). 13 (1): 41–53. doi:10.1089/154099904322836447. PMID 15006277.

139. Sternberg D (2007). The Cholesterol Wars: The Cholesterol Skeptics vs the Preponderance of Evidence. Boston: Academic Press. ISBN 0-12-373979-9.

140. Chowdhury R, Warnakula S, Kunutsor S, Crowe F, Ward HA, Johnson L, Franco OH, Butterworth AS, Forouhi NG, Thompson SG, Khaw KT, Mozaffarian D, Danesh J, Di Angelantonio E (2014). "Association of dietary, circulating, and supplement fatty acids with coronary risk: A systematic review and meta-analysis". Annals of Internal Medicine. 160 (6): 398–406. doi:10.7326/M13-1788. PMID 24723079.

141. Rizos CV, Elisaf MS, Liberopoulos EN (24 February 2011). "Effects of thyroid dysfunction on lipid profile". The Open Cardiovascular Medicine Journal. 5 (1): 76—84. doi:10.2174/1874192401105010076. PMC 3109527 . PMID 21660244.

142. "How To Get Your Cholesterol Tested". American Heart Association. Retrieved 2013-07-10.

143. Stone NJ, Robinson J, Goff DC (2013). "Getting a grasp of the Guidelines". American College of Cardiology. Retrieved 2 April 2014.

144. "Implications of Recent Clinical Trials for the ATP III Guidelines". National Heart, Lungs and Blood Institute. Archived from the originalon 2 February 2014. Retrieved 2014-01-27.

145. Westover EJ, Covey DF, Brockman HL, Brown RE, Pike LJ (December 2003). "Cholesterol depletion results in site-specific increases in epidermal growth factor receptor phosphorylation due to membrane level effects. Studies with cholesterol enantiomers". J. Biol. Chem. 278 (51): 51125–33. doi:10.1074/jbc.M304332200. PMC 2593805 . PMID 14530278.

146. Kristiana I, Luu W, Stevenson J, Cartland S, Jessup W, Belani JD, Rychnovsky SD, Brown AJ (September 2012). "Cholesterol through the looking glass: ability of its enantiomer also to elicit homeostatic responses". J. Biol. Chem. 287 (40):

33897–904. doi:10.1074/jbc.M112.360537. PMC 3460484 . PMID 22869373.

147. Edwards IJ, O'Flaherty JT (2008). "Omega-3 Fatty Acids and PPARgamma in Cancer". PPAR Research. 2008: 358052. doi:10.1155/2008/358052. PMC 2526161 . PMID 18769551.
148. DeCaterina, R; Basta, G (June 2001). "n-3 Fatty acids and the inflammatory response – biological background" (PDF). European Heart Journal Supplements. 3, Suppl D: D42–D49. doi:10.1016/S1520-765X(01)90118-X. Retrieved 2006-02-10.
149. Funk, Colin D. (30 November 2001). "Prostaglandins and Leukotrienes: Advances in Eicosanoid Biology". Science. 294 (5548): 1871–1875. doi:10.1126/science.294.5548.1871. PMID 11729303. Retrieved 2007-01-08.
150. Piomelli, Daniele (2000). "Arachidonic Acid". Neuropsychopharmacology: The Fifth Generation of Progress. Archived from the original on 2006-07-15. Retrieved 2006-03-03.
151. Soberman, Roy J.; Christmas, Peter (2003). "The organization and consequences of eicosanoid signaling". J. Clin. Invest. 111 (8): 1107–1113. doi:10.1172/JCI18338. PMC 152944 . PMID 12697726. Retrieved 2007-01-05.
152. Beare-Rogers (2001). "IUPAC Lexicon of Lipid Nutrition" (PDF). Retrieved June 1, 2006.
153. Prostacyclin—PGI—was previously classified as prostaglandin and retains its old PGI2 identifier.
154. Eicosanoids with different letters have placement of double-bonds and different functional groups attached to the molecular skeleton. Letters indicate roughly the order the eicosanoids were first described in the literature. For diagrams for PG [A–H] see Cyberlipid Center. "Prostanoids". Retrieved 2007-02-05.
155. Rossi AG, Thomas MJ, O'Flaherty JT (1988). "Stereospecific actions of 5-hydroxyeicosatetraenoate". FEBS Letters. 240 (1-2): 163–6. doi:10.1016/0014-5793(88)80360-0. PMID 3191990.
156. Straus DS, Glass CK (2001). "Cyclopentenone prostaglandins: new insights on biological activities and cellular targets". Medicinal Research Reviews. 21 (3): 185–210. doi:10.1002/med.1006.abs. PMID 11301410.
157. Das UN (1983). "Prostaglandins and gene action: possible relevance to the effect of PG system on leukocyte alkaline phosphatase enzyme activity". Medical Hypotheses. 11 (2): 185–94. doi:10.1016/0306-9877(83)90062-2. PMID 6684205.
158. Prasad KN, Hovland AR, Cole WC, Prasad KC, Nahreini P, Edwards-Prasad J, Andreatta CP (2000). "Multiple antioxidants in the prevention and treatment of Alzheimer disease: analysis of biologic rationale". Clinical Neuropharmacology. 23 (1): 2–13. doi:10.1097/00002826-200001000-00002. PMID 10682224.
159. Xu Y, Qian SY (2014). "Anti-cancer activities of ω-6 polyunsaturated fatty acids". Biomedical Journal. 37 (3): 112–9. doi:10.4103/2319-4170.131378. PMC 4166599 . PMID 24923568.
160. Gomolka B, Siegert E, Blossey K, Schunck WH, Rothe M, Weylandt KH (2011). "Analysis of omega-3 and omega-6 fatty acid-derived lipid metabolite formation

in human and mouse blood samples". Prostaglandins & Other Lipid Mediators. 94 (3-4): 81–7. doi:10.1016/j.prostaglandins.2010.12.006. PMID 21236358.

161. Zulfakar MH, Edwards M, Heard CM (2007). "Is there a role for topically delivered eicosapentaenoic acid in the treatment of psoriasis?". European Journal of Dermatology : EJD. 17 (4): 284–91. doi:10.1684/ejd.2007.0201. PMID 17540633.
162. Caramia G (2012). "Essential fatty acids and lipid mediators. Endocannabinoids". La Pediatria Medica E Chirurgica: Medical and Surgical Pediatrics (in Italian). 34 (2): 65–72. doi:10.4081/pmc.2012.2. PMID 22730630.
163. Wiktorowska-Owczarek A, Berezińska M, Nowak JZ (2015). "PUFAs: Structures, Metabolism and Functions". Advances in Clinical and Experimental Medicine. 24 (6): 931–41. doi:10.17219/acem/31243. PMID 26771963.
164. Tanaka N, Yamaguchi H, Furugen A, Ogura J, Kobayashi M, Yamada T, Mano N, Iseki K (2014). "Quantification of intracellular and extracellular eicosapentaenoic acid-derived 3-series prostanoids by liquid chromatography/electrospray ionization tandem mass spectrometry". Prostaglandins, Leukotrienes, and Essential Fatty Acids. 91 (3): 61–71. doi:10.1016/j.plefa.2014.04.005. PMID 24996760.
165. Van Dyke TE, Serhan CN (2003). "Resolution of inflammation: a new paradigm for the pathogenesis of periodontal diseases". J. Dent. Res. 82 (2): 82–90. doi:10.1177/154405910308200202. PMID 12562878.
166. Serhan CN, Gotlinger K, Hong S, Arita M (2004). "Resolvins, docosatrienes, and neuroprotectins, novel omega-3-derived mediators, and their aspirin-triggered endogenous epimers: an overview of their protective roles in catabasis". Prostaglandins Other Lipid Mediat. 73 (3–4): 155–72. doi:10.1016/j.prostaglandins.2004.03.005. PMID 15290791.
167. Anderle P, Farmer P, Berger A, Roberts MA (2004). "Nutrigenomic approach to understanding the mechanisms by which dietary long-chain fatty acids induce gene signals and control mechanisms involved in carcinogenesis". Nutrition (Burbank, Los Angeles County, Calif.). 20 (1): 103–8. doi:10.1016/j.nut.2003.09.018. PMID 14698023.
168. Evans AR, Junger H, Southall MD, et al. (2000). "Isoprostanes, novel eicosanoids that produce nociception and sensitize rat sensory neurons". J. Pharmacol. Exp. Ther. 293 (3): 912–20. PMID 10869392.
169. O'Brien WF, Krammer J, O'Leary TD, Mastrogiannis DS (1993). "The effect of acetaminophen on prostacyclin production in pregnant women". Am. J. Obstet. Gynecol. 168 (4): 1164–9. doi:10.1016/0002-9378(93)90362-m. PMID 8475962.
170. Behrendt H, Kasche A, Ebner von Eschenbach C, Risse U, Huss-Marp J, Ring J (2001). "Secretion of proinflammatory eicosanoid-like substances precedes allergen release from pollen grains in the initiation of allergic sensitization". Int. Arch. Allergy Immunol. 124 (1–3): 121–5. doi:10.1159/000053688. PMID 11306946.
171. Sarau HM, Foley JJ, Schmidt DB, et al. (1999). "In vitro and in vivo pharmacological characterization of SB 201993, an eicosanoid-like LTB4 receptor

antagonist with anti-inflammatory activity". Prostaglandins Leukot. Essent. Fatty Acids. 61 (1): 55–64. doi:10.1054/plef.1999.0074. PMID 10477044.

172. Czerska M, Zieliński M, Gromadzińska J (2016). "Isoprostanes - A novel major group of oxidative stress markers". International Journal of Occupational Medicine and Environmental Health. 29 (2): 179–90. doi:10.13075/ijomeh.1896.00596. PMID 26670350.
173. Friedli O, Freigang S (2016). "Cyclopentenone-containing oxidized phospholipids and their isoprostanes as pro-resolving mediators of inflammation". Biochimica et Biophysica Acta. doi:10.1016/j.bbalip.2016.07.006. PMID 27422370.
174. Cuyamendous C, de la Torre A, Lee YY, Leung KS, Guy A, Bultel-Poncé V, Galano JM, Lee JC, Oger C, Durand T (2016). "The novelty of phytofurans, isofurans, dihomo-isofurans and neurofurans: Discovery, synthesis and potential application". Biochimie. 130: 49–62. doi:10.1016/j.biochi.2016.08.002. PMID 27519299.
175. University of Kansas Medical Center (2004). "Eicosanoids and Inflammation" (PDF). Retrieved 2007-01-05.
176. Gabbs M, Leng S, Devassy JG, Monirujjaman M, Aukema HM (2015). "Advances in Our Understanding of Oxylipins Derived from Dietary PUFAs". Advances in Nutrition (Bethesda, Md.). 6 (5): 513–40. doi:10.3945/an.114.007732. PMC 4561827 . PMID 26374175.
177. Powell WS, Rokach J (2015). "Biosynthesis, biological effects, and receptors of hydroxyeicosatetraenoic acids (HETEs) and oxoeicosatetraenoic acids (oxo-ETEs) derived from arachidonic acid". Biochimica et Biophysica Acta. 1851 (4): 340–55. doi:10.1016/j.bbalip.2014.10.008. PMID 25449650.
178. Capra V, Rovati GE, Mangano P, Buccellati C, Murphy RC, Sala A (2015). "Transcellular biosynthesis of eicosanoid lipid mediators". Biochimica et Biophysica Acta. 1851 (4): 377–82. doi:10.1016/j.bbalip.2014.09.002. PMID 25218301.
179. Cyrus, Tillmann; Witztum, Joseph L.; Rader, Daniel J.; Tangirala, Rajendra; Fazio, Sergio; Linton, Macrae F.; Funk, Colin D. (June 1999). "Disruption of the 12/15-lipoxygenase gene diminishes atherosclerosis in apo E–deficient mice". J Clin Invest. 103 (11): 1597–1604n. doi:10.1172/JCI5897. PMC 408369 . PMID 10359569.
180. Schewe T. (Mar–Apr 2002). "15-lipoxygenase-1: a prooxidant enzyme". Biol Chem. 383 (3–4): 365–74. doi:10.1515/BC.2002.041. PMID 12033428.
181. Korbecki J, Baranowska-Bosiacka I, Gutowska I, Chlubek D (2014). "Cyclooxygenase pathways". Acta Biochimica Polonica. 61 (4): 639–49. PMID 25343148.
182. Claar D, Hartert TV, Peebles RS (2015). "The role of prostaglandins in allergic lung inflammation and asthma". Expert Review of Respiratory Medicine. 9 (1): 55–72. doi:10.1586/17476348.2015.992783. PMC 4380345 . PMID 25541289.
183. Simopoulos AP (2010). "Genetic variants in the metabolism of omega-6 and omega-3 fatty acids: their role in the determination of nutritional requirements

and chronic disease risk". Experimental Biology and Medicine (Maywood, N.J.). 235 (7): 785–95. doi:10.1258/ebm.2010.009298. PMID 20558833.

184. Surh YJ, Na HK, Park JM, Lee HN, Kim W, Yoon IS, Kim DD (2011). "15-Deoxy-$\Delta^{12,14}$-prostaglandin J_2, an electrophilic lipid mediator of anti-inflammatory and pro-resolving signaling". Biochemical Pharmacology. 82 (10): 1335–51. doi:10.1016/j.bcp.2011.07.100. PMID 21843512.
185. Powell, W. S.; Rokach, J (2013). "The eosinophil chemoattractant 5-oxo-ETE and the OXE receptor". Progress in Lipid Research. 52 (4): 651–65. doi:10.1016/j.plipres.2013.09.001. PMID 24056189.
186. Rådmark O, Werz O, Steinhilber D, Samuelsson B (2015). "5-Lipoxygenase, a key enzyme for leukotriene biosynthesis in health and disease". Biochimica et Biophysica Acta. 1851 (4): 331–9. doi:10.1016/j.bbalip.2014.08.012. PMID 25152163.
187. Ahmad S, Thulasingam M, Palombo I, Daley DO, Johnson KA, Morgenstern R, Haeggström JZ, Rinaldo-Matthis A (2015). "Trimeric microsomal glutathione transferase 2 displays one third of the sites reactivity". Biochimica et Biophysica Acta. 1854 (10 Pt A): 1365–71. doi:10.1016/j.bbapap.2015.06.003. PMID 26066610.
188. Pace-Asciak, C. R. (2009). "The hepoxilins and some analogues: A review of their biology". British Journal of Pharmacology. 158 (4): 972–81. doi:10.1111/j.1476-5381.2009.00168.x. PMC 2785520 . PMID 19422397.
189. Dobrian, A. D.; Lieb, D. C.; Cole, B. K.; Taylor-Fishwick, D. A.; Chakrabarti, S. K.; Nadler, J. L. (2011). "Functional and pathological roles of the 12- and 15-lipoxygenases". Progress in Lipid Research. 50 (1): 115–31. doi:10.1016/j.plipres.2010.10.005. PMC 3012140 . PMID 20970452.
190. Ivanov, I; Kuhn, H; Heydeck, D (2015). "Structural and functional biology of arachidonic acid 15-lipoxygenase-1 (ALOX15)". Gene. 573 (1): 1–32. doi:10.1016/j.gene.2015.07.073. PMID 26216303.
191. Wittwer, J; Hersberger, M (2007). "The two faces of the 15-lipoxygenase in atherosclerosis". Prostaglandins, Leukotrienes and Essential Fatty Acids. 77 (2): 67–77. doi:10.1016/j.plefa.2007.08.001. PMID 17869078.
192. Kroetz DL, Xu F (2005). "Regulation and inhibition of arachidonic acid omega-hydroxylases and 20-HETE formation". Annual Review of Pharmacology and Toxicology. 45: 413–38. doi:10.1146/annurev.pharmtox.45.120403.100045. PMID 15822183.
193. Yang, L; Mäki-Petäjä, K; Cheriyan, J; McEniery, C; Wilkinson, I. B. (2015). "The role of epoxyeicosatrienoic acids in the cardiovascular system". British Journal of Clinical Pharmacology. 80 (1): 28–44. doi:10.1111/bcp.12603. PMC 4500322 . PMID 25655310.
194. Spector, A. A.; Kim, H. Y. (2015). "Cytochrome P450 epoxygenase pathway of polyunsaturated fatty acid metabolism". Biochimica et Biophysica Acta (BBA) - Molecular and Cell Biology of Lipids. 1851 (4): 356–65. doi:10.1016/j.bbalip.2014.07.020. PMC 4314516 . PMID 25093613.

195. Fer, M; Dréano, Y; Lucas, D; Corcos, L; Salaün, J. P.; Berthou, F; Amet, Y (2008). "Metabolism of eicosapentaenoic and docosahexaenoic acids by recombinant human cytochromes P450". Archives of Biochemistry and Biophysics. 471 (2): 116–25. doi:10.1016/j.abb.2008.01.002. PMID 18206980.

196. Shahabi, P; Siest, G; Meyer, U. A.; Visvikis-Siest, S (2014). "Human cytochrome P450 epoxygenases: Variability in expression and role in inflammation-related disorders". Pharmacology & Therapeutics. 144 (2): 134–61. doi:10.1016/j.pharmthera.2014.05.011. PMID 24882266.

197. Frömel, T; Kohlstedt, K; Popp, R; Yin, X; Awwad, K; Barbosa-Sicard, E; Thomas, A. C.; Lieberz, R; Mayr, M; Fleming, I (2013). "Cytochrome P4502S1: A novel monocyte/macrophage fatty acid epoxygenase in human atherosclerotic plaques". Basic Research in Cardiology. 108 (1): 319. doi:10.1007/s00395-012-0319-8. PMID 23224081.

198. Fleming, I (2014). "The pharmacology of the cytochrome P450 epoxygenase/soluble epoxide hydrolase axis in the vasculature and cardiovascular disease". Pharmacological Reviews. 66 (4): 1106–40. doi:10.1124/pr.113.007781. PMID 25244930.

199. Westphal, C; Konkel, A; Schunck, W. H. (2011). "CYP-eicosanoids--a new link between omega-3 fatty acids and cardiac disease?". Prostaglandins & Other Lipid Mediators. 96 (1–4): 99–108. doi:10.1016/j.prostaglandins.2011.09.001. PMID 21945326.

200. Matsuoka T, Narumiya S (2007). "Prostaglandin receptor signaling in disease". TheScientificWorldJournal. 7: 1329–47. doi:10.1100/tsw.2007.182. PMID 17767353.

201. Thomas J, Fairclough A, Kavanagh J, Kelly AJ (2014). "Vaginal prostaglandin (PGE2 and PGF2a) for induction of labour at term". The Cochrane Database of Systematic Reviews (6): CD003101. doi:10.1002/14651858.CD003101.pub3. PMID 24941907.

202. Rossi A, Anzalone A, Fortuna MC, Caro G, Garelli V, Pranteda G, Carlesimo M (2016). "Multi-therapies in androgenetic alopecia: review and clinical experiences". Dermatologic Therapy. doi:10.1111/dth.12390. PMID 27424565.

203. Garza LA, Liu Y, Yang Z, Alagesan B, Lawson JA, Norberg SM, Loy DE, Zhao T, Blatt HB, Stanton DC, Carrasco L, Ahluwalia G, Fischer SM, FitzGerald GA, Cotsarelis G (2012). "Prostaglandin D2 inhibits hair growth and is elevated in bald scalp of men with androgenetic alopecia". Science Translational Medicine. 4 (126): 126ra34. doi:10.1126/scitranslmed.3003122. PMC 3319975 . PMID 22440736.

204. Hata AN, Breyer RM (2004). "Pharmacology and signaling of prostaglandin receptors: multiple roles in inflammation and immune modulation". Pharmacology & Therapeutics. 103 (2): 147–66. doi:10.1016/j.pharmthera.2004.06.003. PMID 15369681.

205. Figueiredo-Pereira ME, Corwin C, Babich J (2016). "Prostaglandin J2: a potential target for halting inflammation-induced neurodegeneration". Annals of the New

York Academy of Sciences. 1363: 125–37. doi:10.1111/nyas.12987. PMID 26748744.

206. Hoxha M, Buccellati C, Capra V, Garella D, Cena C, Rolando B, Fruttero R, Carnevali S, Sala A, Rovati GE, Bertinaria M (2016). "In vitro pharmacological evaluation of multitarget agents for thromboxane prostanoid receptor antagonism and COX-2 inhibition". Pharmacological Research. 103: 132–43. doi:10.1016/j.phrs.2015.11.012. PMID 26621246.

207. Cruz JE, Ward A, Anthony S, Chang S, Bae HB, Hermes-DeSantis ER (2016). "Evidence for the Use of Epoprostenol to Treat Raynaud's Phenomenon With or Without Digital Ulcers: A Review of the Literature". The Annals of Pharmacotherapy. 50: 1060–1067. doi:10.1177/1060028016660324. PMID 27465880.

208. O'Connell C, Amar D, Boucly A, Savale L, Jaïs X, Chaumais MC, Montani D, Humbert M, Simonneau G, Sitbon O (2016). "Comparative Safety and Tolerability of Prostacyclins in Pulmonary Hypertension". Drug Safety. 39 (4): 287–94. doi:10.1007/s40264-015-0365-x. PMID 26748508.

209. Cacione DG, Baptista-Silva JC, Macedo CR (2016). "Pharmacological treatment for Buerger's disease". The Cochrane Database of Systematic Reviews. 2: CD011033. doi:10.1002/14651858.CD011033.pub2. PMID 26828199.

210. Citterio A, Arnoldi A, Panzeri E, D'Angelo MG, Filosto M, Dilena R, Arrigoni F, Castelli M, Maghini C, Germiniasi C, Menni F, Martinuzzi A, Bresolin N, Bassi MT (2014). "Mutations in CYP2U1, DDHD2 and GBA2 genes are rare causes of complicated forms of hereditary spastic paraparesis". Journal of Neurology. 261 (2): 373–81. doi:10.1007/s00415-013-7206-6. PMID 24337409.

211. Liu M, Yokomizo T (2015). "The role of leukotrienes in allergic diseases". Allergology International : Official Journal of the Japanese Society of Allergology. 64 (1): 17–26. doi:10.1016/j.alit.2014.09.001. PMID 25572555.

212. Bäck M, Dahlén SE, Drazen JM, Evans JF, Serhan CN, Shimizu T, Yokomizo T, Rovati GE (2011). "International Union of Basic and Clinical Pharmacology. LXXXIV: leukotriene receptor nomenclature, distribution, and pathophysiological functions". Pharmacological Reviews. 63 (3): 539–84. doi:10.1124/pr.110.004184. PMID 21771892.

213. Bäck M, Powell WS, Dahlén SE, Drazen JM, Evans JF, Serhan CN, Shimizu T, Yokomizo T, Rovati GE (2014). "Update on leukotriene, lipoxin and oxoeicosanoid receptors: IUPHAR Review 7". British Journal of Pharmacology. 171 (15): 3551–74. doi:10.1111/bph.12665. PMC 4128057 . PMID 24588652.

214. Cingi C, Muluk NB, Ipci K, Şahin E (2015). "Antileukotrienes in upper airway inflammatory diseases". Current Allergy and Asthma Reports. 15 (11): 64. doi:10.1007/s11882-015-0564-7. PMID 26385352.

215. Nettis E, D'Erasmo M, Di Leo E, Calogiuri G, Montinaro V, Ferrannini A, Vacca A (2010). "The employment of leukotriene antagonists in cutaneous diseases belonging to allergological field". Mediators of Inflammation. 2010: 1–6. doi:10.1155/2010/628171. PMC 2945673 . PMID 20886028.

216. Kanaoka Y, Maekawa A, Austen KF (2013). "Identification of GPR99 protein as a potential third cysteinyl leukotriene receptor with a preference for leukotriene E4 ligand". The Journal of Biological Chemistry. 288 (16): 10967–72. doi:10.1074/jbc.C113.453704. PMC 3630866 . PMID 23504326.
217. Romano M, Cianci E, Simiele F, Recchiuti A (2015). "Lipoxins and aspirin-triggered lipoxins in resolution of inflammation". European Journal of Pharmacology. 760: 49–63. doi:10.1016/j.ejphar.2015.03.083. PMID 25895638.
218. Chiang N, Serhan CN, Dahlén SE, Drazen JM, Hay DW, Rovati GE, Shimizu T, Yokomizo T, Brink C (2006). "The lipoxin receptor ALX: potent ligand-specific and stereoselective actions in vivo". Pharmacological Reviews. 58 (3): 463–87. doi:10.1124/pr.58.3.4. PMID 16968948.
219. Qu Q, Xuan W, Fan GH (2015). "Roles of resolvins in the resolution of acute inflammation". Cell Biology International. 39 (1): 3–22. doi:10.1002/cbin.10345. PMID 25052386.
220. Lim JY, Park CK, Hwang SW (2015). "Biological Roles of Resolvins and Related Substances in the Resolution of Pain". BioMed Research International. 2015: 830930. doi:10.1155/2015/830930. PMC 4538417 . PMID 26339646.
221. Serhan CN, Chiang N, Dalli J, Levy BD (2015). "Lipid mediators in the resolution of inflammation". Cold Spring Harbor Perspectives in Biology. 7 (2): a016311. doi:10.1101/cshperspect.a016311. PMID 25359497.
222. Serhan CN, Chiang N (2013). "Resolution phase lipid mediators of inflammation: agonists of resolution". Current Opinion in Pharmacology. 13 (4): 632–40. doi:10.1016/j.coph.2013.05.012. PMC 3732499 . PMID 23747022.
223. Yang L, Mäki-Petäjä K, Cheriyan J, McEniery C, Wilkinson IB (2015). "The role of epoxyeicosatrienoic acids in the cardiovascular system". British Journal of Clinical Pharmacology. 80 (1): 28–44. doi:10.1111/bcp.12603. PMC 4500322 . PMID 25655310.
224. Clinical trial number NCT00847899 for "Evaluation of Soluble Epoxide Hydrolase (s-EH) Inhibitor in Patients With Mild to Moderate Hypertension and Impaired Glucose Tolerance" at ClinicalTrials.gov
225. Bos C, Richel D, Ritsema T, Peppelenbosch M, Versteeg H (2004). "Prostanoids and prostanoid receptors in signal transduction". Int J Biochem Cell Biol. 36 (7): 1187–205. doi:10.1016/j.biocel.2003.08.006. PMID 15109566.
226. Samuelsson B (May 1983). "Leukotrienes: mediators of immediate hypersensitivity reactions and inflammation". Science. 220 (4597): 568–575. doi:10.1126/science.6301011. PMID 6301011.
227. Haeggström JZ, Funk CD (2011). "Lipoxygenase and leukotriene pathways: biochemistry, biology, and roles in disease". Chemical Reviews. 111 (10): 5866–98. doi:10.1021/cr200246d. PMID 21936577.
228. Anwar Y, Sabir JS, Qureshi MI, Saini KS (2014). "5-lipoxygenase: a promising drug target against inflammatory diseases-biochemical and pharmacological regulation". Current Drug Targets. 15 (4): 410–22. doi:10.2174/1389450114666131209110745. PMID 24313690.

229. Kar M, Altıntoprak N, Muluk NB, Ulusoy S, Bafaqeeh SA, Cingi C (March 2016). "Antileukotrienes in adenotonsillar hypertrophy: a review of the literature". European Archives of Oto-Rhino-Laryngology. 273: 4111–4117. doi:10.1007/s00405-016-3983-8. PMID 26980339.

230. Oussalah A, Mayorga C, Blanca M, Barbaud A, Nakonechna A, Cernadas J, Gotua M, Brockow K, Caubet JC, Bircher A, Atanaskovic M, Demoly P, K Tanno L, Terreehorst I, Laguna JJ, Romano A, Guéant JL (April 2016). "Genetic variants associated with drugs-induced immediate hypersensitivity reactions: a PRISMA-compliant systematic review". Allergy. 71 (4): 443–62. doi:10.1111/all.12821. PMID 26678823.

231. Mitchell S, Balp MM, Samuel M, McBride D, Maurer M (2015). "Systematic review of treatments for chronic spontaneous urticaria with inadequate response to licensed first-line treatments". International Journal of Dermatology. 54 (9): 1088–104. doi:10.1111/ijd.12727. PMID 25515967.

232. Wu SH, Chen XQ, Liu B, Wu HJ, Dong L (2013). "Efficacy and safety of 15(R/S)-methyl-lipoxin A(4) in topical treatment of infantile eczema". The British Journal of Dermatology. 168 (1): 172–8. doi:10.1111/j.1365-2133.2012.11177.x. PMID 22834636.

233. Basil MC, Levy BD (2016). "Specialized pro-resolving mediators: endogenous regulators of infection and inflammation". Nature Reviews. Immunology. 16 (1): 51–67. doi:10.1038/nri.2015.4. PMID 26688348.

234. Feltenmark S, Gautam N, Brunnström A, Griffiths W, Backman L, Edenius C, Lindbom L, Björkholm M, Claesson HE (January 2008). "Eoxins are proinflammatory arachidonic acid metabolites produced via the 15-lipoxygenase-1 pathway in human eosinophils and mast cells". Proc. Natl. Acad. Sci. U.S.A. 105 (2): 680–685. doi:10.1073/pnas.0710127105. PMC 2206596 . PMID 18184802.

235. James A, Daham K, Backman L, Brunnström A, Tingvall T, Kumlin M, Edenius C, Dahlén SE, Dahlén B, Claesson HE (2013). "The influence of aspirin on release of eoxin C4, leukotriene C4 and 15-HETE, in eosinophilic granulocytes isolated from patients with asthma". Int. Arch. Allergy Immunol. 162 (2): 135–42. doi:10.1159/000351422. PMID 23921438.

236. Claesson HE (2009). "On the biosynthesis and biological role of eoxins and 15-lipoxygenase-1 in airway inflammation and Hodgkin lymphoma". Prostaglandins & Other Lipid Mediators. 89 (3-4): 120–5. doi:10.1016/j.prostaglandins.2008.12.003. PMID 19130894.

237. Serhan CN, Chiang N, Dalli J (2015). "The resolution code of acute inflammation: Novel pro-resolving lipid mediators in resolution". Seminars in Immunology. 27 (3): 200–15. doi:10.1016/j.smim.2015.03.004. PMC 4515371 . PMID 25857211.

238. Guichardant M, Calzada C, Bernoud-Hubac N, Lagarde M, Véricel E (2015). "Omega-3 polyunsaturated fatty acids and oxygenated metabolism in atherothrombosis". Biochimica et Biophysica Acta. 1851 (4): 485–95. doi:10.1016/j.bbalip.2014.09.013. PMID 25263947.

239. Calder PC (2014). "Biomarkers of immunity and inflammation for use in

nutrition interventions: International Life Sciences Institute European Branch work on selection criteria and interpretation". Endocrine, Metabolic & Immune Disorders Drug Targets. 14 (4): 236–44. doi:10.2174/187153031466614070909 1650. PMID 25008763.

240. Fritsche, Kevin (August 2006). "Fatty Acids as Modulators of the Immune Response". Annual Review of Nutrition. 26: 45–73. doi:10.1146/annurev.nutr.25.050304.092610. PMID 16848700. Retrieved 2007-01-11.
241. National Institute of Health (2005-08-01). "Omega-3 fatty acids, fish oil, alpha-linolenic acid". Archived from the original on May 3, 2006. Retrieved March 26, 2006.
242. Burr, G.O.; Burr, M.M. (1930). "On the nature and role of the fatty acids essential in nutrition" (PDF). J. Biol. Chem. 86 (587). Retrieved 2007-01-17.
243. Bergström, S.; Danielsson, H.; Samuelsson, B. (1964). "The enzymatic formation of prostaglandin E2 from arachidonic acid". Biochim. Biophys. Acta. 90 (207): 207–10. doi:10.1016/0304-4165(64)90145-x. PMID 14201168.
244. Vane, J. R. (June 23, 1971). "Inhibition of prostaglandin synthesis as a mechanism of action for aspirin-like drugs". Nature New Biol. 231 (25): 232–5. doi:10.1038/newbio231232a0. PMID 5284360.
245. Voet, Donald; Voet, Judith; Pratt, Charlotte (2013). Fundamentals of Biochemistry Life at the Molecular Level (Fourth ed.). Hoboken, NJ: John Wiley & Sons, Inc. ISBN 9781118129180.
246. "Glycolipids". nature. Nature Publishing Group. Retrieved November 2015. Check date values in: |access-date= (help)
247. Aureli, Massimo; et al. (August 2015). "Lipid Membrane domains in the Brain". BBA Molecular and Cell Biology of Lipids. 1851 (8): 1006–1016. doi:10.1016/j.bbalip.2015.02.001. PMID 25677824.
248. Williams, GJ; Thorson, JS (2009). "Natural product glycosyltransferases: properties and applications.". Advances in Enzymology and Related Areas of Molecular Biology. 76: 55–119. doi:10.1002/9780470392881.ch2. PMID 18990828.
249. Sinnott, M. L. "Catalytic mechanisms of enzymatic glycosyl transfer". Chem. Rev. 1990, 90, 1171–1202.
250. Sandhoff, Kondrad (December 2015). "Sphingolipidoses". Journal of Clinical Pathology. 68 (12): 94–105. doi:10.1136/jcp.s3-8.1.94.
251. Schnaar, Ronald (15 June 2004). "Glycolipid-mediated cell–cell recognition in inflammation and nerve regeneration". Archives of Biochemistry and Biophysics. 426 (2): 163–172. doi:10.1016/j.abb.2004.02.019.
252. Cooper GM. The Cell: A Molecular Approach. 2nd edition. Sunderland (MA): Sinauer Associates; 2000. cell–cell Interactions. Available from: http://www.ncbi.nlm.nih.gov/books/NBK9851/
253. Erb IH (1 May 1940). "Blood Group Classifications, a Plea for Uniformity". Canadian Medical Association Journal. 42 (5): 418–21. PMC 537907 . PMID 20321693.

254. Neufeld, Elizabeth (January 1964). "Formation of galactolipids". Biochemical and Biophysical Research. 14 (6): 503–508. doi:10.1016/0006-291X(64)90259-1.

255. Harwood, John L.; Nicholls, Rodney G. (1979). "The plant sulfolipid. A major component of the sulfur cycle". Biochemical Society Transactions. 7 (2): 440–7. doi:10.1042/bst0070440. PMID 428677.

256. Hakomori, S (December 1995). "Functional role of glycosphingolipids in cell recognition and signaling". The Journal of Biochemistry. 118 (6): 1091–1103. PMID 8720120.

257. Jurevics, H; Hostettler, J; Muse, ED; Sammond, DW; Matsushima, GK; Toews, AD; Morell, P (May 2001). "Cerebroside synthesis as a measure of the rate of remyelination following cuprizone-induced demyelination in brain.". Journal of Neurochemistry. 77 (4): 1067–76. doi:10.1046/j.1471-4159.2001.00310.x. PMID 11359872.

258. Role of ganglioside metabolism in the pathogenesis of Alzheimer's disease – a review-JOURNAL OF LIPID RESEARCH Volume: 49 Issue: 6 Pages: 1157–1175 Published: JUN 2008

259. Paulick, Margot G.; Bertozzi, Carolyn R. (8 July 2008). "The Glycosylphosphatidylinositol Anchor: A Complex Membrane-Anchoring Structure for Proteins". Biochemistry. 47 (27): 6991–7000. doi:10.1021/bi8006324. ISSN 0006-2960. PMC 2663890 . PMID 18557633.

CHAPTER 8

Purine Metabolism

Chapter Contents

The chief purines found in the nucleotides and nucleic acids are adenine and guanine. Uric acid is the final oxidation product (in man) of these purines. Purines combine through their 9-nitrogen position with sugar residues →nucleoside. If the sugar residue is also phosphorylated a nucleotide results. Purines are occasionally found as free bases, more usually as nucleosides and nucleotides, and as nucleic acids.

INTRODUCTION

Purine metabolism refers to the metabolic pathways to synthesize and break down purines that are present in many organisms.

BIOSYNTHESIS

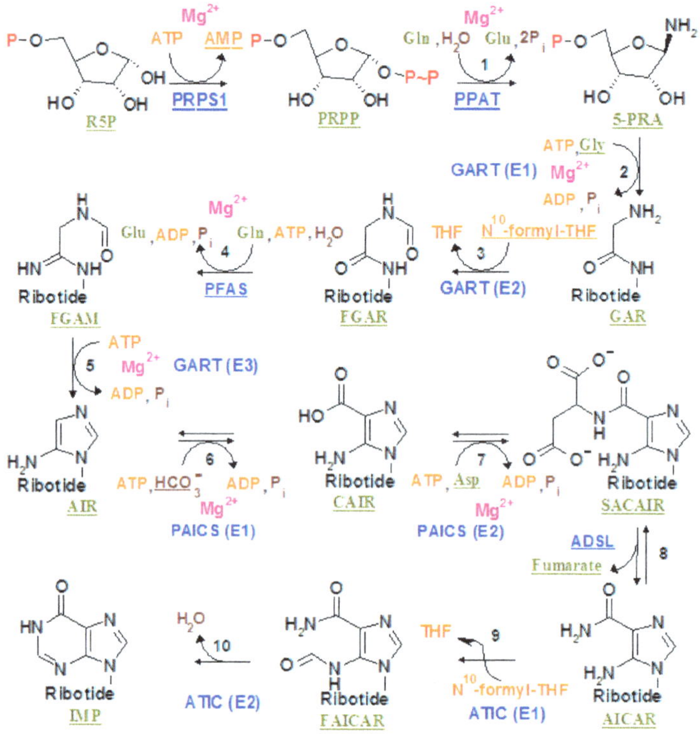

The synthesis of IMP

The color scheme is as follows: enzymes, coenzymes, substrate names, metal ions, inorganic molecules

Purines are biologically synthesized as nucleotides and in particular as ribotides, i.e. bases attached to ribose 5-phosphate. A key regulatory step is the production of 5-phospho-α-D-ribosyl 1-pyrophosphate (PRPP) by ribose phosphate pyrophosphokinase, which is activated by inorganic phosphate and inactivated by purine ribonucleotides. It is not the committed step to purine synthesis because PRPP is also used in pyrimidine synthesis and salvage pathways.

The first committed step is the reaction of PRPP, glutamine and water to 5'-phosphoribosylamine (PRA), glutamate, and pyrophosphate - catalyzed by amidophosphoribosyltransferase, which is activated by PRPP and inhibited by AMP, GMP and IMP.

PRPP + L-Glutamine + H_2O → PRA + L-Glutamate + PPi

In the second step react PRA, glycine and ATP to create GAR, ADP, and pyrophosphate - catalyzed by phosphoribosylamine—glycine ligase (GAR synthetase). Due to the chemical lability of PRA, which has a half-life of 38 seconds at PH 7.5 and 37 °C, researchers have suggested that the compound is channeled from amidophosphoribosyltransferase to GAR synthetase *in vivo.*

PRA + Glycine + ATP → GAR + ADP + Pi

The third is catalyzed by phosphoribosylglycinamide formyltransferase.

GAR + fTHF → fGAR + THF

The fourth is catalyzed by phosphoribosylformylglycinamidine synthase.

fGAR + L-Glutamine + ATP → fGAM + L-Glutamate + ADP + Pi

The fifth is catalyzed by AIR synthetase (FGAM cyclase).

fGAM + ATP → AIR + ADP + Pi + H_2O

The sixth is catalyzed by phosphoribosylaminoimidazole carboxylase.

AIR + CO_2 → CAIR + 2H+

The seventh is catalyzed by phosphoribosylaminoimidazolesuccinocarboxamide synthase.

CAIR + L-Aspartate + ATP → SAICAR + ADP + Pi

The eight is catalyzed by adenylosuccinate lyase.

SAICAR → AICAR + Fumarate

The ninth is catalyzed by phosphoribosylaminoimidazolecarboxamide formyltransferase.

AICAR + fTHF → FAICAR + THF

The last step is catalyzed by Inosine monophosphate synthase.

FAICAR → IMP + H_2O

In eukaryotes the second, third, and fifth step are catalyzed by trifunctional purine biosynthetic protein adenosine-3, which is encoded by the GART gene.

Both ninth and tenth step are accomplished by a single protein named Bifunctional purine biosynthesis protein PURH, encoded by the ATIC gene.

Both adenine and guanine are derived from the nucleotide inosine monophosphate (IMP), which is the first compound in the pathway to have a completely formed purine ring system.

Inosine monophosphate is synthesized on a pre-existing ribose-phosphate through a complex pathway (as shown in the figure on the right). The source of the carbon and nitrogen atoms of the purine ring, 5 and 4 respectively, come from multiple sources. The amino acid glycine contributes all its carbon (2) and nitrogen (1) atoms, with additional nitrogen atoms from glutamine (2) and aspartic acid (1), and additional carbon atoms from formyl groups (2), which are transferred from the coenzyme tetrahydrofolate as 10-formyltetrahydrofolate, and a carbon atom from bicarbonate (1). Formyl groups build carbon-2 and carbon-8 in the purine ring system, which are the ones acting as bridges between two nitrogen atoms.

GMP

- IMP dehydrogenase converts IMP into XMP
- GMP synthase converts XMP into GMP
- GMP reductase converts GMP back into IMP

AMP

- adenylosuccinate synthase converts IMP to adenylosuccinate
- adenylosuccinate lyase converts adenylosuccinate into AMP
- AMP deaminase converts AMP back into IMP

DEGRADATION

Purines are metabolised by several enzymes:

Guanine

- A nuclease frees the nucleotide
- A nucleotidase creates guanosine
- Purine nucleoside phosphorylase converts guanosine to guanine
- Guanase converts guanine to xanthine
- Xanthine oxidase (a form of xanthine oxidoreductase) catalyzes the oxidation of xanthine to uric acid

Adenine

- A nuclease frees the nucleotide
- A nucleotidase creates adenosine, then adenosine deaminase creates inosine
- Alternatively, AMP deaminase creates inosinic acid, then a nucleotidase creates inosine
- Purine nucleoside phosphorylase acts upon inosine to create hypoxanthine
- Xanthine oxidase catalyzes the biotransformation of hypoxanthine to xanthine
- Xanthine oxidase acts upon xanthine to create uric acid

Salvage

Purines from turnover of nucleic acids (or from food) can also be salvaged and reused in new nucleotides.

- The enzyme adenine phosphoribosyltransferase (APRT) salvages adenine.
- The enzyme hypoxanthine-guanine phosphoribosyltransferase (HGPRT) salvages

guanine and hypoxanthine. (Genetic deficiency of HGPRT causes Lesch-Nyhan syndrome.)

Disorders

When a defective gene causes gaps to appear in the metabolic recycling process for purines and pyrimidines, these chemicals are not metabolised properly, and adults or children can suffer from any one of twenty-eight hereditary disorders, possibly some more as yet unknown. Symptoms can include gout, anaemia, epilepsy, delayed development, deafness, compulsive self-biting, kidney failure or stones, or loss of immunity.

Pharmacotherapy

Modulation of purine metabolism has pharmacotherapeutic value.

Purine synthesis inhibitors inhibit the proliferation of cells, especially leukocytes. These inhibitors include azathioprine, an immunosuppressant used in organ transplantation, autoimmune disease such as rheumatoid arthritis or inflammatory bowel disease such as Crohn's disease and ulcerative colitis.

Mycophenolate mofetil is an immunosuppressant drug used to prevent rejection in organ transplantation; it inhibits purine synthesis by blocking inositol monophosphate dehydrogenase. Also Methotrexate indirectly inhibits purine synthesis by blocking the metabolism of folic acid (it is an inhibitor of the Dihydrofolate reductase).

Allopurinol is a drug that inhibits the enzyme xanthine oxidoreductase and, thus, lowers the level of uric acid in the body. This may be useful in the treatment of gout, which is a disease caused by excess uric acid, forming crystals in joints.

NUCLEOTIDE SALVAGE

A salvage pathway is a pathway in which nucleotides (purine and pyrimidine) are synthesized from intermediates in the degradative pathway for nucleotides.

Salvage pathways are used to recover bases and nucleosides that are formed during degradation of RNA and DNA. This is important in some organs because some tissues cannot undergo de novo synthesis.

The salvaged bases and nucleosides can then be converted back into nucleotides.

Substrates

The salvage pathway requires distinct substrates:

Pyrimidines

Uridine phosphorylase or pyrimidine-nucleoside phosphorylase adds ribose 1-phosphate to the free base uracil, forming uridine. Uridine kinase (aka uridine–cytidine kinase) can then phosphorylate this nucleoside into uridine monophosphate (UMP). UMP/CMP kinase (EC 2.7.4.14) can phosphorylate UMP into uridine diphosphate, which nucleoside diphosphate kinase can phosphorylate into uridine triphosphate.

Thymidine phosphorylase or pyrimidine-nucleoside phosphorylase adds 2-deoxy-alpha-D-ribose 1-phosphate to thymine, forming thymidine. Thymidine kinase can then phosphorylate this compound into thymidine monophosphate (TMP). Thymidylate kinase can phosphorylate TMP into thymidine diphosphate, which nucleoside diphosphate kinase can phosphorylate into thymidine triphosphate.

The nucleosides cytidine and deoxycytidine can be salvaged along the uracil pathway by cytidine deaminase, which converts them to uridine and deoxyuridine, respectively. Alternatively, uridine–cytidine kinase can phosphorylate them into cytidine monophosphate (CMP) or deoxycytidine monophosphate (dCMP). UMP/CMP kinase can phosphorylate (d) CMP into cytidine diphosphate or deoxycytidine diphosphate, which nucleoside diphosphate kinase can phosphorylate into cytidine triphosphate or deoxycytidine triphosphate.

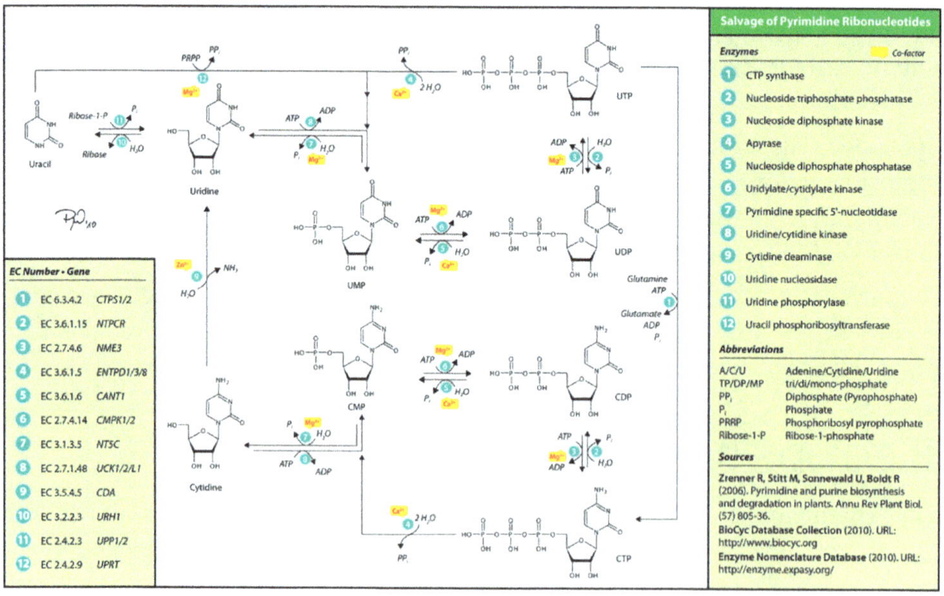

The salvage of pyrimidine ribonucleotides.

Purines

Phosphoribosyltransferases add activated ribose-5-phosphate (Phosphoribosyl pyrophosphate, PRPP) to bases, creating nucleoside monophosphates. There are two types of phosphoribosyltransferases: adenine phosphoribosyltransferase (APRT) and hypoxanthine-guanine phosphoribosyltransferase (HGPRT). It is an important enzyme in Purine pathway metabolism. It is also involved in Lesch-Nyhan syndrome associated with a deficiency of HGPRT.

Nucleobase	Enzyme	Nucleotide
hypoxanthine	hypoxanthine/guanine phosphoribosyl transferase (HGPRT)	IMP
guanine	hypoxanthine/guanine phosphoribosyl transferase (HGPRT)	GMP
adenine	adenine phosphoribosyltransferase (APRT)	AMP

PYRIMIDINE METABOLISM

Pyrimidine biosynthesis occurs both in the body and through organic synthesis.

De Novo Biosynthesis of Pyrimidine

carbamoyl phosphate synthetase II	carbamoyl phosphate	This is the regulated step in the pyrimidine biosynthesis.
aspartic transcarbamolyase (aspartate carbamoyl transferase)	carbamoyl aspartic acid	-
dihhydroorotase	dihydroorotate	Dehydration
dihydroorotate dehydrogenase (the only mitochondrial enzyme)	orotate	Dihydroorotate then enters the mitochondria where it is oxidised through removal of hydrogens. This is the only mitochondrial step in nucleotide rings biosynthesis.
orotate phosphoribosyltransferase	OMP	PRPP is used.
OMP decarboxylase	UMP	Decarboxylation
uridine-cytidine kinase 2	UDP	Phosphorylation. ATP is used.
nucleoside diphosphate kinase	UTP	Phosphorylation. ATP is used.
CTP synthase	CTP	Glutamine and ATP are used.

The first three enzymes are all coded by the same gene in Metazoa (CAD). In Fungi, a similar protein exists but lacks the dihydroorotase function: another protein catalyzes the second step.

In other organisms (Bacteria, Archaea and the other Eukaryota), the first three steps are done by three different enzymes.

Pyrimidine Catabolism

Pyrimidines are ultimately catabolized (degraded) to CO_2, H_2O, and urea. Cytosine can be broken down to uracil, which can be further broken down to N-carbamoyl-β-alanine, and then to beta-alanine, CO_2, and ammonia by beta-ureidopropionase. Thymine is broken down into β-aminoisobutyrate which can be further broken down into intermediates eventually leading into the citric acid cycle.

β-aminoisobutyrate acts as a rough indicator for rate of DNA turnover.

Pharmacotherapy

Modulating the pyrimidine metabolism pharmacologically has therapeutical uses.

Pyrimidine synthesis inhibitors are used in active moderate to severe rheumatoid arthritis and psoriatic arthritis. Examples include Leflunomide and Teriflunomide.

REFERENCES

1. "Substrate specificity of glycinamide ribonucleotide synthetase from chicken liver". The Journal of Biological Chemistry. 271: 8192–5. April 5, 1996. doi:10.1074/jbc.271.14.8192. PMID 8626510.
2. Ansari MY, Equbal A, Dikhit MR, Mansuri R, Rana S, Ali V, Sahoo GC, Das P (Nov 2015). "Establishment of Correlation between In-Silico &In-Vitro Test Analysis against Leishmania HGPRT to inhibitors". International Journal of Biological Macromolecules. 83: 78–96. doi:10.1016/j.ijbiomac.2015.11.051. PMID 26616453.
3. "Entrez Gene: CAD carbamoyl-phosphate synthetase 2, aspartate transcarbamylase, and dihydroorotase".
4. "Entrez Gene: DHODH dihydroorotate dehydrogenase".
5. "Entrez Gene: UMPS uridine monophosphate synthetase".
6. "Entrez Gene: UCK2 uridine-cytidine kinase 2".
7. Nielsen, HR; Sjolin, KE; Nyholm, K; Baliga, BS; Wong, R; Borek, E (1974). "Beta-aminoisobutyric acid, a new probe for the metabolism of DNA and RNA in normal and tumorous tissue". Cancer Research. 34 (6): 1381–4. PMID 4363656.

Index